上海市重点图书

Full View of Yangtze River Pharmaceuticals Group (Taizhou, Jiangsu, China)
扬子江药业集团全景（中国·江苏·泰州）

A Newly Compiled
Practical English-Chinese Library
of Traditional Chinese Medicine
（英汉对照）新编实用中医文库

General Compiler-in-Chief Zuo Yanfu
总主编　左言富
Translators-in-Chief
Zhu Zhongbao Huang Yuezhong Tao Jinwen Li Zhaoguo
总编译　朱忠宝　黄月中　陶锦文　李照国（执行）

Compiled by Nanjing University of
Traditional Chinese Medicine
Translated by Shanghai University
of Traditional Chinese Medicine

南京中医药大学　主编
上海中医药大学　主译

LIFE CULTIVATION AND REHABILITATION OF TRADITIONAL CHINESE MEDICINE

中医养生康复学

Compiler-in-Chief	Wang Xudong
Vice-Compilers-in-Chief	Guo Haiying
	Chen Shoupeng
Translators-in-Chief	Li Yong'an
	Lai Yuezhen
Vice-Translators-in-Chief	Le Yimin
	Li Jingyun

主　编　王旭东
副主编　郭海英
　　　　陈守鹏
主　译　李永安
　　　　赖月珍
副主译　乐毅敏
　　　　李经蕴

PUBLISHING HOUSE OF SHANGHAI UNIVERSITY
OF TRADITIONAL CHINESE MEDICINE
上海中医药大学出版社

Publishing House of Shanghai University of Traditional Chinese Medicine
530 Lingling Road, Shanghai, 200032, China

Life Cultivation and Rehabilitation of Traditional Chinese Medicine
Compiler-in-Chief　Wang Xudong　Translators-in-Chief　Li Yong'an　Lai Yuezhen
(A Newly Compiled Practical English-Chinese Library of Traditional Chinese Medicine
General Compiler-in-Chief　Zuo Yanfu)

All rights reserved. No part of this book may be reproduced, stored in a retrieval system, or transmitted in any form or by any means, electronic, mechanical, photocopying, recording or otherwise, without the prior written permission in writing of the Publisher.

ISBN 7-81010-649-X/R・615　paperback
ISBN 7-81010-682-1/R・647　hardback
Printed in Shanghai Xinhua Printing Works

图书在版编目(CIP)数据

中医养生康复学/王旭东主编；李永安,赖月珍主译.—上海：上海中医药大学出版社,2003

(英汉对照新编实用中医文库/左言富总主编)

ISBN 7-81010-649-X

Ⅰ.中… Ⅱ.①王…②李…③赖… Ⅲ.①养生(中医)—英、汉②中医学：康复医学—英、汉　Ⅳ.①R212 ②R247.9

中国版本图书馆 CIP 数据核字(2003)第 010454 号

中医养生康复学　主编 王旭东　主译 李永安 赖月珍

上海中医药大学出版社出版发行　　　(零陵路530号　邮政编码200032)
新华书店上海发行所经销　　　　　　上海新华印刷厂印刷
开本　787 mm×1092 mm　1/18　印张 24　字数 573 千字　印数 1—3 600 册
版次 2003 年 2 月第 1 版　　　　　　　印次 2003 年 2 月第 1 次印刷

ISBN 7-81010-649-X/R・615　　　　　　定价 53.40 元

Compilation Board of the Library

Honorary Director Zhang Wenkang

General Advisor Chen Keji   Xu Jingren

Advisors (Listed in the order of the number of strokes in the Chinese names)

Gan Zuwang	You Songxin	Liu Zaipeng	Xu Zhiyin
Sun Tong	Song Liren	Zhang Minqing	Jin Shi
Jin Miaowen	Shan Zhaowei	Zhou Fuyi	Shi Zhen
Xu Jingfan	Tang Shuhua	Cao Shihong	Fu Weimin

International Advisors M. S. Khan (Ireland) Alessandra Gulì (Italy) Secondo Scarsella (Italy) Raymond K. Carroll (Australia) Shulan Tang (Britain) Glovanni Maciocia (Britain) David Molony (America) Tzu Kuo Shih (America) Isigami Hiroshi (Japan) Helmut Ziegler (Germany)

Director Xiang Ping

Executive Director Zuo Yanfu

Executive Vice-Directors Ma Jian   Du Wendong   Li Zhaoguo

Vice-Directors Huang Chenghui   Wu Kunping   Liu Shenlin   Wu Mianhua
                   Chen Diping   Cai Baochang

Members (Listed in the order of the number of strokes in the Chinese names)

Ding Anwei	Ding Shuhua	Yu Yong	Wan Lisheng	Wang Xu
Wang Xudong	Wang Lingling	Wang Lufen	Lu Zijie	Shen Junlong
Liu Yu	Liu Yueguang	Yan Daonan	Yang Gongfu	Min Zhongsheng
Wu Changguo	Wu Yongjun	Wu Jianlong	He Wenbin	
He Shuxun (specially invited)		He Guixiang	Wang Yue	
Wang Shouchuan		Shen Daqing	Zhang Qing	Chen Yonghui
Chen Tinghan (specially invited)	Shao Jianmin		Lin Xianzeng (specially invited)	
Lin Duanmei (specially invited)	Yue Peiping		Jin Hongzhu	
Zhou Ligao (specially invited)	Zhao Xia		Zhao Jingsheng	Hu Lie
Hu Kui	Zha Wei	Yao Yingzhi	Yuan Ying	Xia Youbing
Xia Dengjie	Ni Yun	Xu Hengze	Guo Haiying	Tang Chuanjian
Tang Decai	Ling Guizhen (specially invited)		Tan Yong	Huang Guicheng
Mei Xiaoyun	Cao Guizhu	Jiang Zhongqiu	Zeng Qingqi	Zhai Yachun
Fan Qiaoling				

《(英汉对照)新编实用中医文库》编纂委员会

名誉主任 张文康
总 顾 问 陈可冀 徐镜人
顾　　问（按姓氏笔画为序）
　　干祖望　尤松鑫　刘再朋　许芝银　孙 桐　宋立人　张民庆　金 实
　　金妙文　单兆伟　周福贻　施 震　徐景藩　唐蜀华　曹世宏　符为民
外籍顾问
　　萨利姆(爱尔兰)　亚历山大·古丽(意大利)　卡塞拉·塞肯多(意大利)
　　雷蒙特·凯·卡罗(澳大利亚)　汤淑兰(英国)　马万里(英国)
　　大卫·莫罗尼(美国)　施祖谷(美国)　石上博(日本)　赫尔木特(德国)

主　　任 项 平
执行主任 左言富
执行副主任 马 健　杜文东　李照国
副 主 任 黄成惠　吴坤平　刘沈林　吴勉华　陈涤平　蔡宝昌
编　　委（按姓氏笔画为序）
丁安伟	丁淑华	于 勇	万力生	王 旭
王旭东	王玲玲	王鲁芬	卢子杰	申俊龙
刘 玉	刘跃光	严道南	杨公服	闵仲生
吴昌国	吴拥军	吴建龙	何文彬	何树勋(特邀)
何贵翔	汪 悦	汪受传	沈大庆	张 庆
陈永辉	陈廷汉(特邀)	邵健民	林显增(特邀)	
林端美(特邀)	岳沛平	金宏柱	周礼杲(特邀)	
赵 霞	赵京生	胡 烈	胡 葵	查 炜
姚映芷	袁 颖	夏有兵	夏登杰	倪 云
徐恒泽	郭海英	唐传俭	唐德才	凌桂珍(特邀)
谈 勇	黄桂成	梅晓芸	曹贵珠	蒋中秋
曾庆琪	翟亚春	樊巧玲		

Translation Committee of the Library

Advisors   Shao Xundao   Ou Ming

Translators-in-Chief   Zhu Zhongbao   Huang Yuezhong   Tao Jinwen

Executive Translator-in-Chief   Li Zhaoguo

Vice-Translators-in-Chief   (Listed in the order of the number of strokes in the Chinese names)

Xun Jianying   Li Yong'an   Zhang Qingrong   Zhang Dengfeng   Yang Hongying   Huang Guoqi   Xie Jinhua

Translators   (Listed in the order of the number of strokes in the Chinese names)

Yu Xin	Wang Ruihui	Tian Kaiyu	Shen Guang
Lan Fengli	Cheng Peili	Zhu Wenxiao	Zhu Yuqin
Zhu Jinjiang	Zhu Guixiang	Le Yimin	Liu Shengpeng
Li Jingyun	Yang Ying	Yang Mingshan	He Yingchun
Zhang Jie	Zhang Haixia	Zhang Wei	Chen Renying
Zhou Yongming	Zhou Suzhen	Qu Yusheng	Zhao Junqing
Jing Zhen	Hu Kewu	Xu Qilong	Xu Yao
Guo Xiaomin	Huang Xixuan	Cao Lijuan	Kang Qin
Dong Jing	Qin Baichang	Zeng Haiping	Lou Jianhua
Lai Yuezhen	Bao Bai	Pei Huihua	Xue Junmei
Dai Wenjun	Wei Min		

Office of the Translation Committee

Director   Yang Mingshan

Secretaries   Xu Lindi   Chen Li

《(英汉对照)新编实用中医文库》编译委员会

顾　　问　邵循道　欧　明
总 编 译　朱忠宝　黄月中　陶锦文
执行总编译　李照国
副 总 编 译　(按姓氏笔画为序)
　　寻建英　李永安　张庆荣　张登峰　杨洪英　黄国琪　谢金华

编 译 者　(按姓氏笔画为序)
　　于　新　王瑞辉　田开宇　申　光　兰凤利　成培莉　朱文晓
　　朱玉琴　朱金江　朱桂香　乐毅敏　刘升鹏　李经蕴　杨　莹
　　杨明山　何迎春　张　杰　张海峡　张　维　陈仁英　周永明
　　周素贞　屈榆生　赵俊卿　荆　蓁　胡克武　徐启龙　徐　瑶
　　郭小民　黄熙璇　曹丽娟　康　勤　董　晶　覃百长　曾海苹
　　楼建华　赖月珍　鲍　白　裴慧华　薛俊梅　戴文军　魏　敏

编译委员会办公室
主　任　杨明山
秘　书　徐林娣　陈　力

Approval Committee of the Library

Director Li Zhenji

Vice-Directors Shen Zhixiang   Chen Xiaogu   Zhou Zhongying   Wang Canhui
  Gan Zuwang   Jiang Yuren

Members (Listed in the order of the number of strokes in the Chinese names)

Ding Renqiang	Ding Xiaohong	Wang Xinhua	You Benlin
Shi Yanhua	Qiao Wenlei	Yi Sumei	Li Fei
Li Guoding	Yang Zhaomin	Lu Mianmian	Chen Songyu
Shao Mingxi	Shi Bingbing	Yao Xin	Xia Guicheng
Gu Yuehua	Xu Fusong	Gao Yuanhang	Zhu Fangshou
Tao Jinwen	Huang Yage	Fu Zhiwen	Cai Li

General Compiler-in-Chief   Zuo Yanfu

Executive Vice-General-Compilers-in-Chief   Ma Jian   Du Wendong

Vice-General-Compilers-in-Chief   (Listed in the order of the number of strokes in the Chinese names)

Ding Shuhua	Wang Xudong	Wang Lufen	Yan Daonan
Wu Changguo	Wang Shouchuan	Wang Yue	Chen Yonghui
Jin Hongzhu	Zhao Jingsheng	Tang Decai	Tan Yong
Huang Guicheng	Zhai Yachun	Fan Qiaoling	

Office of the Compilation Board Committee

Directors   Ma Jian   Du Wendong

Vice-Directors   Wu Jianlong   Zhu Changren

Publisher   Zhu Bangxian

Chinese Editors   (Listed in the order of the number of strokes in the Chinese names)

Ma Shengying	Wang Lingli	Wang Deliang	He Qianqian
Shen Chunhui	Zhang Xingjie	Zhou Dunhua	Shan Baozhi
Jiang Shuiyin	Qin Baoping	Qian Jingzhuang	Fan Yuqi
Pan Zhaoxi			

English Editors   Shan Baozhi   Jiang Shuiyin   Xiao Yuanchun

Cover Designer   Wang Lei

Layout Designer   Xu Guomin

《(英汉对照)新编实用中医文库》审定委员会

主　　　任　李振吉
副　主　任　沈志祥　陈啸谷　周仲瑛　王灿晖　干祖望　江育仁
委　　　员　（按姓氏笔画为序）
　　　　　　丁仁强　丁晓红　王新华　尤本林　石燕华　乔文雷　衣素梅　李　飞
　　　　　　李国鼎　杨兆民　陆绵绵　陈松育　邵明熙　施冰冰　姚　欣　夏桂成
　　　　　　顾月华　徐福松　高远航　诸方受　陶锦文　黄雅各　傅志文　蔡　丽

总　主　编　左言富
执行副总主编　马　健　杜文东
副 总 主 编　（按姓氏笔画为序）
　　　　　　丁淑华　王旭东　王鲁芬　严道南　吴昌国　汪　悦　汪受传　陈永辉
　　　　　　金宏柱　赵京生　唐德才　谈　勇　黄桂成　翟亚春　樊巧玲
编纂委员会办公室
主　　　任　马　健　杜文东
副　主　任　吴建龙　朱长仁

出　版　人　朱邦贤
中文责任编辑　（按姓氏笔画为序）
　　　　　　马胜英　王玲琍　王德良　何倩倩　沈春晖　张杏洁　周敦华　单宝枝
　　　　　　姜水印　秦葆平　钱静庄　樊玉琦　潘朝曦
英文责任编辑　单宝枝　姜水印　肖元春
美术编辑　王　磊
技术编辑　徐国民

Foreword I

As we are walking into the 21st century, "health for all" is still an important task for the World Health Organization (WHO) to accomplish in the new century. The realization of "health for all" requires mutual cooperation and concerted efforts of various medical sciences, including traditional medicine. WHO has increasingly emphasized the development of traditional medicine and has made fruitful efforts to promote its development. Currently the spectrum of diseases is changing and an increasing number of diseases are difficult to cure. The side effects of chemical drugs have become more and more evident. Furthermore, both the governments and peoples in all countries are faced with the problem of high cost of medical treatment. Traditional Chinese medicine (TCM), the complete system of traditional medicine in the world with unique theory and excellent clinical curative effects, basically meets the need to solve such problems. Therefore, bringing TCM into full play in medical treatment and healthcare will certainly become one of the hot points in the world medical business in the 21st century.

Various aspects of work need to be done to promote the course of the internationalization of TCM, especially the compilation of works and textbooks suitable for international readers. The impending new century has witnessed the compilation of such a

序 一

人类即将迈入21世纪,"人人享有卫生保健"仍然是新世纪世界卫生工作面临的重要任务。实现"人人享有卫生保健"的宏伟目标,需要包括传统医药学在内的多种医学学科的相互协作与共同努力。世界卫生组织越来越重视传统医药学的发展,并为推动其发展做出了卓有成效的工作。目前,疾病谱正在发生变化,难治疾病不断增多,化学药品的毒副作用日益显现,日趋沉重的医疗费用困扰着各国政府和民众。中医药学是世界传统医学体系中最完整的传统医学,其独到的学科理论和突出的临床疗效,较符合当代社会和人们解决上述难题的需要。因此,科学有效地发挥中医药学的医疗保健作用,必将成为21世纪世界卫生工作的特点之一。

加快中医药走向世界的步伐,还有很多的工作要做,特别是适合国外读者学习的中医药著作、教材的编写是极其重要的方面。在新千年来临之际,由南京中医药大学

series of books known as *A Newly Compiled Practical English-Chinese Library of Traditional Chinese Medicine* published by the Publishing House of Shanghai University of TCM, compiled by Nanjing University of TCM and translated by Shanghai University of TCM. Professor Zuo Yanfu, the general compiler-in-chief of this Library, is a person who sets his mind on the international dissemination of TCM. He has compiled *General Survey on TCM Abroad*, a monograph on the development and state of TCM abroad. This Library is another important works written by the experts organized by him with the support of Nanjing University of TCM and Shanghai University of TCM. The compilation of this Library is done with consummate ingenuity and according to the development of TCM abroad. The compilers, based on the premise of preserving the genuineness and gist of TCM, have tried to make the contents concise, practical and easy to understand, making great efforts to introduce the abstruse ideas of TCM in a scientific and simple way as well as expounding the prevention and treatment of diseases which are commonly encountered abroad and can be effectively treated by TCM.

This Library encompasses a systematic summarization of the teaching experience accumulated in Nanjing University of TCM and Shanghai University of TCM that run the collaborating centers of traditional medicine and the international training centers on acupuncture and moxibustion set by WHO. I am sure that the publication of this Library will further promote the development of traditional Chinese med-

主编、上海中医药大学主译、上海中医药大学出版社出版的《（英汉对照）新编实用中医文库》的即将问世，正是新世纪中医药国际传播更快发展的预示。本套文库总主编左言富教授是中医药学国际传播事业的有心人，曾主编研究国外中医药发展状况的专著《国外中医药概览》。本套文库的编撰，是他在南京中医药大学和上海中医药大学支持下，组织许多著名专家共同完成的又一重要专著。本套文库的作者们深谙国外的中医药发展现状，编写颇具匠心，在注重真实、不失精华的前提下，突出内容的简明、实用，易于掌握，力求科学而又通俗地介绍中医药学的深奥内容，重点阐述国外常见而中医药颇具疗效的疾病的防治。

本套文库蕴含了南京中医药大学和上海中医药大学作为WHO传统医学合作中心、国际针灸培训中心多年留学生教学的实践经验和系统总结，更为全面、系统、准确地向世界传播中医药学。相信本书的出版将对中医更好地走向世界，让世界更好地了解中医产生更

icine abroad and enable the whole world to have a better understanding of traditional Chinese medicine.

Professor Zhu Qingsheng

Vice-Minister of Health Ministry of the People's Republic of China

Director of the State Administrative Bureau of TCM

December 14, 2000 Beijing

为积极的影响。

朱庆生教授

中华人民共和国卫生部副部长

国家中医药管理局局长

2000年12月14日于北京

Foreword II

Before the existence of the modern medicine, human beings depended solely on herbal medicines and other therapeutic methods to treat diseases and preserve health. Such a practice gave rise to the establishment of various kinds of traditional medicine with unique theory and practice, such as traditional Chinese medicine, Indian medicine and Arabian medicine, etc. Among these traditional systems of medicine, traditional Chinese medicine is a most extraordinary one based on which traditional Korean medicine and Japanese medicine have evolved.

Even in the 21st century, traditional medicine is still of great vitality. In spite of the fast development of modern medicine, traditional medicine is still disseminated far and wide. In many developing countries, most of the people in the rural areas still depend on traditional medicine and traditional medical practitioners to meet the need for primary healthcare. Even in the countries with advanced modern medicine, more and more people have begun to accept traditional medicine and other therapeutic methods, such as homeopathy, osteopathy and naturopathy, etc.

With the change of the economy, culture and living style in various regions as well as the aging in the world population, the disease spectrum has changed. And such a change has paved the way for the new application of traditional medicine. Besides,

序 二

在现代医学形成之前，人类一直依赖草药和其他一些疗法治病强身，从而发展出许多有理论、有实践的传统医学，例如中医学、印度医学、阿拉伯医学等。中医学是世界林林总总的传统医学中的一支奇葩，在它的基础上还衍生出朝鲜传统医学和日本汉方医学。在跨入21世纪的今天，古老的传统医学依然焕发着活力，非但没有因现代医学的发展而式微，其影响还有增无减，人们对传统医学的价值也有了更深刻的体会和认识。在许多贫穷国家，大多数农村人口仍然依赖传统医学疗法和传统医务工作者来满足他们对初级卫生保健的需求。在现代医学占主导地位的许多国家，传统医学及其他一些"另类疗法"，诸如顺势疗法、整骨疗法、自然疗法等，也越来越被人们所接受。

伴随着世界各地经济、文化和生活的变革以及世界人口的老龄化，世界疾病谱也发生了变化。传统医学有了新的应用，而新疾病所引起的新需求以及现代医学的成

the new requirements initiated by the new diseases and the achievements and limitations of modern medicine have also created challenges for traditional medicine.

WHO sensed the importance of traditional medicine to human health early in the 1970s and have made great efforts to develop traditional medicine. At the 29th world health congress held in 1976, the item of traditional medicine was adopted in the working plan of WHO. In the following world health congresses, a series of resolutions were passed to demand the member countries to develop, utilize and study traditional medicine according to their specific conditions so as to reduce medical expenses for the realization of "health for all".

WHO has laid great stress on the scientific content, safe and effective application of traditional medicine. It has published and distributed a series of booklets on the scientific, safe and effective use of herbs and acupuncture and moxibustion. It has also made great contributions to the international standardization of traditional medical terms. The safe and effective application of traditional medicine has much to do with the skills of traditional medical practitioners. That is why WHO has made great efforts to train them. WHO has run 27 collaborating centers in the world which have made great contributions to the training of acupuncturists and traditional medical practitioners. Nanjing University of TCM and Shanghai University of TCM run the collaborating centers with WHO. In recent years it has, with the cooperation of WHO and other countries, trained about ten thousand international students from over

就与局限又向传统医学提出了挑战，推动它进一步发展。世界卫生组织早在20世纪70年代就意识到传统医学对人类健康的重要性，并为推动传统医学的发展做了努力。1976年举行的第二十九届世界卫生大会将传统医学项目纳入世界卫生组织的工作计划。其后的各届世界卫生大会又通过了一系列决议，要求各成员国根据本国的条件发展、使用和研究传统医学，以降低医疗费用，促进"人人享有初级卫生保健"这一目标的实现。

世界卫生组织历来重视传统医学的科学、安全和有效使用。它出版和发行了一系列有关科学、安全、有效使用草药和针灸的技术指南，并在专用术语的标准化方面做了许多工作。传统医学的使用是否做到安全和有效，是与使用传统疗法的医务工作者的水平密不可分的。因此，世界卫生组织也十分重视传统医学培训工作。它在全世界有27个传统医学合作中心，这些中心对培训合格的针灸师及使用传统疗法的其他医务工作者做出了积极的贡献。南京中医药大学、上海中医药大学是世界卫生组织传统医学合作中心之一，近年来与世界卫生组织和其他国家合作，培训了近万名来自90多个国

90 countries.

In order to further promote the dissemination of traditional Chinese medicine in the world, *A Newly Compiled Practical English-Chinese Library of Traditional Chinese Medicine*, compiled by Nanjing University of TCM with Professor Zuo Yanfu as the general compiler-in-chief and published by the Publishing House of Shanghai University of TCM, aims at systematic, accurate and concise expounding of traditional Chinese medical theory and introducing clinical therapeutic methods of traditional medicine according to modern medical nomenclature of diseases. Undoubtedly, this series of books will be the practical textbooks for the beginners with certain English level and the international enthusiasts with certain level of Chinese to study traditional Chinese medicine. Besides, this series of books can also serve as reference books for WHO to internationally standardize the nomenclature of acupuncture and moxibustion.

The scientific, safe and effective use of traditional medicine will certainly further promote the development of traditional medicine and traditional medicine will undoubtedly make more and more contributions to human health in the 21st century.

Zhang Xiaorui
WHO Coordination Officer
December, 2000

家和地区的留学生。

在南京中医药大学左言富教授主持下编纂的、由上海中医药大学出版社出版的《（英汉对照）新编实用中医文库》，旨在全面、系统、准确、简要地阐述中医基础理论，并结合西医病名介绍中医临床治疗方法。因此，这套文库可望成为具有一定英语水平的初学中医者和具有一定中文水平的外国中医爱好者学习基础中医学的系列教材。这套文库也可供世界卫生组织在编写国际针灸标准术语时参考。

传统医学的科学、安全、有效使用必将进一步推动传统医学的发展。传统医学一定会在21世纪为人类健康做出更大的贡献。

张小瑞
世界卫生组织传统医学协调官员
2000年12月

Preface

The Publishing House of Shanghai University of TCM published *A Practical English-Chinese Library of Traditional Chinese Medicine* in 1990. The Library has been well-known in the world ever since and has made great contributions to the dissemination of traditional Chinese medicine in the world. In view of the fact that 10 years has passed since its publication and that there are certain errors in the explanation of traditional Chinese medicine in the Library, the Publishing House has invited Nanjing University of TCM and Shanghai University of TCM to organize experts to recompile and translate the Library.

Nanjing University of TCM and Shanghai University of TCM are well-known for their advantages in higher education of traditional Chinese medicine and compilation of traditional Chinese medical textbooks. The compilation of *A Newly Compiled Practical English-Chinese Library of Traditional Chinese Medicine* has absorbed the rich experience accumulated by Nanjing University of Traditional Chinese Medicine in training international students of traditional Chinese medicine. Compared with the previous Library, the Newly Compiled Library has made great improvements in many aspects, fully demonstrating the academic system of traditional Chinese medicine. The whole series of books has systematically introduced the basic theory and thera-

前 言

上海中医药大学出版社于1990年出版了一套《(英汉对照)实用中医文库》,发行10年来,在海内外产生了较大影响,对推动中医学走向世界起了积极作用。考虑到该套丛书发行已久,对中医学术体系的介绍还有一些欠妥之处,因此,上海中医药大学出版社特邀南京中医药大学主编、上海中医药大学主译,组织全国有关专家编译出版《(英汉对照)新编实用中医文库》。

《(英汉对照)新编实用中医文库》的编纂,充分发挥了南京中医药大学和上海中医药大学在高等中医药教育教学和教材编写方面的优势,吸收了作为WHO传统医学合作中心之一的两校,多年来从事中医药学国际培训和留学生学历教育的经验,对原《(英汉对照)实用中医文库》整体结构作了大幅度调整,以突出中医学术主体内容。全套丛书系统介绍了中医基础理论和中医辨证论治方法,讲解了中药学和方剂学的基本理论,详细介绍了236味中药、152首常用方剂和100种常用中成药;详述

peutic methods based on syndrome differentiation, expounding traditional Chinese pharmacy and prescriptions; explaining 236 herbs, 152 prescriptions and 100 commonly-used patent drugs; elucidating 264 methods for differentiating syndromes and treating commonly-encountered and frequently-encountered diseases in internal medicine, surgery, gynecology, pediatrics, traumatology and orthopedics, ophthalmology and otorhinolaryngology; introducing the basic methods and theory of acupuncture and moxibustion, massage (tuina), life cultivation and rehabilitation, including 70 kinds of diseases suitable for acupuncture and moxibustion, 38 kinds of diseases for massage, examples of life cultivation and over 20 kinds of commonly encountered diseases treated by rehabilitation therapies in traditional Chinese medicine. For better understanding of traditional Chinese medicine, the books are neatly illustrated. There are 296 line graphs and 30 colored pictures in the Library with necessary indexes, making it more comprehensive, accurate and systematic in disseminating traditional Chinese medicine in the countries and regions where English is the official language.

This Library is characterized by following features:

1. Scientific Based on the development of TCM in education and research in the past 10 years, efforts have been made in the compilation to highlight the gist of TCM through accurate theoretical exposition and clinical practice, aiming at introducing authentic theory and practice to the world.

2. Systematic This Library contains 14 sepa-

264种临床内、外、妇、儿、骨伤、眼、耳鼻喉各科常见病与多发病的中医辨证论治方法；系统论述针灸、推拿、中医养生康复的基本理论和基本技能，介绍针灸治疗病种70种、推拿治疗病种38种、各类养生实例及20余种常见病证的中医康复实例。为了更加直观地介绍中医药学术，全书选用线图296幅、彩图30幅，并附有必要的索引，从而更加全面、系统、准确地向使用英语的国家和地区传播中医学术，推进中医学走向世界，造福全人类。

本丛书主要具有以下特色：
（1）科学性：在充分吸收近10余年来中医教学和科学研究最新进展的基础上，坚持突出中医学术精华，理论阐述准确，临床切合实用，向世界各国介绍"原汁原味"的中医药学术。
（2）系统性：本套丛书包括《中医基础理论》、《中医诊断学》、《中药

rate fascicles, i.e. *Basic Theory of Traditional Chinese Medicine*, *Diagnostics of Traditional Chinese Medicine*, *Science of Chinese Materia Medica*, *Science of Prescriptions*, *Internal Medicine of Traditional Chinese Medicine*, *Surgery of Traditional Chinese Medicine*, *Gynecology of Traditional Chinese Medicine*, *Pediatrics of Traditional Chinese Medicine*, *Traumatology and Orthopedics of Traditional Chinese Medicine*, *Ophthalmology of Traditional Chinese Medicine*, *Otorhinolaryngology of Traditional Chinese Medicine*, *Chinese Acupuncture and Moxibustion*, *Chinese Tuina (Massage)*, and *Life Cultivation and Rehabilitation of Traditional Chinese Medicine*.

3. Practical Compared with the previous Library, the Newly Compiled Library has made great improvements and supplements, systematically introducing therapeutic methods for treating over 200 kinds of commonly and frequently encountered diseases, focusing on training basic clinical skills in acupuncture and moxibustion, tuina therapy, life cultivation and rehabilitation with clinical case reports.

4. Standard This Library is reasonable in structure, distinct in categorization, standard in terminology and accurate in translation with full consideration of habitual expressions used in countries and regions with English language as the mother tongue.

This series of books is not only practical for the beginners with certain competence of English to study TCM, but also can serve as authentic textbooks for international students in universities and colleges of TCM in China to study and practice TCM. For those from TCM field who are going to go

学》、《方剂学》、《中医内科学》、《中医外科学》、《中医妇科学》、《中医儿科学》、《中医骨伤科学》、《中医眼科学》、《中医耳鼻喉科学》、《中国针灸》、《中国推拿》、《中医养生康复学》14个分册,系统反映了中医各学科建设与发展的最新成果。

(3) 实用性:临床各科由原来的上下两册,根据学科的发展进行大幅度的调整和增补,比较详细地介绍了200多种各科常见病、多发病的中医治疗方法,重点突出了针灸、推拿、养生康复等临床基本技能训练,并附有部分临证实例。

(4) 规范性:全书结构合理,层次清晰,对中医各学科名词术语表述规范,对中医英语翻译执行了更为严格的标准化方案,同时又充分考虑到使用英语国家和地区人们的语言习惯和表达方式。

本丛书不仅能满足具有一定英语水平的初学中医者系统学习中医之用,而且也为中医院校外国留学生教育及国内外开展中医双语教学提供了目前最具权威的系列教材,同时也是中医出国人员进

abroad to do academic exchange, this series of books will provide them with unexpected convenience.

Professor Xiang Ping, President of Nanjing University of TCM, is the director of the Compilation Board. Professor Zuo Yanfu from Nanjing University of TCM, General Compiler-in-Chief, is in charge of the compilation. Zhang Wenkang, Minister of Health Ministry, is invited to be the honorary director of the Editorial Board. Li Zhenji, Vice-Director of the State Administrative Bureau of TCM, is invited to be the director of the Approval Committee. Chen Keji, academician of China Academy, is invited to be the General Advisor. International advisors invited are Mr. M. S. Khan, Chairman of Ireland Acupuncture and Moxibustion Fund; Miss Alessandra Gulí, Chairman of "Nanjing Association" in Rome, Italy; Doctor Secondo Scarsella, Chief Editor of YI DAO ZA ZHI; President Raymond K. Carroll from Australian Oriental Touching Therapy College; Ms. Shulan Tang, Academic Executive of ATCM in Britain; Mr. Glovanni Maciocia from Britain; Mr. David, Chairman of American Association of TCM; Mr. Tzu Kuo Shih, director of Chinese Medical Technique Center in Connecticut, America; Mr. Helmut Ziegler, director of TCM Center in Germany; and Mr. Isigami Hiroshi from Japan. Chen Ken, official of WHO responsible for the Western Pacific Region, has greatly encouraged the compilers in compiling this series of books. After the accomplishment of the compilation, Professor Zhu Qingsheng, Vice-Minister of Health Ministry and Director of the State Administrative Bureau of TCM, has set a high value on the books in his fore-

行中医药国际交流的重要工具书。

全书由南京中医药大学校长项平教授担任编委会主任、左言富教授任总主编，主持全书的编写。中华人民共和国卫生部张文康部长担任本丛书编委会名誉主任，国家中医药管理局李振吉副局长担任审定委员会主任，陈可冀院士欣然担任本丛书总顾问指导全书的编纂。爱尔兰针灸基金会主席萨利姆先生、意大利罗马"南京协会"主席亚历山大·古丽女士、意大利《医道》杂志主编卡塞拉·塞肯多博士、澳大利亚东方触觉疗法学院雷蒙特·凯·卡罗院长、英国中医药学会学术部长汤淑兰女士、英国马万里先生、美国中医师公会主席大卫先生、美国康州中华医疗技术中心主任施祖谷先生、德国中医中心主任赫尔木特先生、日本石上博先生担任本丛书特邀外籍顾问。世界卫生组织西太平洋地区官员陈恳先生对本丛书的编写给予了热情鼓励。全书完成后，卫生部副部长兼国家中医药管理局局长朱庆生教授给予了高度评价，并欣然为本书作序；WHO 传统医学协调官员张小瑞对于本丛书的编写给予高度关注，百忙中也专为本书作序。我国驻外教育机构，特别是中国驻英国曼彻斯特领事张益群先生、中国驻美国休斯敦领事严美华

word for the Library. Zhang Xiaorui, an official from WHO's Traditional Medicine Program, has paid great attention to the compilation and written a foreword for the Library. The officials from the educational organizations of China in other countries have provided us with some useful materials in our compilation. They are Mr. Zhang Yiqun, China Consul to Manchester in Britain; Miss Yan Meihua, Consul to Houston in America; Mr. Wang Jiping, First Secretary in the Educational Department in the Embassy of China to France; and Mr. Gu Shengying, the Second Secretary in the Educational Department in the Embassy of China to Germany. We are grateful to them all.

The Compilers
December, 2000

女士、中国驻法国使馆教育处一秘王季平先生、中国驻德国使馆教育处二秘郭胜英先生在与我们工作联系中,间接提供了不少有益资料。在此一并致以衷心感谢!

编　者
2000年12月

Note for compilation

Life Cultivation and Rehabilitation of traditional Chinese medicine (TCM), a monograph systematically introducing the knowledge of TCM life cultivation and rehabilitation, is intended for the readers to learn the theories of life cultivation and rehabilitation and to grasp the various relevant techniques of health care and rehabilitation.

Life cultivation and rehabilitation originally belongs to the different categories of disciplines of the two major branches of traditional Chinese and Western medical systems. The gradual formation of the system of TCM life cultivation and rehabilitation is based on the theories and practice of life cultivation and rehabilitation during the thousands of years of the Chinese people in combination with certain theories and techniques of the modern science of rehabilitation during the second half of the twentieth century. This is just the reason why this book has combined the two disciplines into one science for exposition.

This book is composed of nine chapters. The content includes the basic theories and concepts of life cultivation and rehabilitation of TCM, various effective methods and clinical techniques of life cultivation and rehabilitation, the measures of life cultivation and health care in the light of people groups, seasons, regions of the body as well as the rehabilitation methods of twenty-six commonly-seen diseases.

The book does not offer the sources of the originals cited from the ancient books and expresses the

编写说明

《中医养生康复学》是系统介绍中医养生学和康复学知识的专著,供读者学习中医养生、康复理论,掌握各种相关的保健、康复技术。

养生与康复本属中西医学两大体系不同范畴的分支学科,在中国人数千年养生保健理论与实践基础上,20世纪下半叶又吸收了现代康复医学的某些理论与技术方法,从而逐渐形成了中医养生康复学的理论和技术体系,这也是本书将其合而为一的原因。

全书分为九章。内容包括中医养生康复学基础理论和观念,各种行之有效的养生康复方法和临床技术,针对不同人群、不同季节、不同身体部位的养生保健措施,以及26种常见病证的康复方法。

本书虽源自有数千年历史的中医宝库,但为使读者方便,凡引

originals in simple language instead for the convenience of the readers though it originates from the treasure-house of TCM with a long history of thousands of years. All the names of drugs, acupoints, prescriptions and books in this book are the standard and current ones. As for the names of diseases, we mainly use the names of diseases of modern medicine. In view of the specific characteristics of the discipline of TCM life cultivation and rehabilitation, the first section of chapter nine discusses chiefly symptoms. All the names of diseases of TCM in this book are modern general names.

The science of TCM Life Cultivation and Rehabilitation, a comprehensive practical discipline, is based on the basic theories of TCM, diagnostic techniques, drugs, prescriptions as well as internal medicine, surgery, gynecology and pediatrics. Therefore, the readers can achieve overall mastery through a comprehensive study of this book in combination with other books of the series of books by means of mutual connection and consultation.

述古书内容者，均未标出原文，而是以通俗语言表述。书中涉及的药名、穴名、方名、书名，均使用规范而通行的名称。病名，则以西医病名为主。考虑到中医养生康复学科的特殊性，第九章第一节是以症状为纲叙述的。书中涉及的中医病名，均为现代通用者。所选用的治疗方剂和食疗药膳方，均出自历代中医名著，为节约篇幅，本书未注明出处。

中医养生康复学是一门奠基于中医基础理论、诊断技术、药物、方剂以及内、外、妇、儿各科基础上的综合性实用学科，因此，应注意与本丛书其他分册内容融会贯通，互相联系，互相参照，以便全面理解和掌握。

Contents

1 The Theoretical Basis of Life Cultivation and Rehabilitation of TCM 1
  1.1 **Purpose: Health and longevity** 2
    1.1.1 The integration of life with nature 2
    1.1.2 Health and longevity on harmony 3
    1.1.3 Comprehensive physiological and psychic life cultivation and rehabilitation 3
  1.2 **Basis: Life and life span** 4
    1.2.1 Life 4
    1.2.2 Life span and health 6
    1.2.3 Ageing 7
    1.2.4 Masters' experience in life cultivation and life prolongation in successive dynasties 9
  1.3 **Concept: Conforming to nature** 14
    1.3.1 Man's relevant adaptation to nature 14
    1.3.2 Unity of physique and spirit 16
    1.3.3 Interdependence of movement and motionlessness 17
    1.3.4 Coordination and balance 18
    1.3.5 Healthy qi as the base 19
  1.4 **Principle: Wholism and syndrome differentiation** 20
    1.4.1 Principle of wholism 20
    1.4.2 Principle of syndrome differentiation 21
    1.4.3 Principle of functions 22

2 Natural Therapeutic Methods of Life Cultivation and Rehabilitation 23
  2.1 **Regulating emotions** 23
    2.1.1 Abstaining from anger 23
    2.1.2 Giving vent to depression 24
    2.1.3 Straightening one out with the help of a friend 24
    2.1.4 Diverting emotions 24
    2.1.5 Sports 25

目 录

第一章　中医养生康复学理论基础 ……………………………………… 1
第一节　目标：健康与长寿 …………………………………………… 2
一、生命与自然融为一体 ……………………………………………… 2
二、健康与长寿在于和谐 ……………………………………………… 3
三、生理和心理综合养护 ……………………………………………… 3
第二节　基点：生命与寿限 …………………………………………… 4
一、生命 ………………………………………………………………… 4
二、寿命与健康 ………………………………………………………… 6
三、衰老 ………………………………………………………………… 7
四、历代名家养生延寿经验 …………………………………………… 9
第三节　观念：顺应自然 ……………………………………………… 14
一、天人相应 …………………………………………………………… 14
二、形神合一 …………………………………………………………… 16
三、动静互涵 …………………………………………………………… 17
四、协调平衡 …………………………………………………………… 18
五、正气为本 …………………………………………………………… 19
第四节　原则：整体辨证 ……………………………………………… 20
一、整体原则 …………………………………………………………… 20
二、辨证原则 …………………………………………………………… 21
三、功能原则 …………………………………………………………… 22

第二章　养生康复的自然疗法 …………………………………………… 23
第一节　调节情志法 …………………………………………………… 23
一、遏止 ………………………………………………………………… 23
二、发泄 ………………………………………………………………… 24
三、疏导 ………………………………………………………………… 24
四、移情 ………………………………………………………………… 24
五、运动 ………………………………………………………………… 25

2.1.6	Suggestion	25
2.1.7	Colors	26
2.1.8	Checking one emotion with another	27

2.2 Environments, daily life and clothing ... 29

2.2.1	Environments	30
2.2.2	Daily life	31
2.2.3	Clothing	39
2.2.4	Defecation and urination	41

2.3 Life cultivation and rehabilitation with the diet ... 43

2.3.1	The effects of life cultivation with the diet	43
2.3.2	Principles of rehabilitation with the diet	44
2.3.3	The commonly-used dietary prescriptions for life cultivation	46
2.3.4	Health care with diet	60

2.4 Health care methods in sexual life ... 61

2.4.1	Sexual life and prolonging life	61
2.4.2	Measures for health care in sexual life	61
2.4.3	Taboos on sexual life	62

2.5 Therapies with sports ... 64

2.5.1	The characteristics and applying principles of enhancing health with sports activities in TCM	64
2.5.2	Examples of life cultivation and rehabilitation with classical sports activities	66

2.6 Therapies with recreation ... 71

2.6.1	Musical therapy	71
2.6.2	Singing therapy	73
2.6.3	Dancing therapy	74
2.6.4	Drama therapy	74
2.6.5	Therapies with a musical instrument and chess, practicing paintings and calligraphy	75

2.7 Life cultivation and rehabilitation with loutrotherapy ... 78

2.7.1	Medicated bath	78
2.7.2	Mud bath	82
2.7.3	Sand bath	83

六、暗示 ………………………………………………………… 25
　　七、色彩 ………………………………………………………… 26
　　八、以情制情 …………………………………………………… 27
第二节　环境、起居、服饰法 …………………………………………… 29
　　一、环境 ………………………………………………………… 30
　　二、起居 ………………………………………………………… 31
　　三、服饰 ………………………………………………………… 39
　　四、排便 ………………………………………………………… 41
第三节　食养食疗法 ……………………………………………………… 43
　　一、饮食养生的作用 …………………………………………… 43
　　二、饮食康复的原则 …………………………………………… 44
　　三、常用食养食疗方 …………………………………………… 46
　　四、饮食保健 …………………………………………………… 60
第四节　性生活保健法 …………………………………………………… 61
　　一、性生活与延年益寿 ………………………………………… 61
　　二、性生活的保健措施 ………………………………………… 61
　　三、性生活禁忌 ………………………………………………… 62
第五节　运动疗法 ………………………………………………………… 64
　　一、中医运动健身的特点和运用原则 ………………………… 64
　　二、古典运动养生、康复法举隅 ……………………………… 66
第六节　娱乐疗法 ………………………………………………………… 71
　　一、音乐 ………………………………………………………… 71
　　二、歌咏 ………………………………………………………… 73
　　三、舞蹈 ………………………………………………………… 74
　　四、戏剧 ………………………………………………………… 74
　　五、琴棋书画 …………………………………………………… 75
第七节　沐浴疗法 ………………………………………………………… 78
　　一、药浴 ………………………………………………………… 78
　　二、泥浆浴 ……………………………………………………… 82
　　三、沙浴 ………………………………………………………… 83

3 Techniques of TCM Life Cultivation and Rehabilitation ... 85
3.1 Acupuncture therapy ... 85
3.1.1 Body acupuncture ... 85
3.1.2 Ear acupuncture ... 91
3.1.3 Scalp acupuncture ... 93
3.1.4 Moxibustion for health care ... 94
3.2 Massage therapy ... 105
3.2.1 The applying principles of massage ... 105
3.2.2 Manipulations of self-massage and their application ... 107
3.3 Therapies with traditional Chinese drugs ... 109
3.3.1 Therapies with oral medications ... 110
3.3.2 Life cultivation and rehabilitation with external therapy ... 113
3.3.3 Drugs and prescriptions for promoting longevity ... 118
3.4 Nursing of TCM Rehabilitation ... 125
3.4.1 Nursing with the concept of wholism ... 125
3.4.2 Differentiating syndrome to decide nursing ... 127
3.4.3 Comprehensive nursing ... 128
3.4.4 The nursing methods of attaching equal importance to somatic and psychic health ... 130

4 Forbidden Points for Life Cultivation and Rehabilitation ... 132
4.1 Abstinence from smoking and drinking ... 132
4.1.1 Smoking is harmful to health ... 132
4.1.2 Drinking and health ... 134
4.2 Abstinence from food preference ... 135
4.3 Abstinence from overstrain ... 137
4.3.1 Abstinence from mental overstrain ... 137
4.3.2 Abstinence from physical overstrain ... 138
4.3.3 Abstinence from sexual overstrain ... 140
4.4 Abstinence from extreme emotional activities ... 141

5 Examples of TCM Life Cultivation in Accordance with Individual Differences ... 143
5.1 Constitutional cultivation ... 143
5.1.1 Constitution with yin deficiency ... 144
5.1.2 Constitution with yang deficiency ... 146

第三章 养生康复的中医技术 85
第一节 针灸疗法 85
一、体针 85
二、耳针 91
三、头针 93
四、保健灸 94
第二节 推拿疗法 105
一、推拿的应用原则 105
二、自我推拿手法及其运用 107
第三节 中药疗法 109
一、内服法 110
二、外治法 113
三、长寿药物 118
第四节 中医康复护理 125
一、整体护理 125
二、辨证护理 127
三、综合护理 128
四、心身并重的护理法 130

第四章 养生康复禁忌 132
第一节 戒烟酒 132
一、吸烟有害健康 132
二、饮酒与健康 134
第二节 戒偏嗜 135
第三节 戒过劳 137
一、戒神劳 137
二、戒体劳 138
三、戒房劳 140
第四节 戒情志偏激 141

第五章 因人制宜的养生实例举隅 143
第一节 体质养生 143
一、阴虚体质 144
二、阳虚体质 146

5.1.3	Constitution with qi deficiency	148
5.1.4	Constitution with blood deficiency	148
5.1.5	Constitution with excessive yang	149
5.1.6	Constitution with blood stasis	151
5.1.7	Constitution with phlegm and dampness	151
5.1.8	Constitution with qi depression	153
5.2	**Life cultivation in the pregnant women**	**154**
5.2.1	Prenatal conditioning	154
5.2.2	Regulating the diet	156
5.2.3	Living a normal daily life	157
5.2.4	Proper balance between work and rest	158
5.2.5	Abstinence from sexual life	159
5.2.6	Using drugs with caution	159
5.3	**Health care for children**	**160**
5.3.1	Early education	160
5.3.2	Reasonable diet	161
5.3.3	Rearing the children carefully	166
5.3.4	Training physique	168
5.3.5	Developing good habits	169
5.3.6	Benefiting intelligence with traditional Chinese drugs	170
5.4	**Health care for women**	**172**
5.4.1	Health care during the menstrual period	172
5.4.2	Health care during the puerperium	173
5.4.3	Health care during the breast feeding period	175
5.4.4	Health care during the climacterium	176
5.5	**Health care for old people**	**177**
5.5.1	Establishing the psychological state of being optimistic, open-minded, kind and enterprising	177
5.5.2	Taking the nutritious, bland, well-cooked, soft and various diet	178
5.5.3	Sports activities	180
5.5.4	Reasonable administration	180
5.6	**Health care for mental workers**	**181**
5.6.1	Scientific use of the brain	181
5.6.2	Protecting eyesight	182
5.6.3	Living in a suitable environment	182

三、气虚体质 ··· 148
　　四、血虚体质 ··· 148
　　五、阳盛体质 ··· 149
　　六、血瘀体质 ··· 151
　　七、痰湿体质 ··· 151
　　八、气郁体质 ··· 153
第二节　胎孕养生 ··· 154
　　一、胎教 ··· 154
　　二、饮食调养 ··· 156
　　三、起居宜慎 ··· 157
　　四、劳逸适度 ··· 158
　　五、戒房事 ··· 159
　　六、审慎用药 ··· 159
第三节　少儿保健 ··· 160
　　一、早期教育 ··· 160
　　二、合理膳食 ··· 161
　　三、精心养护 ··· 166
　　四、体格锻炼 ··· 168
　　五、培养良好习惯 ··· 169
　　六、中药益智 ··· 170
第四节　妇女保健 ··· 172
　　一、经期保健 ··· 172
　　二、产褥期保健 ··· 173
　　三、哺乳期保健 ··· 175
　　四、更年期保健 ··· 176
第五节　老年保健 ··· 177
　　一、建立乐观、豁达、善良、进取的心理状态 ··············· 177
　　二、保持营养、清淡、熟软、多样的饮食 ··················· 178
　　三、适宜运动 ··· 180
　　四、合理用药 ··· 180
第六节　脑力劳动者的保健 ····································· 181
　　一、科学用脑 ··· 181
　　二、保护目力 ··· 182
　　三、居处适宜 ··· 182

5.6.4	Tonifying the brain with drugs	182
5.6.5	Eyesight-protecting drugs and foods	184
5.6.6	Brain-tonifying and intelligence-benefiting drugs	185
5.6.7	Health care with sports and massage	188

5.7 Health care for physical workers ... 189

5.7.1	Moving the limbs	189
5.7.2	Balancing the diet	190
5.7.3	Reasonable use of the brain	193

5.8 Life cultivation for handicapped people ... 194

5.8.1	Health care for visual disabilities	194
5.8.2	Health care for hearing disabilities	199
5.8.3	Health care for linguistic disabilities	204
5.8.4	Health care for disabilities of limbs and the body	207
5.8.5	Health care for intellectual disabilities	211
5.8.6	Health care for mental disabilities	216

6 Examples of TCM Life Cultivation in Accordance with Seasonal Conditions ... 220

6.1 Life cultivation in spring ... 221

6.1.1	Regulating the daily life	221
6.1.2	Regulating emotions	222
6.1.3	Regulating the diet	224
6.1.4	Physical training	225

6.2 Life cultivation in summer ... 225

6.2.1	Regulating the daily life	226
6.2.2	Regulating emotions	227
6.2.3	Regulating the diet	228
6.2.4	Physical training	229

6.3 Life cultivation in autumn ... 230

6.3.1	Regulating the daily life	230
6.3.2	Regulating emotions	232
6.3.3	Regulating the diet	232
6.3.4	Physical training	234

6.4 Life cultivation in winter ... 235

6.4.1	Regulating the daily life	235

四、食物补脑 ··· 182
　　五、护眼药食 ··· 184
　　六、健脑益智药物 ··· 185
　　七、运动按摩保健 ··· 188
第七节　体力劳动者的保健 ··· 189
　　一、活动肢体 ··· 189
　　二、平衡膳食 ··· 190
　　三、合理用脑 ··· 193
第八节　残疾人群的养生 ··· 194
　　一、视力残障 ··· 194
　　二、听力残障 ··· 199
　　三、语言残障 ··· 204
　　四、肢体残障 ··· 207
　　五、智力残障 ··· 211
　　六、精神残障 ··· 216

第六章　因时制宜的养生实例举隅 ··································· 220
第一节　春季养生 ··· 221
　　一、起居调养 ··· 221
　　二、情志调节 ··· 222
　　三、饮食调养 ··· 224
　　四、运动锻炼 ··· 225
第二节　夏季养生 ··· 225
　　一、起居调养 ··· 226
　　二、情志调节 ··· 227
　　三、饮食保健 ··· 228
　　四、运动锻炼 ··· 229
第三节　秋季养生 ··· 230
　　一、起居调养 ··· 230
　　二、情志调节 ··· 232
　　三、饮食调养 ··· 232
　　四、运动锻炼 ··· 234
第四节　冬季养生 ··· 235
　　一、起居调养 ··· 235

6.4.2	Regulating emotions	236
6.4.3	Regulating the diet	237
6.4.4	Physical training	238

7 Examples of TCM Health Care for Specific Regions — 240

7.1 Oral health care — 240
- 7.1.1 Consolidating the teeth — 240
- 7.1.2 Swallowing saliva — 242

7.2 Facial health care — 243
- 7.2.1 Massage and acumox — 243
- 7.2.2 Diet — 245
- 7.2.3 Drugs — 245

7.3 Health care of the hair — 247
- 7.3.1 Combing the hair and massaging the scalp — 247
- 7.3.2 Diet — 248
- 7.3.3 Drugs — 249

7.4 Health care of the eyes — 251
- 7.4.1 Exercising the eyes — 251
- 7.4.2 Massage — 252
- 7.4.3 Sitting in repose with the eyes closed — 252
- 7.4.4 Diet — 253
- 7.4.5 Drugs — 253

7.5 Health care of the ears — 254
- 7.5.1 Massage — 255
- 7.5.2 Avoiding the drug allergy — 256

7.6 Health care of the nose — 256
- 7.6.1 Bathing the nose — 256
- 7.6.2 Massage — 257
- 7.6.3 Drugs — 257

7.7 Health care of the extremities — 258
- 7.7.1 Health care of the upper limbs — 258
- 7.7.2 Health care of the lower limbs — 260

7.8 Health care of the chest, back, waist and abdomen — 262
- 7.8.1 Health care of the chest — 262
- 7.8.2 Health care of the back — 263

二、精神调养 …………………………………… 236
　　三、饮食保健 …………………………………… 237
　　四、运动锻炼 …………………………………… 238
第七章　特定部位的养生实例举隅 ………………… 240
　第一节　口腔保健 ………………………………… 240
　　一、固齿 ………………………………………… 240
　　二、咽津 ………………………………………… 242
　第二节　颜面保健 ………………………………… 243
　　一、按摩、针灸 ………………………………… 243
　　二、饮食 ………………………………………… 245
　　三、药物 ………………………………………… 245
　第三节　头发保健 ………………………………… 247
　　一、梳理、按摩 ………………………………… 247
　　二、饮食 ………………………………………… 248
　　三、药物 ………………………………………… 249
　第四节　眼睛保健 ………………………………… 251
　　一、运目 ………………………………………… 251
　　二、按摩 ………………………………………… 252
　　三、闭目养神 …………………………………… 252
　　四、饮食 ………………………………………… 253
　　五、药物 ………………………………………… 253
　第五节　耳部保健 ………………………………… 254
　　一、按摩 ………………………………………… 255
　　二、避免药物过敏 ……………………………… 256
　第六节　鼻部保健 ………………………………… 256
　　一、浴鼻 ………………………………………… 256
　　二、按摩 ………………………………………… 257
　　三、药物 ………………………………………… 257
　第七节　四肢保健 ………………………………… 258
　　一、上肢保健 …………………………………… 258
　　二、下肢保健 …………………………………… 260
　第八节　胸背腰腹保健 …………………………… 262
　　一、胸部保健 …………………………………… 262
　　二、背部保健 …………………………………… 263

7.8.3	Health care of the waist		264
7.8.4	Health care of the abdomen		265

8 Rehabilitation Examples of Commonly-Seen Diseases ... 266

8.1 Rehabilitation for sequelae ... 266

8.1.1	Low fever		266
8.1.2	Cough		270
8.1.3	Edema		273
8.1.4	Hypodynamia		277
8.1.5	Polyhidrosis		280
8.1.6	Insomnia		283
8.1.7	Anorexia		287
8.1.8	Palpitation due to fright		289
8.1.9	Constipation		293
8.1.10	Diarrhea		297

8.2 Rehabilitation for senile diseases ... 301

8.2.1	Hypertension		302
8.2.2	Sequelae of apoplexy		308
8.2.3	Hypotension		314
8.2.4	Coronary heart disease		318
8.2.5	Chronic obstructive pulmonary disease		323
8.2.6	Diabetes		329
8.2.7	Senile dementia		335
8.2.8	Senile pruritus		338

8.3 Rehabilitation for malignant tumor ... 342

8.3.1	Cancer of digestive tract		343
8.3.2	Pulmonary carcinoma		354
8.3.3	Cerebroma		359
8.3.4	Mammary cancer		364

8.4 Rehabilitation for commonly-seen internal diseases ... 370

8.4.1	Chronic nephritis		370
8.4.2	Chronic hepatitis and cirrhosis		374
8.4.3	Gastroptosis		380
8.4.4	Pulmonary tuberculosis		384
8.4.5	Posthemorrhagic syndromes		388

Postscript ... 392

三、腰部保健 ········· 264
四、腹部保健 ········· 265

第八章 常见病证的康复实例举隅 ········· 266
第一节 疾病后遗症状的康复 ········· 266
一、低热 ········· 266
二、咳嗽 ········· 270
三、浮肿 ········· 273
四、乏力 ········· 277
五、多汗 ········· 280
六、失眠 ········· 283
七、食少 ········· 287
八、惊悸 ········· 289
九、便秘 ········· 293
十、泄泻 ········· 297

第二节 老年病证的康复 ········· 301
一、高血压病 ········· 302
二、中风后遗症 ········· 308
三、低血压症 ········· 314
四、冠心病 ········· 318
五、慢性阻塞性肺病 ········· 323
六、糖尿病 ········· 329
七、老年性痴呆 ········· 335
八、老年性瘙痒症 ········· 338

第三节 恶性肿瘤的康复 ········· 342
一、消化道癌症 ········· 343
二、肺癌 ········· 354
三、脑肿瘤 ········· 359
四、乳腺癌 ········· 364

第四节 常见内科病症的康复 ········· 370
一、慢性肾炎 ········· 370
二、慢性肝炎和肝纤维化 ········· 374
三、胃下垂 ········· 380
四、肺结核 ········· 384
五、失血后诸证 ········· 388

后记 ········· 392

1 The Theoretical Basis of Life Cultivation and Rehabilitation of TCM

Life cultivation is to achieve the purposes of conserving health, preventing diseases, enhancing health and prolonging life span by means of various health care measures such as cultivating the mind, regulating the diet, exercising constitution of the human body, moderating sexual life and adapting oneself to cold and heat. In short, all the activities of promoting health and prolonging life span belong to those of health preservation. Life cultivation of TCM, a practical science, is to explore and study Chinese psychological and physiological health care measures through the ages as well as enhancement of physique, prevention of diseases and prolongation of life under the guidance of TCM theories.

Rehabilitation is to improve the life quality of patients and the handicapped by treating the functional decline or dysfunction of body due to various congenital or postnatal factors by way of mental regulation, proper diet, physical training, acumox and massage, administration as well as bathing, recreation, etc. It is mainly applicable to the patients with pathogenic handicap and maim. Rehabilitation of TCM is a science to study the basic theories, therapeutic methods and their application under the guidance of TCM theories.

The science of life cultivation and rehabilitation of

第一章 中医养生康复学理论基础

养生,是指合理选用养精神、调饮食、练形体、慎房事、适寒温等保健方法,通过长期的锻炼和修习,达到保养身体、减少疾病、增进健康、延年益寿的目的。简而言之,所有促进健康,延长寿命的活动都是养生活动。中医养生学,则是在中医理论的指导下,探索和研究中国历代心理、生理保健以及增强体质,预防疾病,延长寿命的实用科学。

康复,是指采用精神调节、合理饮食、体育锻炼、针灸推拿、药物以及沐浴、娱乐等各种措施,对先天或后天各种因素造成的机体功能衰退或障碍进行恢复,达到提高或改善病残者生命质量的目的。它主要适用于病残、伤残患者。中医康复学,则是在中医学理论指导下,研究借鉴和吸收现代康复医学基本理论、医疗方法及其应用而形成的一门学科。

传统中医养生学大体类

traditional Chinese medicine is similar to the first medicine (preventive medicine) in modern medicine, while rehabilitation medicine belongs to the category of the third medicine. During the history of TCM development, the two medical branches are closely connected with each other in the aspects of academic sources, theoretical basis, methods and techniques though both of them differ in the objects of study, areas of application and disciplinary names. This is one major characteristic of TCM, and embodies the holistic concept of combination of prevention with treatment and integration of treatment with health preservation.

1.1 Purpose: Health and longevity

TCM Life Cultivation and Rehabilitation is a science based on the summarization of the practical experience of thousands of years. It, a comprehensive academic system with health and longevity as its purposes, includes multidisciplinary knowledge like preventive medicine, psychological medicine, behavior medicine, medical health care, astrometeorology, geomedicine and social medicine. It is based on Chinese five-thousand-year civilization with its unique oriental features and national style.

1.1.1 The integration of life with nature

TCM believes that man lives amidst the universe and his vital activities are inevitably influenced by the natural laws of material movement. Therefore, all the activities of the human body inevitably has formed close patterns with nature. The relationship between vital activities of

似于现代医学指称的第一医学（预防医学），康复医学则属于第三医学范畴。尽管两者研究的对象、适应的范围及其学科的名称有所不同，但在中医学的历史上，两者的学术渊源、理论基础、方法技能却是共通互用的。这是中医学的一大特色，体现了防治结合、治养结合的整体观念。

第一节 目标：健康与长寿

中医养生康复学是从几千年实践经验中总结出来而不断有所发展的一门学科，其内容包括预防医学、心理医学、行为医学、保健医学、天文气象学、地理医学、社会医学等学科知识，中医养生康复学是以健康长寿为目的的综合学术体系，具有独特的中国文化色彩和民族风格。

一、生命与自然融为一体

中医学认为，人生活在宇宙之间，生命活动必然会受到自然界物质运动规律的影响，因此，人体的所有活动必然与自然息息相关。人体生命活

the human body and nature as well as society should be harmonious and orderly. Otherwise, it is not good for health. This is the thought of "man's relevant adaptation to nature" and "unity of physique and spirit."Accordingly, special emphasis is placed on the harmony between man and natural and social environments.

1.1.2 Health and longevity on harmony

The theories of TCM stress the significance of harmony and balance. It holds that the substance metabolism of the human body should include ascension and descension, that psychology and physiology should be mutually harmonious and that psychological disorders may be regulated with visceral movement while body diseases may be cured with psychological therapeutic methods.

TCM life cultivation and rehabilitation follows the patterns of natural changes so that the pace of life process is accordingly adjusted with the changes of time, space, four seasons and climate. For example, emotional health care should be neither supercilious nor obsequious, but mean and moderate; sleep neither excessive nor insufficient; sexual life neither ignored nor excessive while the body needs labor but should not be exhausted, etc. All these are based on the unique theories and methods of health and longevity.

1.1.3 Comprehensive physiological and psychic life cultivation and rehabilitation

TCM has numerous life cultivation methods, but it emphasizes comprehensive regulation so that people should not focus on or have partiality for one method only. Meanwhile, perseverance is required to achieve more

动与自然、社会的关系,必须是和谐有序的,反之,会对健康不利。这就是"天人相应"、"形神合一"的思想。因此,中医养生学和中医康复学特别强调人与自然环境和社会环境的协调。

二、健康与长寿在于和谐

中医理论强调和谐、平衡,认为体内的物质代谢必须有升有降,心理与生理应该互相协调,心理疾病可以通过脏腑活动来调整,生理疾病也可以运用心理疗法来治愈。

中医养生、康复遵循自然变化的规律,使生命过程的节奏,随着时间、空间的移易和四时气候的改变而进行调整。例如,情绪保健要求不卑不亢,中和适度;睡眠不能偏多偏少;性生活不可无也不可多;形体需要劳动但不能疲倦等,都是立足于健康长寿的独特理论和方法。

三、生理和心理综合养护

中医养生和康复的方法很多,但强调综合调理,不可以偏执偏信于一方一法。同时还要持之以恒,从自然环境

overall and comprehensive prevention of diseases and health care as well as functional rehabilitation from natural environment to food, clothing, shelter and transportation, from life preference to mental hygiene, from enhancement of physique with drugs to health care through sports, etc.

The principle of treatment based on the individual physique, seasonal conditions and local conditions in the basic TCM theories is also applicable to health preservation activities and rehabilitation treatment. People differ in sex and age; time includes the four seasons of spring, summer, autumn and winter while geography varies in south and north as well as high and low. All these should not be lumped together. Different methods of health preservation and rehabilitation should be reasonably adopted on the basis of differentiation of the similarity and difference according to the following discussion in each chapter to achieve the best health care.

1.2 Basis: Life and life span

1.2.1 Life

TCM classic *Huangdi Neijing*, or *Canon of Medicine*, holds that life consists of "qi" ("qi" belongs to the classical philosophical category, referring to the basic element which constitutes everything in the world). The balance and harmony of the internal environment of the human body, the wholism and unity of the human body and the external surroundings are the foundation for man to live and exist. In normal cases, the adjustment of the human body can adapt the internal environment to the changes of the external natural environment to maintain normal physiological functions. If human activities violate the patterns of natural changes, or abnormal and violent changes occur in the external natural surroundings, the regulatory function of the human body will fail to adapt itself to the situation, destroying the relative balance of the internal and external surroundings and consequently giving rise to disease. Therefore, "conforming to nature" is the first requirement for health preservation.

Essence, qi and spirit are the basic substances essential to vital activities.

Essence is the basic material constituting the human body and promoting the growth and development of the human body. Essence is divided into "congenital essence" and "acquired essence". Congenital essence is inherited from the parents. After birth, the nutritious cream derived form the diet is called acquired essence. Congenital essence and acquired essence can be transformed into each other and supplement mutually to form the dynamic foundation of vital activities. If essence is deficient, vital activities will decline, causing premature ageing and susceptibility to diseases.

Qi is the important substance constituting life, too. The sufficiency or deficiency of qi determines the strength of the life force and the length of the life span. The vital phenomena are the ascending, descending, coming-in and coming-out of the functional activities of qi.

Spirit is a general term for vital activities of body and also the outward manifestation of vital activities of the human body. It includes mentality, consciousness, thinking, movement, perception, etc. Essence and blood are the material foundation for spirit. And sufficient essence and qi bring on prosperous spirit. Therefore, whether life is healthy or not can be judged by inspecting the state of spirit.

常的生理功能。如果人的活动违反自然变化的规律,或外界自然环境发生反常的剧变,而人的自我调节功能又不能与之相适应时,可因内、外环境的相对平衡遭到破坏而导致疾病。因此,"顺应自然"是养生的首要条件。

精、气、神是生命活动所需的基本物质。

精,是构成人体及促进人体生长发育的基本物质,有"先天之精"与"后天之精"之分。"先天之精"来自父母;人出生之后,从饮食中获得的营养精华称为"后天之精",先天、后天之精互相转化,互相补充,成为生命活动的动力基础。精的不足或亏虚,可导致生命活动减退,或导致早衰、多病。

气,也是构成生命的重要物质。人体生命力的强弱、生命的寿夭,在于气的盛衰。生命现象,就是气机的升降出入。

神,是机体生命活动的总称,也是人体生命活动的外在表现,包括精神意识、思维活动、运动、知觉等。神以精血为物质基础,精、气充盈,神就健旺,所以,生命的健康与否,可以通过神的状况来判断。

It can be seen from the above that vital activities are determined by the conditions of essence, qi, spirit and visceral functions. Abundant essence, qi and spirit, the balance of visceral qi and blood ensure good health and freedom from diseases, insusceptibility to ageing, and extension of life span.

1.2.2　Life span and health

In ancient China, life span was called "tiannian", which means "the life span endowed by Heaven for existence in the world." Ancient medical professionals believed that the normal human life span is 100 years to 120 years. According to the biological laws, the life span of mammary animals is 5 times to 7 times that of the period of growth. The life span of human is calculated according to the time of dentition of the last tooth (at the age of 20 to 25). Accordingly, the life span of human should be 120 or so. However, due to natural and man-made calamities, poverty and diseases, most people suffer from shorter life and cannot reach the normal life expectancy. The average life span of the Chinese is about 70, 50 years shorter or so theoretically.

Life span is determined by the human health conditions while the main factors affecting health are ageing and diseases. Accordingly, preserving and restoring health are the essential requirements for longevity.

Inspecting "spirit" can judge whether the human body is healthy or not. The signs of "having spirit" are as follows: the general appearance is sturdy, neither fat nor thin; the beard and hair are black, bright and lustrous; the complexion is ruddy with delightful expression; the eyes are expressive and full of vividness; the respiration is

由此可见,生命活动,是由精、气、神以及脏腑功能状态决定的。精、气、神充足,脏腑气血平衡,人体才会健康无病,不易衰老,寿命才能得以延长。

二、寿命与健康

中国古代将人的寿命称为"天年",意指先天赋予的"寿数"。古代医家认为正常人的寿命在100～120岁之间。按照生物学的原理,哺乳动物的寿命是其生长期的5至7倍,人的生长期是以最后一颗牙齿长出来的时间(20～25岁)来计算,因此人的寿命应该是120岁左右。但由于天灾人祸,贫病横夭,大多会折损年寿,达不到预期寿命。中国人的平均寿命为70岁左右,比理论寿命少了50年左右。

寿命的长短由人体的健康状况所决定,而影响健康的主要因素是衰老和疾病,维护健康、恢复健康是长寿的必要条件。

人体健康与否,可通过对"神"的观察来判断。"有神"的标志为:

形体壮实,肥瘦恰当;须发润泽,黑亮有光;面色红润,表情欢畅;眼睛有神,灵气荡

calm and neither rapid nor slow; the appetite is good with three meals deliciously eaten; the teeth are hard and firm without caries and injury; the sense of hearing is acute without tinnitus; the voice is loud and clear with long breath; the waist and legs are flexible without pain and soreness; the urination and defecation are smooth with normal discharges; the tongue is red with thin fur while the pulse is even and slow.

The above discussion includes the two parts of physiological and psychological health states. In fact, TCM has held that psychological health is as important as physiological health since ancient times. The theory of "seven emotions" in the etiology requires emotional regulation and spiritual happiness. This is also the external manifestation of good visceral functions.

1.2.3 Ageing

Ageing is the natural law of normal human vital activities. Reasonable health preservation measures may delay the occurrence of physiological ageing, block the progress of pathological ageing so as to prolong human life span. Premature ageing mainly includes the following causes.

1.2.3.1 Deficiency of essence and qi

Essence is stored in the kidney. "The kidney is the congenital base of life." If renal essence is deficient, life will age prematurely. The deficiency of essence and qi originates mainly from congenital insufficiency, excessive sexual life, exhaustion of diseases, physical overstrain, etc.

1.2.3.2 Malnutrition

The diet is the source for the human body to obtain nutrients. Malnutrition includes the two aspects of insufficient ingestion and malabsorption. Insufficient ingestion is seldom seen in modern people while malabsorption is more common. If the nutrients required by the human body cannot be instantly supplemented, this will affect the health of human body, speed up ageing, even result in death.

1.2.3.3 Impairment of the five zang organs

The heart stores spirit and controls blood circulation. It is the dominator of vital activities. If the heart suffers from diseases, it will affect blood circulation and mental functions, consequently accelerating ageing. The liver stores blood, governs smoothing and regulating the flow of qi and blood, regulates emotions, promotes digestion as well as regulates blood volume. If the liver suffers from diseases, it will affect various physiological functions of blood, emotions, digestion, etc., accordingly giving rise to ageing of the human body. The lung dominates qi of the general body. Deficiency and impairment or obstruction of the lung qi may affect the functions of the general body. In these cases, ageing manifestations like unendurance to physical labor, gradual functional decline of respiration and blood circulation will occur.

1.2.3.4 Excessive emotional stimuli

If persistent emotional stimuli or sudden violent psychic trauma occur beyond the range of adjustment of physiological activities of the human body, it will cause disorders of qi and blood inside the human body, functional disturbances of viscera, meridians and collaterals, thus speeding up ageing.

1.2.3.5 Maladjustment of work and rest

Overstrain and overrest are both harmful to health. The so-called overstrain refers to not only excessive and heavy mental labor and physical labor, but also abnormal life style such as frequent sexual life, excessive food ingestion and recreation, etc. On the contrary, excessively

人摄入不足已很少见,而吸收不足则较多见,若人体所需要的营养得不到及时补充,便会影响机体健康,加速衰老,甚至导致死亡。

3. 五脏受损

心藏神,主血脉,是生命活动的主宰,心脏患病,会影响血脉的运行及神志功能,从而加速衰老。肝藏血,主疏泄,调节情志,帮助消化,又有贮存和调节血量的作用。肝脏患病会影响到血液、情志、消化等众多方面的生理功能,故能导致人体衰老。肺主一身之气,肺气虚损或肺气阻塞,全身功能都会受到影响,出现不耐劳作,呼吸及血液循环功能逐渐减退等衰老表现。

4. 情志过激

长期持久的精神刺激或突然受到剧烈的精神创伤,超过人体生理活动所能调节的范围,就会引起体内阴阳气血失调,脏腑经络功能紊乱,从而加速衰老。

5. 劳逸失度

过劳或者过逸都对健康不利。所谓过劳,不仅指脑力劳动、体力劳动过于繁重,也包括不正常的生活方式,如过于频繁的性生活、过度的饮食

comfortable life is not good for health and longevity, either.

1.2.3.6 Heredity

Ageing is closely related to heredity. Good heredity results in strong physique full of vigor and insusceptibility to ageing. Conversely, poor heredity brings on wan and sallow complexion and listlessness. Consequently, ageing will occur early or acceleratively.

1.2.3.7 Social environment

Dramatic changes in social position may bring about mental and physical impairment to people. Thus, premature ageing will appear. Besides, rich life is replaced by poverty or respectable status is followed by low one, both of which may result in premature ageing, even death at a young age. Also, irrational social systems, unhealthy social customs, backward ideology, intense and acute competition for existence as well as complicated interpersonal relationships may all result in metabolic disorders of the human body, giving rise to premature ageing.

1.2.3.8 Natural surroundings

Residents in mountainous areas with cold climate possess relatively long life; dwellers have relatively short life in flatlands and low-lying lands as well as in the south with high temperature throughout the year. Besides, environmental pollution in cities is more serious than that in rural areas, this can affect health and promote premature ageing.

1.2.4 Masters' experience in life cultivation and life prolongation in successive dynasties

China is a country with longer average life span in the world, and a history of studying the theory and methods of longevity for more than 2,000 years. During each historical period, there exist famous typical longevous masters. They have not only lived a long life, but also accumulated much experience in strengthening health and prolonging life.

1.2.4.1 Lao Zi: "Cherish no worries and keep away from fame and gain"

During the periods of the Spring and Autumn and the Warring States, Lao Zi, the originator of Taoism, put forward his ideas about life cultivation: "Cherish no worries and keep away from fame and gain", "Man restores the pure and innocent nature of the ancients", "Conform to nature", "cherish mild character" and "train the body to remove depression". The chief gist of these ideas lies in mental tranquilization and abstinence from improper personal desires. Only in this way, can human spirit be cultivated, essence and qi internally stored. Consequently, health and longevity can be obtained. Experts on life cultivation throughout the ages have attached importance to the thought on life cultivation of "cherishing no worries and keeping away from fame and gain." It is the theoretical source of TCM life cultivation. According to the record of historical literature, the life span of Lao Zi exceeded 160 years.

1.2.4.2 Confucius: "Be benevolent to achieve longevity"

Confucius was the academic founder of Confucianism. As far as life cultivation and longevity are concerned, Confucius advocated moral life cultivation, stressed the importance of cultivation of the mind, that material desires should be reduced as much as possible and that human behavior should be restrained by social norms. Of these social norms, the philosophical concepts of "benevolence" and "the doctrine of the mean" were also embodied in his life cultivation practice such as "three kinds of

一个不同的历史时期都有著名的长寿典型,他们不仅自己能够得以长生,而且创造了很多健体延寿的经验。

1. 老子:"清静无为"

春秋战国时期,道家鼻祖老子提出了"清静无为"、"返朴归真"、"顺应自然"、"贵柔"、"动形达郁"的养生观。其主要精神是:心神宁静,少私寡欲,这样,人的精神才能得到润养,精气能够内藏,由此而健康长寿。清静无为以养神长寿的思想,一直为历代养生家所重视,是中医养生理论的源头之一。传说老子寿命为160岁以上。

2. 孔子:"仁爱多寿"

孔子是儒家学术的奠基人。在养生长寿方面,孔子提倡道德养生,强调精神调摄,尽量减少物质欲望,以社会准则来规范人的行为,其"仁爱"、"中庸"的哲学观念,也体现在养生实践之中,如"君子三戒"(即戒色、戒斗、戒得)。此外,注意生活规律,不过劳

abstinence for gentlemen" (Namely: "abstinence from sexual life, abstinence from fights and abstinence from worrying about personal gains and losses.) " In addition, people should live a regular life and avoid overstrain and overrest; dietary requirements should be nutritious, fresh, clean, meticulously cooked and delicious. Though Confucius lived in an age of chaos caused by war, his life span also reached 72 years. Menicus, another representative figure of Confucianism who was good at cultivating noble spirit, died at the age of 83.

1.2.4.3　Hua Tuo: "Ageing does not occur with the movement of the body"

Hua Tuo, the noted doctor in the Han Dynasty, theoretically expounded life cultivation with the bodily movement. He thought "movement" promotes easy digestion and smooth blood circulation, and that in this way, people can enjoy long life just as "Running water is never stale and a door hinge never gets worm-eaten." On this basis, he invented the famous "Wuqinxi", or the five mimic-animal games. It is an easy, convenient and effective keep-fit exercise which imitates the motions of the five animals of tiger, dear, bear, monkey and bird. Hua Tuo lived to be over 80. Hua Tuo should have been a longevous man if he had not been detained and killed.

1.2.4.4　Tao Hongjing: "Cultivate the mind to nourish the body"

Tao Hongjing, the famous expert on life cultivation in the Southern Dynasty, had a good command of medicine and was well versed in Buddhism and Taoism. His book *Records on Cultivating Character and Prolonging Life* is the earliest extant treatise on life cultivation in China. The book discusses a great number of life cultivation principles and methods, the main ones of which include conformity to seasonal changes, regulation of emotions,

过逸；在饮食上，要求营养丰富，新鲜洁净，烹调精细，味道鲜美。孔子生活在战乱时代，其寿命亦达72岁。另一位善养"浩然正气"的儒家代表人物孟子则享年83岁。

3. 华佗："动则不衰"

汉代名医华佗，从理论上阐述了动形养生的道理，认为"动"能够消化食物，流通血脉，"流水不腐，户枢不蠹"，所以健康长寿。在此基础上，他创编了著名的"五禽戏"，即模仿虎、鹿、熊、猿、鸟五种动物动作的健身体操，方法简便，行之有效。若非他惨遭拘禁刑戮，华佗也应该是一位高寿者。

4. 陶弘景："调神养形"

南朝的著名养生家陶弘景，精于医学，通晓佛、道，所著《养性延命录》一书，为中国现存最早的养生学专著。书中论述的养生法则和方术甚多，大致有：顺四时、调情志、动诸节、调气息、节饮食、宜小劳、慎房事等，其中"调神养

movement of every joint, regulation of respiration, moderate amount of food intake, light physical labor, proper sexual life, etc. Of all the principles and methods, "cultivate the mind to nourish the body" is the dominant idea. Tao Hongjing also died at the age of 80.

1.2.4.5 Sun Simiao: "Cultivate the disposition to preserve health"

Sun Simiao, a great expert on medicine and life cultivation, wrote a great work *Qian Jin Fang*, or *Valuable Prescriptions*, which has been handed down. Besides, he wrote treatises on life cultivation such as *Sheyang Zhenzhong Fang*, or *Handy Prescriptions for Life Cultivation*. The comprehensive regulation methods are adopted in his life cultivation techniques such as dietary therapy for life cultivation, promotion of health with moderate sexual life (Sexual life promotes health.), regulation of the mind for promotion of activities, massage, etc. The content is very rich. The application of these life cultivation methods is based on the theory of "cultivation of disposition" (regulating emotions, taking prevention before the onset of diseases). Sun Simiao lived to be 101.

1.2.4.6 Li Dongyuan: "Regulate the spleen and stomach"

Li Dongyuan, the founder of the School of Nourishing Earth (Spleen) of the four medical schools in the Jin and Yuan Dynasties, also emphasized that the protection of splenogastric functions is the important principle for prolonging life. This means: firstly, regulation of diet protects and nourishes the spleen and stomach; secondly, emotional regulation protects the spleen and stomach; thirdly, in preventing and treating diseases, protection of the spleen and stomach should be taken into consideration. This theory has laid a foundation for health preservation, especially for senile life cultivation. Li Dongyuan

形"是其主导思想。陶弘景亦为 80 高寿之长者。

5. 孙思邈:"养性摄生"

唐代大医学家、养生家孙思邈,有巨著《千金方》存世,另著有《摄养枕中方》等养生专著。其养生术采用综合调理的方法,诸如食疗调养、房中补益(性生活对健康的促进作用)、调神动形、推拿按摩等,内容丰富。这些养生方法的使用,建立在"养性"(调摄情志,未病先防)学说的基础上。孙思邈高龄至 101 岁。

6. 李东垣:"调理脾胃"

金元四大家中"补土派"的李东垣,亦强调维护脾胃功能是延年益寿的重要原则:一是调节饮食护养脾胃;二是调摄情志保护脾胃;三是防病治病顾护脾胃。该理论为养生学,尤其是老年养生奠定了基础。李东垣的年寿为 71 岁。

died at the age of 71.

1.2.4.7 Zhu Danxi: "Nourish and protect yin"

Zhu Danxi put forth a well-known theory concerning the human health — "Yang is usually in excess while yin is constantly insufficient in the human body." He especially emphasized the importance of protecting essence. Particularly, he warned people time and again of the impairment of yin due to excessive sexual life. The specific measures for protecting yin include conforming to seasonal variations to regulate and nourish the mind and qi, eating bland diet to avoid promoting fire and promoting dampness, abstinence from sexual desires for conservation of essence to extinguish renal fire and eliminate lust. Zhu Danxi died at the age of 77.

1.2.4.8 Li Shizhen: "Stand hard work to extend life span"

Li Shizhen of the Ming Dynasty is not only famous for *Bencao Gangmu*, or *Compendium of Materia Medica*, but also had a good command of the comprehensive application of life cultivation techniques. He had very rich discussions concerning life cultivation with drugs and the diet, collected many dietary therapeutic methods. Li Shizhen advocated that senior citizens should reinforce and tonify primordial qi, regulate the spleen and stomach, use prescriptions with warming and tonic actions to prolong life. He himself earnestly practiced his advocation of "standing hard work to prolong life." On the one hand, he made nothing of hardships, traveled across mountains and rivers to seek for medical materials. On the other hand, he also strengthened his constitution in this way. Li Shizhen lived to be 75.

1.2.4.9 Zhang Jingyue: "The interdependence of yin and yang"

Zhang Jingyue, a medical expert of the Ming Dynasty, believed that yang qi and yin essence are rooted in the kidney. Therefore, he advocated that life cultivation should concentrate on enhancing the kidney with simultaneous consideration of yin and yang. And he also established a set of tonic prescriptions with the actions of mutual tonification of yin and yang which have been handed down up to now. In addition, he also put forward the theory of "life cultivation in the middle-aged" (which attaches importance to life cultivation in middle-aged people). This has a positive significance for prevention of premature ageing and senile diseases. He died at the age of 77.

1.3 Concept: Conforming to nature

Conforming to nature is the important content of the concept of holism in Chinese medical system. All the methods and functions both in life cultivation and health care and the rehabilitation of diseases are embodied in the feature of conforming to nature.

1.3.1 Man's relevant adaptation to nature

TCM believes man and universe, all vital activities and nature are closely related to each other, and man should keep harmony with nature at any time in anywhere. This is the thought of "man's relevant adaptation to nature." Only when the concept of man's harmony and unity with nature is constantly observed, can good effects of life cultivation and rehabilitation be achieved. This point is specifically expounded as follows.

1.3.1.1 Adaptation to seasons

Seasonal variations influence the human body greatly. In spring and summer, yang qi releases and qi and blood easily tend to reach the surface. Therefore, the skin is loosened and sweat comes out. In autumn and winter, yang qi turns constricted and stored. At this time, qi and blood tend to reach the interior, thus, it manifests as tight skin, scanty sweat and profuse urine. Because of the above points, there exists the theory of "nourishing yang in spring and summer and yin in autumn and winter." Seasonal changes should also be taken into account in modifying drugs to achieve better effects during rehabilitation."

Seasons have direct influences on the five zang organs and six fu organs. Relative excess of qi and blood may occur in different viscera, meridians and collaterals in different seasons. For example, "relative excess of qi and blood exists in the liver in spring"; "relative excess of qi and blood exists in the heart in summer"; "relative excess of qi and blood exists in the spleen in late summer"; "relative excess of qi and blood exists in the lung in autumn" and "relative excess of qi and blood exists in the kidney in winter". Reasonable application of this principle may get twice the result with half the effort in life cultivation or rehabilitation. This principle can also be applied in selecting acupoints according to the syndrome differentiation in acumox and massage.

1.3.1.2 Conforming to geography

Dampness prevails in the east, heat in the south, dryness in the west and cold in the north in the Chinese geographical environment. People in different regions differ from one another in physique and susceptibility to diseases. Accordingly, different treatment should be based on specific situations during the daily life cultivation and rehabilitation of diseases.

1.3.1.3 Conforming to society

Chinese life cultivation experts throughout the history believe that healthy and longevous people view the world optimistically and positively. They do not approach society pessimistically and negatively. There exist conflicts of interests, unstable or unfair affairs in society everywhere at anytime. If viewing society pessimistically, people may get angry every day. This has bad effects on health. If approaching society optimistically, people may form a good spiritual environment. This is beneficial to life cultivation and rehabilitation. A Chinese saying goes like this "One is always happy if one is content with one's lot." The classic *Yang Sheng Yao Yu*, or *Essential Words for Life Cultivation*, says: "If one smiles, one will become a little younger; if one is angry, one will become a little older; if one struggles with others, one will get a little thinner; if one yields, one will become a little stronger."

1.3.2 Unity of physique and spirit

Physique refers to the configuration and constitution of the human body consisting of the tissues and organs of muscle, blood vessels, tendons, bones, viscera, etc. as the material base of man; spirit refers to the mental activities such as emotions, consciousness and thinking. It also denotes the outward manifestations of all vital activities as the reflections of the functions of the human body.

1.3.2.1 Physique as the base

"Physique" is the material base of "spirit". TCM believes "the five types of spirit" (vitality, soul, vigor, will and consciousness) and five emotions (joy, anger, sorrow, anxiety and fear) are produced by the five zang organs (the heart, liver, spleen, lung and kidney) respectively. "Spirit" requires the nourishment of qi, blood and food essence. In case of spiritual disorders, the treatment should be based on the five zang organs. This is the

二、形神合一

形，指形体，即肌肉、血脉、筋骨、脏腑等组织器官，是人的物质基础；神，指情志、意识、思维等精神活动，又指生命活动的全部外在表现，是人体功能的反映。

1. 形为基础

"形"是"神"的物质基础，中医的"五神"（神魂魄志意）、"五志"（怒喜思忧恐）分别由五脏（心肝脾肺肾）所生成。"神"需要大量的气血精微濡养，如果神志方面出现疾患，要从五脏论治，这就是中医形神统一、形为基础观的具体

specific manifestation of unity of physique and spirit, and physique as the material base of spirit.

1.3.2.2 Spirit as the commander

The cardiac spirit functions as the commander and coordinator of the human body. The wholeness of characteristics, functions, behavior and principles reflected in vital activities are all managed, coordinated and unified by spirit. Thus, there exist the measures of putting "cultivation of disposition" and "regulation of the mind" first in life cultivation. These methods of life cultivation with regulation of the mind are also applicable to physical diseases.

1.3.2.3 Simultaneous cultivation of spirit and physique

This means that people should not only pay attention to conserving their physique, but also to the cultivation of spirit. The two aspects supplement each other and promote mutually to achieve the harmonious and unified development of the body and spirit.

1.3.3 Interdependence of movement and motionlessness

1.3.3.1 Movement of yang and motionlessness of yin

Viscera belong to yin, characterized by motionlessness. Functional activities pertain to yang, marked by movement. The coordination of movement with motionlessness of visceral functions of organism completes all the absorption, transportation and transformation of food, the circulation and metabolism of water, the flow of qi and blood, the transportation and excretion of digested stuff, mutual transformation of material and function, etc. Therefore, maintaining proper harmony between movement and motionlessness can make every organ function vigorously. As a result, the ageing and changes of each organ are delayed.

1.3.3.2 Coordination between movement and motionlessness

Of Chinese experts on life cultivation in successive dynasties, some relatively attached importance to movement, some to tranquility. However, most of them advocated the combination of movement and motionlessness. According to different people and situations, relative emphasis is placed on one aspect to gain the effect of simultaneous nourishment of physique and spirit. Life cultivation with concurrent movement and motionlessness, proper adjustment of movement and motionlessness and equal stress on both are the important principles of traditional Chinese life cultivation and rehabilitation.

1.3.4 Coordination and balance

Coordination of physiological functional states of the human body and the relationships with the external environment, balance of the normal functions of each system and tissues and organs of the organism as well as exchanges of material between functions of organism and nature are the important academic content of traditional Chinese life cultivation and rehabilitation.

1.3.4.1 Balance of elements

The interpromotion and restraint of the five elements maintain ecological balance in nature and the physiological coordination and balance of the human body. Besides, the human body should have the balance and coordination of chemical elements in nature. For instance, iodine deficiency gives rise to thyroid enlargement and zinc deficiency to infertility. According to the concept of balance of elements in TCM, imbalance of elements inside the human

官充满活力,从而推迟各器官的衰老改变。

2. 动静相济

中国历代养生家有的偏重于运动,有的偏重于静养,但大多数养生家提倡动静结合,根据不同对象和情况各有侧重,以达到形神共养的效果。动静兼修,动静适宜,运动和静养并重,是中国传统养生和康复的重要原则。

四、协调平衡

协调人体自身的生理功能状态及其与外在环境之间的相互关系,平衡机体各系统和组织器官间的正常功能,以及机体与外界的物质交换,也是中国养生、康复学术的重要内容。

1. 元素平衡

五行元素的"生克制化",维持着自然界的生态平衡和人体生理的协调平衡。人体还必须与自然界化学元素平衡协调。例如,缺碘导致甲状腺肿,缺锌可致不育等。依照中医元素平衡的观念,必须纠正体内元素的失调,维持体内

body should be remedied to keep the coordination and balance of various elements inside the body.

1.3.4.2 Coordinative balance

Dysfunctions, loss of symmetry and unstable states of the human body are the important causes giving rise to physiological hypofunction, premature ageing and diseases of the human body. There exist the theory and methods of coordinative balance in the medical techniques of life cultivation and rehabilitation in TCM. For example, there are such methods as "treating diseases in the upper part by managing the lower", "treating diseases in the lower by managing the upper", "treating diseases in the left by managing the right" and "treating diseases in the right by managing the left"in acumoxi and massage as well as "alternation of physical labor and mental one" and "alternation of movement and motionlessness"in life cultivation.

1.3.5 Healthy qi as the base

"The congenital base lies in the kidney and the postnatal base in the spleen." The nutritional essence coming from the two zang organs of the spleen and kidney is the motive power of the visceral functions of the whole human body. Thus, the concept of healthy qi as the base should first aim at the two zang organs of the spleen and kidney.

Reinforcing essence and qi is the key to the tonification of the kidney, and strengthening transportation and transformation is the key to enhancement of the spleen, both of which promote and supplement mutually. Of all activities of life cultivation and rehabilitation, the conservation and promotion of functions of the spleen and kidney are the important content which cannot be ignored.

各种元素的协调平衡。

2. 调节平衡

人体的功能失调、对称失衡、状态失稳，是导致人体生理功能低下和早衰、疾病的重要原因。中医养生学和康复技术手段中有调节平衡的理论和方法，如针灸、推拿中的"上病下取"、"下病上取"、"左病右取"、"右病左取"等方法，养生学中的"体脑交替"、"动静交替"等。

五、正气为本

"先天之本在肾，后天之本在脾"，脾、肾两脏产生的营养精微，是全身脏腑功能的动力，因此，正气为本的观念，首先要落实在脾、肾两脏。

培补精气是补肾的关键，增强运化是健脾的关键，两者还有相互促进，相互补充的作用。在所有的养生、康复活动中，脾肾功能的维护和促进，是切不可忽视的重要内容。

1.4 Principle: Wholism and syndrome differentiation

1.4.1 Principle of wholism

The human body is an organic whole. The medicine of TCM life cultivation and rehabilitation should guide or help patients to be in harmony with nature and society. Besides, it should also make all component parts of the human body harmonious and unified mutually, physique and spirit harmonious and unified. These are the principles of wholism in the science of life cultivation and rehabilitation.

1.4.1.1 Component parts in harmony with the organic whole, equal stress on physique and spirit

During rehabilitation, local dysfunctions should be unified with the organic whole. In addition, attention should be constantly paid to the regulation of relationships between physique and spirit to restore the unified and harmonious states.

1.4.1.2 Unity between functions and nature, blood and qi in step with four seasons

The activities of life cultivation and rehabilitation should conform to seasonal and climatic changes as well as geographical differences, etc. This book constantly pays attention to principles of "treatment in accordance with geographical conditions" and "treatment in accordance with seasonal conditions", the purposes of which are to conform to the laws of seasonal and climatic changes and regional differences during regulation of viscera, promotion of qi flow and blood circulation and cultivation of the mind. In doing so, people can adapt themselves to the natural changes of germination, growth, reaping and storing so as to keep the relative balance of yin and yang inside and outside the human body. As a result, the aim of health and longevity will be reached.

Social environments may also influence physiological functions and pathological changes of the human body. For example, due to the social development, industrialization and urbanization speed up. This causes environmental pollution (including air pollution, soil pollution and noise pollution). As a result, some new diseases occur. The changes of life style and increase of work pressure give rise to more and more "modern civilization diseases". A large number of the currently widespread psychosomatic diseases are associated with social environments such as coronary heart disease, hypertension, peptic ulcer and bronchial asthma. Therefore, guiding patients to adapt themselves to changes of social environments, correcting their bad life styles and behaviors, greatly enhancing the control over and prevention of environmental pollution belong to the important content of the science of TCM rehabilitation as well.

1.4.2 Principle of syndrome differentiation

Differentiating syndrome to decide treatment is the greatest characteristic of TCM. During life cultivation and rehabilitation, the result of syndrome differentiation should be applied to determine the corresponding principles and methods of life cultivation and rehabilitation. Under the guidance of differentiating syndrome to decide treatment, same disease with different syndromes is also rehabilitated differently while different diseases with the same syndrome are rehabilitated in the same way, too. Besides, the principle of combination of syndrome differentiation with disease differentiation should be concurrently taken into consideration in guiding rehabilitation.

社会环境的变化也会影响人体的生理功能及病理变化,如由于社会发展的工业化和都市化趋势的加快,导致环境(空气、土壤、噪声)污染,可以引发一些新的疾病;生活方式的改变,工作压力的增大,造就"现代文明病"日益严重。当今时代大量流行的心身疾病,如冠心病、高血压、消化性溃疡、支气管哮喘等的发生,都与社会环境有关。因此,帮助患者适应社会环境的变化,纠正其不良生活方式与行为,加大对环境污染的治理与防护等,也都属于中医康复学的重要内容。

二、辨证原则

辨证论治是中医学最大的特色。养生措施和康复医疗必须根据辨证的结果来确定相应的养生、康复原则和方法,在辨证论治理论的指导下,病同证异,康复亦异;病异证同,康复亦同。此外,还要兼顾辨证与辨病相结合的原理来指导康复医疗。

1.4.3 Principle of functions

The physiological activities of the human body are the ascending, descending, exiting and entering of the functional activities of qi. The science of life cultivation requires that these normal functional states should be maintained and restored in rehabilitation. Besides, attention should be paid to functional training, movement of physique to promote circulation of healthy qi, and harmonization of physiological functions of viscera and tissues. In this way, patients' abilities to adapt themselves to their individual life, family and social life as well as professional work can be to the greatest extent restored.

1.4.3.1 Normal visceral functions mainly lie in coordination

Convalescent patients still suffer from residual pathogenic factors and deficiency of healthy qi after recovery from wounds, handicap and diseases. Their visceral functions are not completely restored. Comprehensive measures should be taken to restore visceral functions as quickly as possible, and to coordinate other viscera according to the pathological features. For instance, as for a patient with liver disease during convalescence, not only dampness and heat in the liver meridian should be cleared away, but also the injury of the spleen and stomach should be taken into account.

1.4.3.2 The significance of viability mainly lies in quality

Viability chiefly refers to daily living ability and professional working ability. Various ways should be adopted to train, conserve and restore functions in the fields of bodily movement, perception, lingual communication, life and profession, etc. to improve the life quality.

三、功能原则

人体生理活动,是气机的"升降出入"有序。养生学要求维护生理功能;康复医疗的目的是恢复正常的功能状态。它注重功能训练,运动形体,促使精气流通,使脏腑组织的生理功能得以协调,最大限度地恢复个人生活、家庭和社会生活以及职业工作的适应能力。

1. 脏腑功能重在协调

康复患者,伤残病后余邪未尽,正气尚虚,脏腑功能未完全恢复正常,必须针对其病理特点,采取综合措施,促使脏腑功能尽快恢复,并且能与其他脏腑协调。如肝病患者康复期不仅要消除其肝经湿热,也要顾及脾胃功能的损伤。

2. 生存能力重在质量

生存能力主要指日常生活能力和职业工作能力,要采取多种方式进行功能训练,保存和恢复其身体运动、感知、言语交流、生活和职业等方面的功能,提高生活质量。

2 Natural Therapeutic Methods of Life Cultivation and Rehabilitation

2.1 Regulating emotions

The ancient Chinese medical staff have pointed out long before: Healthy human body means not only freedom from diseases and weakness, but also sound mental condition and social adaptive capacity. In modern society, psychic factors give rise to more and more psychosomatic diseases. Psychological diseases will become the frequent and widespread diseases of human being in the 21st century.

Under normal circumstances, seven emotional activities play a role of coordinating the physiological functions of the five zang organs. But excessive seven emotions beyond the scope of the self-adjustment of the human body can cause disturbance of visceral qi and blood. Consequently, diseases occur.

2.1.1 Abstaining from anger

"Anger" has been the emotional taboo for experts on life cultivation throughout the history. It impairs not only the liver, but also the heart, stomach and brain, etc., which leads to cause various diseases. Accordingly, anger, the bad emotion, should be possibly controlled in life

第二章 养生康复的自然疗法

第一节 调节情志法

中国古代医学家们很早以前就已经指出：健康的人体，不仅是没有疾病和虚弱现象，而且还要有良好的精神状态和社会适应能力。现代社会中，精神因素引起的心身疾患越来越普遍，21世纪，精神类疾病将成为人类的多发病和流行病。

在正常情况下，七情活动对五脏生理功能起着协调作用，但若七情太过，超过人体自身调节的范围，使脏腑气血紊乱，则能导致疾病。

一、遏止

"怒"是历代养生家最忌讳的一种情绪，它不仅伤肝脏，还可伤心、伤胃、伤脑等，导致各种疾病。因此怒是养生、康复最应节制的不良

cultivation and rehabilitation.

Restraining one's anger means that one should rationally overcome emotional impulses. When anything irritating comes up, one should first think of its bad consequence so as to rationally restrain and control one's bad and violent emotions. For instance, ancient and modern wise people often hang up aphorisms such as "restraining anger" and "ceasing to be angry" over their desks to remind them of abstinence from anger.

2.1.2　Giving vent to depression

One may adopt proper methods to give vent to one's bad emotions when meeting setbacks, or being wronged, or confronting troublesome and grief affairs. For instance, one may cry aloud in a place where there are no people when meeting with a misfortune or being extremely grieved; one may go to an open field and shout loudly to let off his depression and emotions when encountering setbacks and feeling constrained.

2.1.3　Straightening one out with the help of a friend

When bad emotions occur, one should find two or three intimate friends to air one's depression and follow friend's advice, eventually to overcome bad emotions.

2.1.4　Diverting emotions

Diverting emotions means overcoming emotions and changing the directionality of emotions to get rid of distracting thoughts and depression and to change bad emotions and habits. When met with depression, one might as well "read books to divert oneself from boredom, listen to

情绪。

制怒，就是要以理性克服感情上的冲动，平时遇到可怒之事，要想到不良后果，以理智驾驭并控制粗暴的情绪反应。如古今明理之人常在案头悬挂"制怒"、"息怒"之类警句，提醒自己戒怒。

二、发泄

在遭遇挫折，或蒙受冤屈，或遇见烦闷、悲愤之事时，应采取适当的方式发泄不良情绪。如：遇到不幸事件，悲痛万分时，在无人处大哭一场；遭逢挫折，心情压抑时，去空旷处大声喊叫，将郁结情绪发泄出来。

三、疏导

出现不良情绪时，相约三二知心朋友，宣泄心中郁闷，并接受友人的劝解疏导，可以借此化解或排遣不良情绪。

四、移情

移情，即排遣情思，改变情绪的指向性，以排除内心杂念和抑郁，改变其不良情绪和习惯。当遇到情绪郁闷时，不妨"看书解闷，听曲消愁"，利

music to dispel melancholy." In addition, the musical instrument, chess, painting and calligraphy may be utilized to divert emotions and mould one's temperament.

2.1.5 Sports

Bad emotions due to mental stimuli can be let off by sports activities and also by diverting one's attention and regulating the balance of the human body. Various activities such as playing balls, walking, mountaineering, practicing Taijiquan and performing a sword dance can all divert or let off mental stress and discomfort. Especially, traditional physical training emphasizes the combination of movement with motionlessness, which can make the body comfortable and people happy. It is very effective for eliminating bad emotions. In addition, people may also take part in physical labor to get rid of mental tension, anger and grief with physical exercises.

2.1.6 Suggestion

Suggestion therapy is a method to promote the patient's rehabilitation by means of suggestion. The ancient Chinese idiom "mistaking the reflection of a bow in the cup for a snake—extremely suspicious" is a typical example of this suggestion. The ancient Chinese pray for recovery also includes some elements of suggestion therapy.

Suggestion has both positive suggestion and negative suggestion. Positive suggestion means the patient accepts other people's ideas completely, unconditionally, uncritically and without analysis no matter the ideas are correct or not. It exerts positive effects on psychosomatic health. Negative suggestion, however, denotes that the patient thoroughly negates and rejects other people's ideas. It has negative effects on psychosomatic health. Suggestion therapy makes use of the positive effects of suggestion to promote psychosomatic health of the human body. Meanwhile, attention should be paid to avoiding the negative effects of suggestion.

Suggestion therapy may be conducted on two occasions: one is performed in complete waking state without hypnotization; the other means suggestion is given to the patient after he or she enters hypnosis. The latter excels the former in effects. Besides, the patient also may perform positive self suggestion and repeatedly intensify the consciousness of "excellent health and recovery from the disease". In this way, visceral functions can be consequently induced to develop along an orderly direction.

2.1.7　Colors

According to the effects of colors on the human body and emotions, certain colors are selected to exert direct effects on the mind and emotions via eyes. This is the so-called pleasing the eyes and refreshing the mind. Besides, the color tones, color temperatures, etc. may also be used to regulate emotions.

The method, under the guidance of the theory of "the five colors corresponding to the five zang organs and five emotions", is used to arrange the colors of the patient's living surroundings such as living rooms, utensils, furnishings, clothes, quilts, window curtains and lights as well as the dresses of doctors and nurses of rehabilitation according to the requirements. Also, rooms of rehabilitation with colors and "color instruments" are installed in hospitals and sanitariums to rehabilitate the corresponding diseases. Colors and their indications are as follows.

2.1.7.1　Warm colors

Red and orange, with warm feeling, possess the

暗示的积极作用而促使人体身心的康复,同时应注意避免暗示的消极作用。

暗示疗法可在两种场合下进行:一种是不经任何催眠过程,而在完全觉醒状态下进行;另一种是先使患者进入催眠状态,然后予以暗示。后者的效果优于前者。此外,患者还可以进行积极的自我暗示,反复强化"身体健康,疾病痊愈"的意识,从而诱导脏腑功能向有序的方向发展。

七、色彩

根据色彩对人体神志的影响,选定一定的色彩,通过眼睛直接作用于精神情志,即所谓悦目爽神,还可以通过色调、色温等调节精神。

该法以"五色配五脏、五志"的理论为指导,在病人居住环境,如居室、用具、陈设、衣被、窗帘、灯光以及与病人接触的康复医护人员的衣着上,按需要的颜色布置和穿戴,或者在医院或疗养院设置色彩疗法康复室和"颜色仪",来对适合的病种进行康复调理。色彩及其适应证:

1. 暖色

红色、橙色,具有温暖的

actions of making people excited and joyful. The colors are applicable to depression, depressive psychosis, lethargy, dementia, etc.

2.1.7.2 Cold colors

Among indigo blue, blue, purple and green, one may select one color, or two, or three. The colors have the actions of cooling, tranquilizing and making people restrained. Cold colors are applicable to dysphoria, irascibility, insomnia, terror and fear as well as mania, epilepsy, etc.

2.1.7.3 Joyful colors

Red and pink make people happy and have the action of restraining grief. The colors are applicable to people with low spirits, susceptibility to grief and cry, and depression.

2.1.7.4 Sad colors

Black is mainly applied or white may also be used to restrict anger. Both colors are applicable to susceptibility to anger, overjoy, etc.

2.1.7.5 Fearful color

Black has the action of restricting overjoy. The color is applicable to mania, endless laughing, etc.

2.1.7.6 Anxious colors

Yellow, light blue and light green possess the actions of restricting fear and benefiting thinking. The colors are applicable to terror, fear, distraction, etc.

The flexible selection of either single color or multiple colors, either light colors or rich colors, is used to form the proper compatibility according to the requirement of the patient's in applying the colors.

2.1.8 Checking one emotion with another

This is the method mentioned more than 2000 years ago in "Discussion on Principles of Yin-Yang Doctrine and its Relations with Natural Things and Phenomena", a chapter of *Plain Questions*. The content includes "anger impairs the liver while grief restricts anger"; "joy impairs the heart while fear restricts joy"; "anxiety impairs the spleen while anger restricts anxiety"; "melancholy impairs the lung while joy restricts melancholy" and "fear impairs the kidney while anxiety restricts fear." This method of checking one emotion with another is based on the principle of excess curing excess. Zhang Zihe, a medical expert of the Jin and Yuan Dynasties, introduced it specifically as follows: "Checking anger with grief means using sorrowful words to move one; checking grief with joy using crack jokes to please one; checking joy with fear using fear and death to frighten one; checking anxiety with anger using insulting language to excite one; checking fear with anxiety using worrying words to make one forget the fear."

2.1.8.1 Fear restricts joy

This is a method to restrain great joy impairing the heart and restore mental functions by applying fearful factors to astringe the dissipated cardiac spirit. The method is often applicable to diseases of scattered cardiac qi due to endless laughing as well as emotional disorders due to excessive joy.

2.1.8.2 Anger restricts anxiety

This is a method to restore functions of the heart and spleen by using irritating factors to restrain excessive anxiety. The method is often applicable to melancholia, insomnia, epilepsy, etc. caused by impairment of the spleen and consumption of spirit due to excessive anxiety.

2.1.8.3 Joy restricts grief

This is a method to overcome excessive grief by utilizing funny factors. The method often makes use of romantic, very witty and humorous language, and amusing

的方法,其内容是"怒伤肝,悲胜怒";"喜伤心,恐胜喜";"思伤脾,怒胜思";"忧伤肺,喜胜忧";"恐伤肾,思胜恐"。这种"以情制情"的方法,基于"以偏救偏"的原理。金元医家张子和具体地介绍:"以悲制怒,以怆恻苦楚之言感之;以喜治悲,以谑浪戏狎之言娱之;以恐治喜,以恐惧死亡之言怖之;以怒制思,以污辱欺罔之言触之;以思治恐,以虑彼忘此之言夺之。"

1. 恐胜喜

是通过恐惧因素来收敛耗散的心神,克制大喜伤心,恢复心神功能的方法。本法常用于喜笑不休,心气涣散的病证以及因过喜而致的情志失调。

2. 怒胜思

是通过忿怒因素来克制思虑太多,恢复心脾功能的方法。本法常用于思虑太多,伤脾耗神所致的郁证、失眠、癫痫等病证。

3. 喜胜悲

是通过喜乐因素来消除悲哀太过的方法。本法常利用轻松浪漫、妙趣横生的语言

performance, telling jokes, listening to xiangsheng (a traditional Chinese comic dialogue) and watching plays. And even sometimes, the doctor intentionally makes a ridiculous diagnosis to satisfy the patient's eagerness. In doing all these, the purposes are to free the patient from the difficult positions and consequently achieve the effect of joy restricting grief. The method is often clinically applicable to crying with grief and hysteria as well as diseases due to excessive grief.

2.1.8.4 Grief restricts anger

This is a method to restrain excessive anger by making use of grievous factors. The method is commonly applicable to other diseases with accompanying emotional excitement such as vertigo, mania and epilepsy.

2.1.8.5 Anxiety restricts fear

This is a method to restrain fright and fear by adopting anxious factors. The method is commonly applied in rehabilitation to get rid of the patient's fearful mood.

In applying the method of "checking one emotion with another", pay attention to the intensity of emotional stimuli. The intensity has to exceed that of the pathogenic emotional factors. For instance, sudden stimuli or continuous intensification of stimuli may be applied. Moreover, modern people may adopt other relevant methods as long as they grasp the essence of the above-mentioned methods. Mechanical application of these methods is not advisable.

2.2 Environments, daily life and clothing

The life cultivation methods of environments, daily life, clothing mainly discuss the environmental influences on human health, the scientific arrangement of daily life including food, clothing, shelter and transportation, standing, lying, suffering, enjoyment, strain, rest, etc. as well as adoption of a set of measures, the purposes of which are to eliminate diseases, strengthen health and prolong life.

2.2.1 Environments

Environments include natural environments and artificial environments. Natural environments include air, water, soil, rocks, living things, etc. on the earth; artificial environments refer to the urban and rural living residential environments built by man for collective life. The indoor environment is included in the artificial environments.

The ancient Chinese fengshuishu (geomancy) was the theory and art which studies how to establish an ideal environment beneficial to prolonging life and life cultivation. It was the comprehensive theory of ancient architectural planning and design integrating geography, ecology, architecture, ethics, aesthetics, etc. into an organic whole. Synthesizing the essentials of the above aspects, the ancient Chinese feugshuishu believed that the natural environment suitable for man is the one with clear and plentiful water source, fresh air, sufficient sunlight, good vegetation as well as a quiet secluded and beautiful landscape. This type of natural environment not only satisfies the basic human need of material life, but also suits the special human psychological requirement.

Because of geographical causes in certain places, "goiter prevails in the mountain area" and "malaria prevails in the south of the Five Ridges (the area covering

的影响,对日常生活中衣食住行、站立坐卧、苦乐劳逸等各个方面进行科学安排并采取一系列健身措施,以达到祛病强身、益寿延年的目的。

一、环境

环境包括自然环境和人工环境。自然环境包括地球上的空气、水、土壤、岩石和生物等;人工环境指人类为从事社会集居生活而建立的城乡生活居住环境,室内环境包括在人工环境中。

中国古代的风水术,是一种探讨如何创造有益于延年益寿、养生保健的理想环境的理论和艺术,它强调人与自然的和谐相处,是一种集地质学、地理学、生态学、建筑学、伦理学、美学等于一体的综合性的古代建筑规划设计理论。综合其中要点,它认为人类适宜的自然环境应该是:洁净而充足的水源,新鲜的空气,充沛的阳光,良好的植被以及幽静秀丽的景观等。这种自然环境,不仅能满足人类基本的物质生活需求,还适应人类特殊的心理需求。

某些地方由于地理条件的原因,出现"山区多瘿瘤"、"岭南多瘴气"等地方病,中医

Guangdong and Guangxi"), etc. Many TCM treatises have realized these phenomena long before. In addition, the trace elements essential for the human body also distribute differently under different geographical conditions. For example, endemic goiter easily occurs in iodine deficiency areas while fluorine deficiency gives rise to dental caries, etc. Apart from the above, certain radioactive substances are also harmful to the human body such as uranium ore and phosphorus ore. Powerful radioactive sources may give rise to increased incidences of anemia, leukemia and cancer in local people.

Therefore, people should try their best to avoid the areas and ores, which are not beneficial to human health, high tension lines and strong magnetic field as well as the locally built living areas with supersonic waves and radioactive rays.

Besides, harnessing pollution of air, water sources and noises is the basic conditions to ensure health. It needs the joint efforts of the government, society, families and individuals for the establishment of an environment beneficial to health and longevity.

2.2.2 Daily life

2.2.2.1 Regular work and rest

One basic requirement of TCM life cultivation is "normal daily life" which means regular work, rest and daily life. This is an important principle for strengthening health and prolonging life.

If there exist irregular daily life, work and rest and unscrupulous behavior, ageing phenomena may occur such as declined adaptive capacity and body resistance, increased incidence. As a result, premature ageing may occur to affect life span.

The most helpful and correct life style for life cultivation and longevity is the reasonable arrangement of daily life, work and rest which requires that people should sleep, get up, eat, work, study, exercise the body, defecate, urinate, bathe, etc. at fixed times. However, the so-called "at fixed times" should still be flexibly handled according to the specific conditions (the differences in ages, seasons, regions and physiques) and mechanical application should be avoided.

2.2.2.2　Proper balance between work and rest

The ancients advocated that the criteria for work and rest were "moderation", regular and moderate adjustment without excess in either one. Only when the integration of movement and motionlessness, and moderation of work and rest are adopted, can tendons and bones be exercised, qi and blood flow smooth, physique strong, willpower enhanced and vigorous life-force conserved.

Work and rest include not only the consumption of physical strength, but also the moderate use of the brain. In other words, the use of the brain should include moderation of work and rest and the advocation of scientific use of the brain. Mental labor without tiredness keeps the constant use of the brain without decline. Regular and reasonable use of the brain can prevent ageing, increase intelligence, especially prevent senile dementia.

The criteria for moderation of work and rest vary in persons. In general, the following may be used for reference. ① Physical labor should be proper in intensity; ② mental labor should be integrated with physical activities; ③ rest and health conservation should be various. Not only should rest in sleeping way be adopted, but also rest in other ways should be applied such as listening to music, chatting, playing chess, walking, enjoying the sight of scenery, fishing, composing poems, painting and practicing Taijiquan.

2.2.2.3 Scientific sleeping

Sleeping plays an extremely important role in one's life time. If one wants health and longevity, he or she should adopt reasonable sleeping habits, ensure sleeping quality, restore the body from fatigue and store up energy to prevent and treat diseases, strengthen health and benefit longevity. The effects of sleeping on health and longevity manifest in the following five fields: ① eliminating fatigue to restore strength; ② protecting brain to conserve intelligence; ③ strengthening immunity to increase body resistance; ④ promoting infantile development and increasing body height; ⑤ making the skin healthy and aesthetical and excreting the waste. In the case of abnormal sleeping, the above-mentioned five aspects may change for the worse, and affect the health of human body and longevity.

2.2.2.3.1 **Sleeping time**　Chinese life cultivation experts have created quite a number of beneficial and very effective sleeping methods for life cultivation which are simple and convenient and easy to practice. For instance, "Sleeping at Midnight and Noon" is one of the sleeping methods for life cultivation. The method is as follows: Go to sleep at midnight (11 p.m. to 1 a.m.) and noon (11 a.m. to 1 p.m.) respectively, because at midnight and noon are the time for the alternation of yin and yang, the moment yin and yang change from excess to extreme deficiency or from extreme deficiency to excess, and qi, blood, yin and yang inside the body are extremely imbalanced. At this time, peaceful lying can avoid the impairment of qi and blood. It has been proved by practice that the quality and efficiency of sleeping at midnight and noon are both good. As for old people, the sleeping method can also reduce the sick rates of cardiovascular and cerebro-vascular diseases. It conforms to the principle of life cultivation.

Good sleeping regularity should be developed in sleeping time. The ancients summarized the regularity in sleeping as: "Man should rise early in spring and summer and late in autumn and winter, but not as early as before the cock crows in the morning or as late as after the sun rises."

2.2.2.3.2 Sleeping postures "Sleeping like a bow" is the requirement of sleeping posture. This is a beneficial sleeping posture for the human body. Medical experts both in the past and at present have chosen the right lateral position. The right lateral position can increase cardiac output, strengthen digestion of food, absorption of nutrients and metabolism. Besides, man himself feels more comfortable, too.

As for females, supination and pronation are not advisable, because pronation may increase facial wrinkles, and supination is harmful to pelvic blood circulation which easily gives rise to emmeniopathy. Right lateral position is suitable for normal people while left lateral position is advisable for pregnant women, because right lateral position may constrict veins of lower abdominal cavity and affect blood return, which is harmful to fetal development and delivery. Nevertheless, left lateral position is beneficial to fetal growth and may greatly reduce complications of pregnancy.

As far as infants are concerned, the posture should be constantly changed with the help of adults, because prolonged lateral position or supination and pronation easily cause asymmetrical development of skull, or deformity of five sense organs of the face. Generally, infants should be turned over once every 1 to 2 hours.

在睡眠时间上,要训练良好的睡眠规律。古人将睡眠的时间规律总结为:"春夏宜早起,秋冬任晏眠,晏忌日出后,早忌鸡鸣前。"

(2) 睡眠姿态　在睡眠姿态方面,要求"卧如弓"。这是一种对人体有益的卧姿。古今医家都选择右侧卧为最佳卧姿。右侧卧时心输出量增多,食物的消化和营养物质的吸收与代谢得到加强,人自身感觉也比较舒适。

对于女性来说,不宜仰卧和俯卧,因为俯卧会增加颜面皱纹,仰卧对盆腔血液循环不利,易致各种月经病。正常人宜右侧卧,而孕妇宜取左侧卧,因为右侧卧会压迫腹部下腔静脉,影响血液回流,不利于胎儿发育和分娩。而左侧卧有利于胎儿生长,可以大大减少妊娠并发症。

对婴幼儿来说,应该在大人的帮助下经常地变换体位。因为长时间一侧卧或仰卧、俯卧,易使头颅发育不对称,或面部五官畸形。一般每隔1～2小时翻一次身。

Semilateral position or semi-sitting position is advisable for patients with heart failure and patients with attack of cough and asthma. Meanwhile, the pillow and postdorsal region are high padded. Lateral position is suitable for patients with thoracoabdominal dropsy due to pulmonary diseases. Left lateral position or prone position is not suitable for patients with heart diseases with symptoms of blood stasis. The same is true of patients with pulmonary heart disease in case cardiac load is too heavy. Lying position with low head and high feet easily results in renal diseases.

It should be pointed out that though the above sleeping postures are beneficial to life cultivation and health care, keeping the postures unchanged after falling asleep is not required, for it is impossible to realize this.

2.2.2.3.3 Sleeping articles

(1) Pillow　The pillow should be slightly lower than the distance from the shoulder to the neck of the same side. If it is too high, it may affect the smoothing and regulating functions of the liver meridian, and also induce cerebral ischemia, snoring and stiff neck; if it is too low, it may affect the dispersing and descending of the lung qi, and also cause congestion of the head and resultant edema of eyelids and the face. The pillow is not advisably very wide, with the width of 15 to 20 cm. But being slight long is not harmful. The material of loose and soft texture with proper hardness and slight elasticity should be selected for pillow core.

There exists the habit of using medicinal pillows for life cultivation and rehabilitation in TCM. A medicinal pillow is the one with the medicinal core prepared with different traditional Chinese drugs. This type of pillows has therapeutic and health care actions. The commonly-used

对于心衰病人及咳喘发作病人宜取半侧位或半卧位，同时将枕与后背垫高。对于肺病造成的胸腹积液患者，宜取患侧卧位。有瘀血症状的心脏病人，如肺心病人等一般不宜取左侧卧或俯卧，以防心脏负荷过重。头低足高位置睡觉，易得肾脏疾患。

应该指出的是，上述睡眠姿势虽然有利于养生保健，但并不要求睡着后姿势永远不变，因为这是无法做到的。

（3）卧具选择

①枕头　枕高以稍低于肩至同侧颈部距离为宜，过高影响肝脉疏泄，还会诱发脑缺氧、打鼾和落枕；过低则影响肺气宣降，还会使头部充血，易造成眼睑和颜面浮肿。枕头不宜过宽，以15～20 cm为好，但稍长不妨。枕芯应选质地松软之物，软硬适度，稍有弹性。

中医有使用药枕养生、康复的习惯。药枕是采用不同药物加工制成枕芯做成的枕头。这种枕头既有治疗作用，又具保健作用。常用的单味

medicinal pillows with one ingredient include:

1) Pillow padded with Juhua (*Flos Chrysanthemi*): It is applicable to patients with headache, conjunctival congestion and dizziness or acute catarrhal conjunctivitis, insomnia with asthenic dysphoria as well as hypertension.

2) Pillow padded with Bohe (*Herba Menthae*): It is applicable to headache, toothache, rhinitis, laryngopharyngitis, hypertension, etc. and also has the actions of preventing summer-heat and lowering the temperature.

3) Pillow padded with Sangye (*Folium Mori*): It is applicable to headache, vertigo, and hypertension, etc.

4) Pillow padded with tea leaves: The pillow is padded with the used and dried tea leaves. It is applicable to the prevention and treatment of hypertension, neurasthenia, dizziness due to summer-heat, etc.

5) Pillow padded with Qiaomai (*Semen Fagopyri Esculenti*): It is applicable to insomnia, headache, vertigo, and infantile night cry, etc.

6) Pillow padded with Lüdou (*Semen Phaseoli Radiati*): It is applicable to the prevention and treatment of headache and wind syndrome of the head, and improves sight, induces resuscitation, removes summer-heat and dysphoria.

7) Pillow padded with Dengxin (*Medulla Junci*): It is applicable to insomnia, vexation, amnesia, and infantile night cry, etc. and benefits intelligence.

8) Pillow padded with Juemingzi (*Semen Cassiae*): It is applicable to constipation, ocular diseases, hypertension, and infantile night cry, etc.

9) Pillow padded with Cebaiye (*Cacumen Biotae*): It is applicable to persistent oral and nasal bleeding, chronic pharyngitis, congestion of throat, chronic cough and patients with mild baldness.

10) Pillow padded with Cansha (*Excrementa Bom-*

药枕有：

菊花枕：适用于头痛目赤、头晕或患风火赤眼、虚烦失眠及高血压病患者。

薄荷枕：适用于头痛、牙痛、鼻炎、咽喉炎、高血压等疾病，并有防暑降温作用。

桑叶枕：适用于头痛、眩晕、高血压等疾病。

茶叶枕：用饮后晒干的茶叶装枕。适用于防治高血压、神经衰弱、暑热头晕等。

荞麦枕：适用于失眠、头痛眩晕、小儿夜啼等病症。

绿豆枕：适用于防治头痛头风，可令人明目开窍，解暑除烦。

灯芯枕：适用于失眠、心烦、健忘、小儿夜啼等证，并有益智作用。

决明子枕：适用于患有便秘、目疾、高血压和小儿夜啼等。

侧柏叶枕：适用于口鼻经常出血，慢性咽炎，咽部充血，慢性咳嗽及轻度脱发者。

蚕沙枕：适用于头风、落

bycum): It is applicable to wind syndrome of the head, stiff neck, arthritis of cervical vertebrae and mandible.

The above are the medicinal pillows made of a single ingredient. If made into compound medicinal pillows, they have better therapeutic effects.

1) Insomnia: The pillow core is padded with Heidou (*Semen Sojae Nigrum*) and powder of magnetitum.

2) Rhinitis and nasosinusitis: The pillow core is padded with equal shares of Baizhi (*Radix Angelicae Dahuricae*) and Xinyi (*Flos Magnoliae*).

3) Glaucoma and distending ocular pain: The pillow core is padded with equal shares of Xiakucao (*Spica Prunellae*), Heye (*Folium Nelumnbinis*), Baizhi (*Radix Angelicae Dahuricae*) and Caojueming (*Semen Cassiae*).

4) Pillow for hypertension: ① The pillow core is padded with Caojueming (*Semen Cassiae*) and Juhua (*Flos Chrysanthemi*). ② The pillow core is padded with 100 g of Juhua (*Flos Chrysanthemi*), 100 g of Chuanxiong (*Rhizoma Ligustici Chuanxiong*), 100 g of Mudanpi (*Cortex Moutan Radicis*) and 200 g of Baizhi (*Radix Angelicae Dahuricae*).

5) Pillow for Eliminating Summer-heat: The pillow core is padded with 200 g of the covering of Lüdou (*Semen Phaseoli Radiati*), 200 g of the covering of Biandou (*Semen Dolichoris*), 150 g of Heye (*Folium Nelumbinis*), 200 g of Bohe (*Herba Menthae*) and 100 g of Qiaomaike (the shell of *Semen Fagopyri Esculenti*).

6) Sight-Improving Pillow: The pillow core is padded with 200 g of the covering of Qiaomai (*Semen Fagopyri Esculenti*), 200 g of the covering of Heidou (*Semen Sojae Nigrum*), 80 g of Caojuemingzi (*Semen Cassiae*) and 150 g of Juhua (*Flos Chrysanthemi*).

7) Soporific Pillow: The pillow core is padded with

枕、颈椎关节痛及下颌关节痛。

以上为单味药制成的药枕,如根据病证情况适用复方药枕,则疗效更佳:

失眠:用黑豆、磁石粉装枕芯。

鼻渊(鼻炎、鼻窦炎):白芷、辛夷各等分装药枕。

青光眼、眼胀痛:夏枯草、荷叶、白芷、草决明各等分,装枕。

高血压患者用枕:① 用草决明子、菊花装入枕芯。② 菊花100 g,川芎100 g,牡丹皮100 g,白芷200 g,装枕。

解暑枕:绿豆衣200 g,扁豆衣 200 g,荷叶 150 g,薄荷200 g,荞麦壳100 g,装枕。

明目枕:荞麦皮200 g,黑豆皮200 g,草决明子80 g,菊花150 g,装枕。

安眠枕:夜交藤200 g,合

200 g of Yejiaoteng (*Caulis Polygoni Multiflori*), 60 g of Hehuanhua (*Flos Albiziae*), 30 g of Suanzaoren (*Semen Ziziphi Spinosae*), 30 g of Baiziren (*Semen Biotae*) and 30 g of Wuweizi (*Fructus Schisandrae*).

Besides, the ancient Taoists had a well-known medicinal pillow for longevity called the "Revered Mr. Ding's Celestial Pillow". The prescription is composed of 30 g of Chuanjiao (*Pericarpium Zanthoxyli*), Jiegeng (*Citri Reticulatae Fructus*), Jingshizi (*Herba Schizonepetae*), Baiziren (*Semen Biotae*), Jianghuang (*Rhizoma Curcumae Longae*), Wuzhuyu (*Fructus Evodiae*), Baizhu (*Rhizoma Atractylodis Macrocephalae*), Bohe (*Herba Menthae*), Rougui (*Herba Cistanchis*), Chuanxiong (*Rhizoma Ligustici Chuanxiong*), Yizhiren (*Fructus Alpiniae Oxyphyllae*), Zhishi (*Fructus Aurantii Immaturus*), Danggui (*Radix Angelicae Sinensis*), Chuanwutou (*Radix Aconiti*), Qiannianjian (*Rhizoma Homalomenae*), Wujiapi (*Cortex Acanthopancis Radicis*), Baijili (*Fructus Tribuli*), Qianghuo (*Rhizoma seu Radix Notopterygii*), Fangfeng (*Radix Ledebouriellae*), Xinyi (*Flos Magnoliae*), Baizhi (*Radix Angelicae Dahuriae*), Fuzi (*Radix Aconiti Praeparata*), Baishaoyao (*Radix Paeoniae Alba*), Gaoben (*Rhizoma Ligustici*), Congrong (*Herba Cistanchis*), Beixixin (*Herba Asari Mandshurici*), Zhuyazao (*Fructus Gleditsiae Abnormalis*), Wuyi (*Flos Magnoliae*), Gancao (*Radix Glycyrrhizae*), Jingjie (*Herba Schizonepetae*), Juhua (*Flos Chrysanthemi*), Duzhong (*Cortex Eucommiae*), Wuyao (*Radix Linderae*) and Banxia (*Rhizoma Pinelliae*) respectively.

All the above ingredients are ground into powder. Then fill the pillow core with the powder. Use the pillow every night. One dose can be used for about half a year.

欢花 60 g，酸枣仁、柏子仁、五味子各 30 g，装枕。

此外，古代道家有一著名延年益寿药枕方，名为"丁公仙枕"：川椒、桔梗、荆实子、柏子仁、姜黄、吴茱萸、白术、薄荷、肉桂、川芎、益智仁、枳实、当归、川乌头、千年健、五加皮、白蒺藜、羌活、防风、辛夷、白芷、附子、白芍药、藁本、苁蓉、北细辛、猪牙皂、芜荑、甘草、荆芥、菊花、杜仲、乌药、半夏各 30 g。

以上药物粉碎成粗末，装入布袋或绢袋，充为枕芯，每夜枕之。一剂药料可用半年左右。

The medicinal pillow has better therapeutic effects on diseases of the head, face, five sense organs, shoulders, and neck, etc., but it is not applicable to diseases of the chest, abdomen and limbs. The application should be stopped if the patient is allergic to the drugs.

(2) Bedding   Soft material such as fine cotton cloth, cotton yarn and fine gunny cloth is preferred for the underneath side of the quilt while the material of chemical fibre with electrostatic charge such as acrylic fibres, nylon and dacron is not advisable. It is best to select cotton, silk floss and eiderdown for the wadding of the quilt. Light and big quilt is preferable, but heavy one is not suitable. Soft and thick mattress is advisable. The modification is made with the changes of temperature.

(3) Night clothes and nightcap   The large night clothes without collars and buttons are preferable. Cotton velvet and towelling are advisable in autumn and winter while silk and nuslin are suitable in spring and summer. In winter, it is suitable for old people to wear the cotton nightcap, the size of which is proper to cover the whole head. Wearing the abdominal wrapper is advisable for old people no matter whether it is in winter or summer, especially for old people above the age of 70.

2.2.2.3.4 "Ten forbidden points" for sleeping

Our Chinese ancients had ten forbidden points for sleeping which include: ① supination; ② anxiety; ③ anger before bed time; ④ ingestion before bed time; ⑤ speaking during sleeping; ⑥. facing the lamplight; ⑦ opening the mouth during sleeping; ⑧ covering the head during sleeping; ⑨ facing the draught during sleeping; ⑩ facing the stove during sleep.

2.2.3　Clothing

TCM life cultivation has accumulated more experi-

药枕对头面、五官、肩颈等部位的疾病疗效较好,而胸、腹及肢体疾患则不宜用。如患者对药物过敏,应停止使用。

② 被、褥　被里宜柔软,可选细棉布、棉纱、细麻布等,不宜用腈纶、尼龙、的确良等带静电荷的化纤品。被胎宜选棉花、丝棉、羽绒为最好。被宜轻不宜重,宜宽大;褥宜软而厚,随天气冷暖变化加减。

③ 睡衣、帽等　睡衣宜宽大无领无扣,秋冬宜棉绒、毛巾布,春夏宜丝绸、薄纱。老人冬日睡卧宜带棉布睡帽,以能遮盖住整个头顶为宜;不论冬夏,睡卧时宜带肚兜,70岁以上老人更应如此。

(4) 睡眠"十忌"　我国古人有"睡眠十忌":一忌仰卧;二忌忧虑;三忌睡前恼怒;四忌睡前进食;五忌睡卧言语;六忌睡卧对灯光;七忌睡时张口;八忌夜卧覆首;九忌卧处当风;十忌睡卧对炉火。

三、服饰

中医养生学对四季服饰

ence in the modification of clothing in the four seasons. It demands that dressing and undressing should keep with seasonal changes. For example, in spring, cold does not disappear completely and yang qi increases gradually. Accordingly, it is advisable to wear less upper garments and usual trousers to promote the rising of yang qi. In summer, though yang and heat are excessive, people still need proper dressing to consolidate and protect healthy qi. In autumn, it turns cool, people should also pay attention to the addition of clothing. However, too many garments at a time should be avoided. As the saying goes, "muffle the body in spring and freeze the body in autumn." This means that man should keep himself warm in spring and wear less so as to feel a bit cool in autumn. In winter, more clothing should be added with the increasing intensity of cold. The "once and for all" in dressing cannot be reached and excessively heavy clothing should be avoided.

Keeping the body extremely warm or excessively cold is not advisable. Otherwise, the body will lose its ability to endure wind and cold, consequently causing the declined body resistance against pathogenic factors and weakened ability to prevent diseases. As for old people and people with weak physique, their tolerance of cold and heat is relatively poor. Thus, undressing should be as cautious as possible to avoid the invasion of wind, cold, summer-heat and dampness.

In the case of profuse sweating, undressing is shunned from wind. Otherwise, the body is susceptible to attack by pathogenic wind and cold which consequently gives rise to diseases. Wet clothes with sweat should not be worn long, for after perspiration, the striae of skin are loose and the wet garments are not easily dried. If the sweat and dampness stay on the skin long, they will im-

的增减方面有较多经验,要求脱、添衣服时必须不失四时之节。如：春季阴寒未尽,阳气渐生,早春宜减衣不减裤,以助阳气的升发。夏季尽管阳热炽盛,仍需适当穿着衣服,才能固护正气。秋季气候转凉,亦要注意增衣,但要避免一次添衣过多。俗有"春捂秋冻"之说,即春季宁稍暖,秋季可稍凉。冬季衣物要随寒冷而渐增,不能"一步到位",穿着过厚。

穿衣不宜过暖过寒,否则机体缺乏耐受风寒的能力,而使抗邪防病之力减弱。至于老人和身体虚弱的人对寒热的耐受性较差,应尽量慎于脱、添,以免风寒暑湿之侵。

大汗之时忌当风脱衣,否则易受风寒之邪侵袭而致病。汗湿之衣不得久穿,因为汗后腠理虚,湿衣不易干,汗湿滞留肌肤,伤害人体阳气,易产生风寒湿之类的病变。

pair the yang qi of the human body, easily giving rise to pathological changes of wind, cold and dampness.

2.2.4　Defecation and urination

Cultivating good habits of defecation and urination is of a great significance for health and longevity.

2.2.4.1　Keeping free movement of the bowels

The ancient life cultivation experts attached extreme importance to free movement of the bowels. It is regarded as a symbol of longevity that an old person defecates regularly two times a day. Constant constipation may cause the ascending of turbid qi, adverse and disorderly qi flow and blood circulation, and visceral dysfunctions, consequently giving rise to or inducing many diseases such as headache, toothache, anal and intestinal diseases, coronary heart disease, cerebrovascular accident and intestinal cancer. The methods of keeping free movement of the bowels include: ① cultivating the habit of defecation at fixed time; ② defecating naturally without forced control if there exists stool and no forced defecation if there is no stool; ③ catharsis with massage; clockwise massage can enhance enterogastric functions, digestive and excretory functions while massaging abdominal region regularly promotes catharsis; ④ paying attention to the perianal hygiene and recuperation after defecation. The toilet paper used should be thin and soft. Every night before bed time, the anus is washed with warm and clean water. Sitz-bath with warm water is adopted to keep the anus clean and to maintain good blood circulation.

As for food, oats gruel is better for catharsis, especially for old people. Oats not only relieves constipation, but also reduces cholesterol and triglyceride. Therefore, it has slimming effect as well.

Healthcare after defecation should not be ignored, either. For example, it is advisable to eat some soup or drink some beverage in the case of defecation after overeating to strengthen the stomach qi and promote digestion. In the case of starvation, sitting position is advisable for defecation. Ingestion of a small amount of food is proper after defecation. Besides, drawing up anal muscle may be conducted for 3 to 5 times, the purpose of both is to supplement and consolidate healthy qi.

2.2.4.2 Maintaining clear and smooth urination

The ancient life cultivation experts attached great importance to hygiene of urination. Maintaining clean urine and smooth urination is the important content of conserving the health of the body. The specific methods are mainly as follows. ① Reasonable diet: Small amount of ingestion, vegetarian diet, no immediate drinking after meal, drinking in the case of thirst, etc. are the experience of the ancients for ensuring clean urination. ② diuresis with massage: Massage of the waist: Assume the erectly sitting position. Place the hands on the back to push and rub upwards to the back and downwards to the sacrococcygeal region for 30 to 50 times until the back gets warm. It may be performed at bed time at night and at the time to get up in the morning. Massage of the abdomen: Assume the supine position and regulate breathing. Rub the palms against each other until they get warm. Then, place the palm on the abdomen. Firstly, push and rub the two sides of the abdomen; then, push the middle of the lower abdomen, both of which are done for 30 times. The movements should shift gradually from gentle ones to forceful ones and the force should be mild, slow and even. It is performed in the morning and at night. ③ Forced control over urination should be avoided. Uri-

肥效果。

便后保健亦不能忽视。如饱食后大便，便后宜稍喝一些汤或饮料，以助胃气而利消化。若在饥饿时大便，则排便时宜取坐位，便后稍进食物，还可做提肛动作3～5次，以补固正气。

2. 维持小便清利

古代养生家十分重视小便卫生。保持小便清洁、通利，是维持身体健康的重要内容。其具体方法主要有：① 合理饮食。少食、素食、食后不要立即饮水、感到口渴才饮水等，是古人从实践中得出的保证小便清利的经验。② 按摩利尿。摩腰：取端坐位，两手置于背后，上下推搓30～50次，上至背部，下至骶尾，以腰背部发热为佳，可在晚上就寝时和早晨起床时进行练习。摩腹：取仰卧位，调匀呼吸，将掌搓热，置于下腹部，先推摩下腹部两侧，再推下腹部中央，各做30次。动作要由轻渐重，力量要和缓均匀。早晚练习。③ 切忌忍尿。有尿时要及时排出，忍尿会损伤肾与膀胱之气，引起病变。

nation should be timely when there exists urine. Forced control over urination may impair the kidney and the urinary bladder qi, causing pathological changes.

In addition, emotions, sexual life and movements also influence urination to a certain degree. Therefore, people should keep optimistic, regulate sexual life and exercise properly.

2.3 Life cultivation and rehabilitation with the diet

2.3.1 The effects of life cultivation with the diet

2.3.1.1 Supplementing the supply of nutrients in the human body to strengthen health and prevent diseases. For example, eating animal livers can nourish the liver and prevent night blindness; ingestion of kelp can not only supplement iodine and vitamin, but also prevent goiter; intake of fruit and fresh vegetables can supplement nutrition and prevent scurvy, etc. Besides, the special effects of certain food may be directly utilized to prevent certain diseases. For instance, garlic is used to prevent affection by exopathogen and diarrhea; green gram soup is applied to prevent summer-heat; Congbai (*Bulbus Allii Fistulosi*) and Shengjiang (*Rhizoma Zingiberis Recens*) are adopted to prevent common cold due to invasion by wind, etc.

2.3.1.2 Prolonging life, resisting and preventing ageing. Many types of food have the anti-ageing actions, such as sesame, mulberry, Gouqizi (*Fructus Lycii*), Guiyuanrou (*Arillus Longan*), Hutao (*Semen Juglandis*), bee milk, Huaishanyao (*Rhizoma Dioscoreae*), human milk, milk, soft-shelled turtle, the regular ingestion of which is beneficial to health and longevity.

2.3.2 Principles of rehabilitation with the diet

2.3.2.1 Differentiating syndrome to decide the diet

Different diets are selected for different syndromes. For example, in the case of the exterior syndrome of affection by exogenous wind and cold with the manifestations such as headache, nasal obstruction, aversion to cold, general pain, anhidrosis, warm-and hot-natured food such as Shengjiang (*Rhizoma Zingiberis Recens*), Congbai (*Bulbus Allii Fistulosi*) and brown sugar should be selected and decocted for oral administration. Take it while the decoction is warm. Or minced garlic shredded with warm noodles, soup of coriander and soybean may be ingested to induce diaphoresis, relieve the exterior syndrome and expel cold. In the case of renal yang deficiency with the symptoms such as lassitude in loins and legs, cold limbs, aversion to cold, cramping sensation of the lower abdomen, frequent or unsmooth urination, diets of supplementing fire to remove yin should be selected such as dog meat, sparrow meat and mutton, or renal soup of a white sheep and chicken cooked with Dongchongxiacao (*Cordyceps*).

2.3.2.2 Differentiating disease to decide the diet

Different diets also should be selected according to the differences of diseases on the basis of differentiating syndrome to decide the diet. For instance, in the case of palpitation, Danggui (*Radix Angelicae Sinensis*) and Renshen (*Radix Ginseng*) may be selected to be cooked with the pork heart; in the case of night blindness, various animal livers may be decocted with Gouqizi (*Fructus*

二、饮食康复的原则

1. 辨证用膳

根据临床所辨证型，施以不同的饮食。如外感风寒表证，有头痛、鼻塞、畏寒、全身酸痛、无汗等表现，应选用生姜、葱白、红糖等温热食品煎汤热服，或吃大蒜末拌热面、芫荽黄豆汤发汗解表以散寒。若肾阳不足证，见腰酸膝软、肢冷畏寒、少腹拘急、尿频或不利等症状，应选用狗肉、雀肉、羊肉等食品，或白羊肾羹、冬虫夏草鸡等益火消阴的膳食。

2. 辨病用膳

在辨证施食的基础上，还应根据病种不同而选用不同的饮食。如心悸怔忡，可选用当归、人参煮猪心；雀盲，可选多种动物肝脏与枸杞子、桑椹子等同用；肺虚咳嗽，可选用麻油炒猪肺或猪肺粥；肾虚腰

Lycii), Sangshenzi (*Semen Mori*), etc. for oral administration; the pork lung fried with sesame oil or soup of the pork lung may be used for cough due to pulmonary asthenia; bone marrow and cerebral marrow powder of the pig or gruel of Taoren (*Semen Persicae*) may be selected for senile dementia; the pig pancreas may be selected for diabetes mellitus; more milk, etc. may be drunken for osteoporosis.

2.3.2.3 Scientific selection of diets

The scientific use of diets can be defined by the proverb "The diet should include coarse and fine food grains without being too sweet and salty. People should have three, or four or five meals a day with being 70 to 80 percent full." The first sentence refers to the advocation of a proper proportion between coarse and fine food grains in TCM life cultivation. Coarse food grains include maize, soybean, sweet potato and the like; fine food grains, nonglutinous rice, flour and so on. In the second sentence, "three, or four or five meals" means the times people should have meals a day; "70 to 80 percent full" is the experience of becoming longevous which has been proven by history.

The dietary style of being "70 to 80 percent full" has proven to be the effective method of promoting longevity by the public at all times and in all countries. This is similar to the modern theory of "low caloric diet". There are two methods to measure the so-called "70 to 80 percent full": one is that people feel a little hungry and still want to eat when leaving the dinning table; the other is that people have the sense of hunger when it is not the time for the next meal yet. There exists a saying in TCM life cultivation: "If you want to be healthy, you should always feel 30 percent cold and hungry." This has already be verified by numerous longevous people.

2.3.3 The commonly-used dietary prescriptions for life cultivation

2.3.3.1 Prescriptions for supplementing healthy qi

These prescriptions have tonic, roborant, anti-ageing and life-prolonging actions. They are applicable to patients with weak constitution and deficiency of healthy qi due to prolonged diseases.

2.3.3.1.1 Prescriptions for supplementing qi

Paste of Huangqi (*Radix Astragali seu Hedysari*): 12 g of Shenghuangqi (fresh *Radix Astragali seu Hedysari*), 12 g of Shengshigao (*Gypsum Fibrosum*), 12 g of Xianmaogen (fresh *Radix Curculiginis*), 6 g of the fine powder of Gancao (*Radix Glycyrrhizae*), 10 g of the powder of Huaishanyao (*Rhizoma Dioscoreae*) and 30 g of honey. At first, decoct Huangqi (*Radix Astragali seu Hedysari*), Shigao (*Gypsum Fibrosum*) and Xianmaogen (fresh *Radix Curculiginis*) until the decoction boils for more than 10 times. Then, remove the dregs to leave two cups of the clear decoction. At this time, add Gancao (*Radix Glycyrrhizae*) and Huaishanyao (*Rhizoma Dioscoreae*) powder to the decoction and stir the decoction constantly to prevent the sedimentation of the medicinal powder. Boil the decoction for one more time and the paste forms. Next, pour the honey into the decoction. The whole process comes to an end when the decoction boils. Take all the paste in 3 divided times within a day.

Gruel for Strengthening healthy Qi: 30 to 60 g of prepared Huangqi (*Radix Astragali seu Hedysari*), 3 to 5 g of Renshen (*Radix Ginseng*) or 15 to 30 g of Dangshen (*Radix Codonopsis Pilosulae*), a small amount of white sugar and 100 g of Jingmi (*Semen Oryzae Sativae*). At first, cut Huangqi (*Radix Astragali seu Hedysari*)

三、常用食养食疗方

1. 补益正气类

有滋补强壮、抗衰益寿的作用,适用于久病体虚,正气亏损者。

（1）补气类

黄芪膏：生黄芪12 g,生石膏12 g,鲜白茅根12 g,甘草细末6 g,怀山药细末10 g,蜂蜜30 g。先将黄芪、石膏、鲜茅根煎煮十余沸,去渣澄清汁2杯,再调入甘草、怀山药细末同煮,并不断搅拌,以免药粉沉底。煮一沸其膏即成,再调入蜂蜜,煮令沸即可。分3次食用,1日服完。

补虚正气粥：炙黄芪30~60 g,人参3~5 g(或党参15~30 g),白糖少许,粳米100 g。先将黄芪、人参(或党参)切成薄片,用冷水浸泡半小时,煎取药汁,分早晚2次同粳米煮

and Renshen (*Radix Ginseng*) or Dangshen (*Radix Codonopsis Pilosulae*) into slices and soak them in cold water for half an hour. Then, decoct the ingredients to get the decoction. Use the decoction to cook gruel with Jingmi (*Semen Oryzae Sativae*) in two divided times in the morning and evening for ingestion.

Gruel of Renshen (*Radix Ginseng*) and Lianrou (*Semen Nelumbinis*): 10 g of Renshen (*Radix Ginseng*), 10 g of Lianzi (*Semen Nelumbinis*) and 30 g of Bingtang (*Saccharum*). The common method is used to cook gruel for ingestion.

2.3.3.1.2 Prescriptions for tonifying blood

Hen Stewed with Danggui (*Radix Angelicae Sinensis*): 15 g of Danggui (*Radix Angelicae Sinensis*), 15 g of Dangshen (*Radix Codonopsis Pilosulae*), one hen (roughly 1,500 g), proper amount of green onion, fresh ginger, cooking wine and salt respectively. After butchering the hen, remove the feather and internal organs. Then, wash the hen clean. Next, put Danggui (*Radix Angelicae Sinensis*) and Dangshen (*Radix Codonopsis Pilosulae*) into the abdomen. At this time, add green onion, ginger, cooking wine and a proper amount of clear water. At first, boil the water with strong fire. Afterwards, change the fire into slow fire to decoct until the meat is thoroughly cooked. Eat the meat and drink the soup.

Soup of Chinese dates (*Fructus Ziziphi Jujubae*) and Black Edible Fungus: Five Chinese dates (*Fructus Ziziphi Jujubae*) and 15 g of black edible fungus. Stew the two thoroughly to be eaten.

Gruel of Gouqi (*Fructus Lycii*): 100 g of fresh Gouqizi (*Fructus Lycii*) and 60 g of Jingmi (*Semen Oryzae Sativae*). The two are used to cook gruel. Drink the gruel with salty fermented soybeans as the assistant food.

粥服食。

人参莲肉粥：人参10 g，莲子10 g，冰糖30 g。以常法熬粥食用。

（2）补血类

当归炖母鸡：当归15 g，党参15 g，母鸡1只（约重1 500 g），葱、生姜、料酒、食盐各适量。宰杀母鸡后，去净毛及内脏，洗净，将当归、党参置鸡腹内，放入沙锅中，加入葱、姜、料酒、食盐及适量清水，置灶上先武火煮沸，再改文火慢煎，直至烂熟即成。吃肉、喝汤。

红枣黑木耳汤：红枣5个，黑木耳15 g，炖烂食用。

枸杞粥：鲜枸杞子100 g，粳米60 g，煮粥，粥成以咸豆豉佐餐食用。

2.3.3.1.3 Prescriptions for supplementing qi and tonifying blood

Paste of Guiyuan Shenmi (Paste of Arillus Longan, Radix Codonopsis Pilosulae and Milk): 250 g of Dangshen (*Radix Codonopsis Pilosulae*), 120 g of Beishashen (*Radix Glehniae*) and 120 g of Guiyuanrou (*Arillus Longan*). At first, soak the above ingredients in a proper amount of water until they thoroughly ferment. Decoct the drugs for 30 minutes after the water boils. Decoct the ingredients in 3 different times. Then, mix the decoctions got in the 3 times. Next, decoct the mixed decoction to be condensed with slow fire until the paste forms. At this time, add double amount of honey. Afterwards, decoct them until boiling appears again. Finally, stop decocting and wait until the paste is cold. Store the paste in a bottle for later use. Dissolve a spoonful of the paste in boiling water to be taken at a draught each time, three times a day.

Gruel of Longyanrou (*Arillus Longan*): 15 g of Longyanrou (*Arillus Longan*), 10 g of Fuling (*Poria*), 3 to 5 Chinese dates and 100 g of Jingmi (*Semen Oryzae Sativae*). All the ingredients are used to cook gruel. Add a bit white sugar to the gruel to be eaten.

2.3.3.1.4 Prescriptions for nourishing yin

Wine of Gouqizi (*Fructus Lycii*): 200 g of Gouqizi (*Fructus Lycii*) and 600 ml of white spirit. First, wash Gouqizi (*Fructus Lycii*) clean in clear water. Then, cut the ingredient into small pieces to be kept in a bottle. Afterwards, add about 400 ml of white spirit into the bottle. Next, keep the mouth of the bottle airtight. Vibrate and shake the bottle once every day. The wine can be drunken after a week's soakage. Drink 10 to 20 ml before supper or bed time every day. The wine in the bottle may be added continuously (altogether about 200 ml). Gouqizi

（3）气血双补类

桂圆参蜜膏：党参250 g，北沙参120 g，桂圆肉120 g，先将上药以适量水浸泡，发透以后加热煎煮，沸腾后再煎30分钟，煎煮3次，合并3次煎汁，以文火浓缩，至成稠膏状时加入1倍量的蜂蜜，再煎沸即可停火，待冷后装瓶备用。每服1汤匙，以沸水冲化，顿服，每日3次。

龙眼肉粥：龙眼肉15 g，茯苓10 g，红枣3～5枚，粳米100 g，同煮为粥，可加白糖少许食用。

（4）补阴类

枸杞子酒：枸杞子200 g，白酒600 ml，将枸杞子用清水洗净，剪碎放入瓶中，加白酒约400 ml，瓶口密封，每日振摇1次，浸泡1星期以后即可供饮用。每日晚餐或临睡前饮用10～20 ml。瓶中酒可边饮边加（约共加200 ml），枸杞子可拌糖食用。

(*Fructus Lycii*) may be mixed with sugar for eating.

Pork Liver Stewed with Xuanshen (*Radix Scrophulariae*): 15 g of Xuanshen (*Radix Scrophulariae*), 500 g of pork liver, a proper amount of rapeseed oil, ginger, green onion, soy sauce, millet wine and bean powder respectively. At first, wash the pork liver clean, and place it and Xuanshen (*Radix Scrophulariae*) together in a pot. Then, add a proper amount of water to the pot and cook the ingredients for an hour. Next, take out the pork liver and cut it into slices for later use. In addition, parch the green onion and ginger with a bit of rapeseed oil and put them into the slices of the pig liver. Afterwards, put the soy sauce, white sugar and a small amount of cooking wine into the above decoction and cook the decoction with these ingredients again. After that, put some bean powder into the decoction to make the decoction transparent. Finally, pour the slices of pork liver into the juice and stir the juice evenly. Now, it is ready for use.

Soft-Shelled Turtle Steamed with Ermu (*Bulbus Fritillariae* and *Rhizoma Anemarrhenae*): One soft-shelled turtle (approximately 500 g in weight), 5 g of Beimu (*Bulbus Fritillariae*), Zhimu (*Rhizoma Anemarrhenae*), Qianhu (*Radix Peucedani*), Chaihu (*Radix Bupleuri*) and Xingren (*Semen Armeniace Amarum*) respectively, a proper amount of millet wine and a bit of salt. At first, butcher the soft-shelled turtle and remove the head and internal organs. Then, wash the turtle clean to be cut into cubes. Next, add Beimu (*Bulbus Fritillariae*), Zhimu (*Rhizoma Anemarrhenae*), Qianhu (*Radix Peucedani*), Chaihu (*Radix Bupleuri*) and Xingren (*Semen Armeniacae Amarum*) as well as a proper amount of millet wine and a bit of salt. Add water to inundate the meat cubes. Finally, all the ingredients are steamed in a steamer for an hour. Eat the meat while it is

玄参炖猪肝：玄参15 g，猪肝500 g，菜油、姜、葱、酱油、黄酒、豆粉各适量。将猪肝洗净，与玄参同置锅内，加水适量煮1小时，取出猪肝切成薄片备用。另将葱、姜加菜油稍炒，放入猪肝片中，再将酱油、白糖、料酒少量，兑加煮玄参、猪肝之原汤少许，收汁，勾入豆粉，使汁液透明，倒入猪肝片中，拌匀即成。

二母元鱼：元鱼（鳖）1只（约重500 g），贝母、知母、前胡、柴胡、杏仁各5 g，黄酒适量，食盐少许，宰杀元鱼，去头、内脏，洗净切块，加入贝母、知母、前胡、柴胡、杏仁及适量黄酒、少许食盐，加水没过肉块，置蒸锅中蒸1小时，于蒸熟后趁热食用。

still warm.

Gruel of Baihe (*Bulbus Lilii*): 30 g of the powder of dried Baihe (*Bulbus Lilii*) (doubled in case of fresh one), 100 g of Jingmi (*Semen Oryzae Sativae*) and a proper quantity of Bingtang (*Saccharum*). All the ingredients are used to cook gruel. Eat it in the morning and in the evening respectively.

2.3.3.1.5 Prescriptions for strengthening yang

Wine of Lurong (*Cornu Cervi Pantotrichum*): 3 to 6 g of Lurong (*Cornu Cervi Pantotrichem*), 30 to 60 g of Huaishanyao (*Rhizoma Dioscoreae*) and 500 ml of white spirit. Soak Lurong (*Cornu Cervi Pantotrichum*) and Huaishanyao (*Rhizoma Dioscoreae*) in the spirit. Keep the container airtight. Vibrate and shake the container occasionally. It may be drunken in 7 days. Drink 10 ml every night before bed time.

Kidney Soup of White Sheep: 50 g of Roucongrong (*Herba Cistanchis*), 10 g of Biba (*Fructus Piperis Longi*), Caoguo (*Fructus Tsaoko*) (ten in number), 5 g of Chenpi (*Pericarpium Citri Reticulatae*), 10 g of Hujiao (*Fructus Piperis Nigri seu Albi*), two pairs of white sheep kidneys, 200 g of white sheep fat, salt, green onion, soy sauce, fermented flour, etc. The common methods are adopted to cook soup with the above ingredients. Eat the sheep liver and drink the soup.

Chicken Stewed with Dongchongxiacao (*Cordyceps*): One cock, Dongchongxiacao (*Cordyceps*) (5 to 10 in number), a bit of ginger, green onion and salt respectively. At first, butcher the cock. Then, get rid of the feathers and internal organs to be washed clean. Afterwards, put the cock into a pot and add the Dongchongxiacao (*Cordyceps*), ginger, green onion, salt as well as a proper quantity of water. Finally, stew all the above together until the meat is thoroughly cooked for eating.

百合粥：干百合研粉30 g（鲜品加倍），粳米100 g，加冰糖适量，煮粥早晚服食。

（5）补阳类

鹿茸酒：鹿茸3～6 g，怀山药30～60 g，白酒500 ml。将鹿茸、怀山药浸入酒中，封固，时时振摇，7天后即可供饮用。每晚临睡前饮服10 ml。

白羊肾羹：肉苁蓉50 g，荜茇10 g，草果10 枚，陈皮5 g，胡椒10 g，白羊肾2 对，白羊脂200 g，食盐、葱、酱油、发酵面等，如常法作羹。食用时，吃羊肾、喝羹。

冬虫夏草鸡：雄鸡1 只，冬虫夏草5～10 枚，姜、葱、食盐少许。宰杀雄鸡。去净毛及内脏，洗净后放锅中，加入冬虫夏草及姜、葱、食盐、适量水，用小火慢炖，直至鸡肉烂熟即可供食用。

2.3.3.2 Prescriptions for nourishing the heart and tonifying the brain

These prescriptions have the actions of nourishing the heart, tranquilizing the mind and tonifying the brain to benefit intelligence.

Gruel of Hetaoren (*Semen Juglandis*): 50 g of Hetaoren (*Semen Juglandis*) and a proper amount of rice. Pound the Hetaoren (*Semen Juglandis*) into pieces. Then, wash the rice clean. Next, add a proper quantity of water. All the ingredients are used to cook gruel in the common ways. The gruel is used for assistant food.

Ganmai Dazao Decoction(*Decoction of Radix Glycyrrhizae, Wheat and Chinese Dates*): 30 g of wheat, 10 Chinese dates and 6 g of Gancao (*Radix Glycyrrhizae*). First, wash the Chinese dates and wheat clean. Then, decoct the two together with Gancao (*Radix Glycyrrhizae*) for 2 to 3 times. Remove the dregs to get the decoction. Take the decoction in the morning and in the evening, or drink it as tea.

Gruel of Guiyuanrou (*Arillus Longan*): 15 g of Guiyuanrou (*Arillus Longan*), 3 to 5 Chinese dates and 100 g of Jingmi (*Semen Oryzae Sativae*). The ingredients are used together to cook gruel. A bit of white sugar may be added for eating.

2.3.3.3 Prescriptions for promoting the production of body fluids to quench thirst

These prescriptions possess the functions of clearing away heat, removing dysphoria, nourishing yin, moistening dryness, promoting the production of body fluids to quench thirst, benefiting the rehabilitation of patients with diabetes.

Five-Juice Drink: The juice of pear, juice of water chestnut, juice of lotus root, juice of Maimendong

2. 养心健脑类

有养心安神、健脑益智的功效。

核桃仁粥：核桃仁50 g，粳米适量。将核桃仁捣碎，粳米淘洗干净，加水适量，如常法煮粥。

甘麦大枣汤：小麦30 g，大枣10枚，甘草6 g。先将大枣洗净，将小麦淘洗干净。再与甘草一同煎煮2～3次，去渣取汁，每日早晚饮用，或代茶饮用。

桂圆肉粥：桂圆肉15 g，红枣3～5枚，粳米100 g，同煮为粥，可加白糖少许食用。

3. 生津止渴类

有清热除烦，滋阴润燥，生津止渴作用，有益于消渴病人的康复。

五汁饮：梨汁、荸荠汁、藕汁、麦门冬汁、鲜芦根汁，将生

(*Radix Ophiopogonis*) and juice of fresh Lugen (*Rhizoma Phragmitis*). First, peel the pear (with the kernel removed), water chestnut and fresh lotus root. Then, wash the fresh Lugen (*Rhizoma Phragmitis*) and Maimendong (*Radix Ophiopogonis*) and cut them into pieces. Next, wrap the five ingredients in a piece of clean gauze to squeeze the juice for drinking. The drinking time and quantity may not be fixed. If the patient doesn't prefer cool drink, just warm it with hot water.

Decoction of Pig Pancreas: One pig pancreas, 30 g of Yiyiren (*Semen Coicis*), 60 g of Huangqi (*Radix Astragali seu Hedysari*) and 120 g of Huaishanyao (*Rhizoma Dioscoreae*). Wash the pig pancreas clean. Then, all the ingredients are decocted together for use. Cook the decoction. Drink the clear decoction. The time may not be fixed for drinking.

Crucian Carp Steamed with Tea: Crucian carp and green tea leaves. Take one crucian carp with the weight of 500 g. Then, remove the gills, intestines and internal organs (with the scales remained). Next, fill the abdomen with green tea leaves. Afterwards, place the crucian carp in a dish and put it in a steamer. Finally, steam the crucian carp until it is thoroughly cooked. Eat the bland meat.

2.3.3.4 Prescriptions for rheumatic and rheumatoid arthralgia

These prescriptions are mainly applicable to patients with arthralgia due to wind, cold and dampness, inflexible movement of joints, clonic spasm and contracture of muscle as well as arthralgia.

Decoction of Chinese Flowering Quince: Four Chinese flowering quinces and 1 000 g of white honey. First, steam the Chinese flowering quinces until they are cooked. Then, grind them into paste. Besides, refine the

梨去皮核,荸荠去皮,鲜藕去皮节、鲜芦根、麦门冬洗净,切碎或剪碎,以洁净纱布绞挤取汁,供饮用。不拘时、量饮服。若不喜凉,可水浴令温饮服。

猪胰汤:猪胰1具,生薏苡仁30 g,黄芪60 g,怀山药120 g。先将猪胰洗净,入群药煎煮作汤供用。煮汤,澄汁饮用,不拘时。

清蒸茶鲫鱼:鲫鱼、绿茶。取500 g重鲫鱼1条,去鳃、肠、内脏(留下鱼鳞),腹内装满绿茶,置盘中,放蒸锅内清蒸,熟透即可供用,淡食肉。

4. 蠲痹止痛类

主要用于风寒湿痹、关节不利、筋挛急痛者。

木瓜汤:木瓜4个,白沙蜜1 000 g,先将木瓜蒸熟去皮,研烂如泥。另将白沙蜜炼净。再将两者调和均匀,放入

white honey clean. Finally, mix the two evenly to be stored in a clean chinaware for later use. Mix the prepared paste with boiling water, 1 to 2 spoonfuls each time. Drink the soup on an empty stomach every morning after getting up.

Wine of Wujiapi (*Cortex Acanthopancis*): 50 g of Wujiapi (*Cortex Acanthopancis*), 500 g of Glutinous rice and a proper amount of yeast. First, wash Wujiapi (*Cortex Acanthopancis*) clean. Then, decoct the drug after soaking it thoroughly in a proper quantity of water. Take out the decoction 30 minutes after boiling. Altogether, take out the decoction for two times. Mix the two decoctions. The decoction and clean-washed Jingmi (*Semen Oryzae Sativae*) are used to cook rice. When the rice is cool, add a proper amount of yeast to stir the two evenly. Finally, fermented glutinous rice forms after fermentation. Drink it every day in a proper amount.

Gruel of Chuanwu (*Radix Aconiti*): 3 to 5 g of raw Chuanwutou (*Radix Aconiti*), 30 g of Jingmi (*Semen Oryzae Sativae*), 10 drops of ginger juice and a proper amount of honey. First, pound the raw Chuanwutou (*Radix Aconiti*) into pieces and grind them into very fine powder. Then, use the Jingmi (*Semen Oryzae Sativae*) to cook gruel. When the gruel boils, add the powder of Chuanwutou (*Radix Aconiti*) and change into slow fire to cook. When the gruel is down, add the juice of fresh ginger and honey and stir them evenly. The gruel is finished after another one to two times of boiling. Drink the warm gruel in the morning and in the evening. It is contraindicated for heat syndromes and pregnant women as well as the simultaneous use with Banxia (*Rhizoma Pinelliae*), Beimu (*Bulbus Fritillariae*), Gualou (*Fructus Trichosanthis*), Baiji (*Rhizoma Bletillae*), and Bailian (*Radix Ampelopsis*), etc.

洁净瓷器中盛贮备用，每日晨起空腹，用沸水冲调1～2汤匙，食用。

五加皮酒酿：五加皮50 g，元米500 g，酒曲适量，先将五加皮洗净，加适量水泡透后煎煮，煮沸后每30分钟滤取煎液1次，共取煎液两次。合并两次煎液，与淘净元米共烧元米饭。待冷，加适量酒曲，搅拌均匀，发酵成酒酿。每日适量。

川乌粥：生川乌头3～5 g，粳米30 g，姜汁约10滴，蜂蜜适量。先将生川乌头捣碎，碾为极细粉末。另将粳米煮粥。待粥沸，即加入川乌粉，并改文火缓慢熬煮。粥熟加入生姜汁，调入蜂蜜，搅匀，再稍煮1～2沸，即可。早晚温服。热证及孕妇忌服，不可与半夏、贝母、瓜蒌、白及、白蔹等同用。

2.3.3.5 Prescriptions for promoting qi flow and activating blood circulation

These prescriptions have the actions of promoting qi flow and activating blood circulation, removing blood stasis and activating collaterals. They are applicable to patients with cardiovascular and cerebrovascular diseases such as myocardiac infarction and the sequelae of apoplexy during the stage of recovery.

Gruel of Xiebai (*Bulbus Allii Macrostemi*): 10 to 15 g (or 30 to 45 g fresh one) of Xiebai (*Bulbus Allii Macrostemi*) and 100 g of Jingmi (*Semen Oryzae Sativae*). The two are used together to cook gruel. The warm gruel may be used for breakfast and supper.

Wine of Danshen (*Radix Salviae Miltiorrhizae*): 60 g of Danshen (*Radix Salviae Miltorrhizae*) and 500 ml of high quality wine. Danshen (*Radix Salviae Miltiorrhizae*) is washed clean and pounded into pieces. Then, put the piece into the wine. The wine is finished after a month of soakage.

Gruel of Shanzha (*Fructus Crataegi*): 30 to 40 g (or 60 g fresh one) of Shanzha (*Fructus Crataegi*), 100 g of Jingmi (*Semen Oryzae Sativae*) and 10 g of granulated sugar. First, decoct Shanzha (*Fructus Crataegi*) in an earthenware pot. Then, take out the thick decoction and remove the dregs. Finally, add Jingmi (*Semen Oryzae Sativae*) and granulated sugar to the decoction to cook gruel.

2.3.3.6 Prescriptions for suppressing hyperactive yang to eliminate wind

These prescriptions possess the actions of calming the liver and suppressing hyperactive yang, nourishing yin and eliminating wind. They are applicable to patients with hypertension, mental disease, Parkinson's syndrome, etc. at the stage of recovery.

5. 行气活血类

有行气活血,化瘀通络的作用,适用于心肌梗死、中风后遗症等心脑血管病患者的康复期。

薤白粥:薤白10～15 g(鲜品30～45 g),粳米100 g。取薤白、粳米一同煮粥,可供早点、晚餐服食用,温热食之。

丹参酒:丹参60 g,好酒500 ml。将丹参洗净晾干打碎,放入酒内泡1个月即可。

山楂粥:山楂30～40 g(鲜品60 g),粳米100 g,砂糖10 g。先将山楂用沙锅煎取浓汁,去渣,再入粳米、砂糖煮粥。

6. 潜阳熄风类

有平肝潜阳,育阴熄风的作用,适用于高血压病、癫狂、震颤麻痹综合征等病证患者的康复期。

Gruel of Yuzhu (*Rhizoma Polygonati Odorati*): 15 to 20 g (or 30 to 60 g fresh one) of Yuzhu (*Rhizoma Polygonati Odorati*), a bit of crystal sugar and 100 g of Jingmi (*Semen Oryzae Sativae*). First, wash Yuzhu (*Rhizoma Polygonati*) clean and cut it into pieces. Then, decoct the pieces to keep the thick decoction and to remove the dregs. Next, add Jingmi (*Semen Oryzae Sativae*) into the decoction to cook thin gruel. Finally, add crystal sugar to the gruel. The gruel is finished after one to two times of boiling. Drink the gruel in the morning and in the evening.

Gruel of Lotus Leaf: A large lotus leaf. Wash it clean and decoct it. Then, take out about 500 ml of the decoction. Next, add 100 g of Jingmi (*Semen Oryzae Sativae*) and a proper quantity of white sugar to the decoction to cook gruel. Drink the gruel in the morning and in the evening.

Noodle of Gefen (powder of *Radix Puerariae*): 250 g of Gefen (powder of *Radix Puerariae*), 50 g of Jingjiesui (*Spica Schizonepetae*) and 150 g of Dandouchi (*Semen Sojae Praeparatum*). First, decoct Jingjiesui (*Spica Schizonepetae*) and Dandouchi (*Semen Sojae Praeparatum*) until the decoction boils for 6 to 7 times. Then, remove the dregs to take out the decoction. Next, make Gefen (powder of *Radix Puerariae*) into noodles. Afterwards, put the noodles into the decoction and decoct it. Eat it on an empty stomach.

2.3.3.7 Prescriptions for relieving cough and asthma and eliminating phlegm

These prescriptions possess the functions of relieving cough and asthma and eliminating asthma, etc. They may be applicable to the health care and rehabilitation of diseases of respiratory tract.

Soup of Yanwo (*Nidus Collocaliae*): 3 g of Yanwo

玉竹粥：玉竹 15～20 g（鲜品 30～60 g），冰糖少许，粳米100 g。先将玉竹洗净切碎，煎取浓汁后去渣，入粳米煮为稀粥，放入冰糖，稍煮一二沸即可，早晚服食。

荷叶粥：新鲜荷叶 1 大张，洗净煎取汁约500 ml，加粳米100 g，白糖适量煮粥，早晚服食。

葛粉面：葛粉250 g,荆芥穗50 g、淡豆豉150 g。先煮荆芥穗、淡豆豉 6～7 沸，去渣滤取煎汁。将葛粉做成面条，放入芥穗、豆豉汤中煮熟。空腹食用。

7. 止咳、祛痰、平喘类

具有止咳、祛痰、平喘等作用，可用于呼吸道疾患的保健康复。

燕窝汤：燕窝3 g,冰糖

(*Nidus Collocaliae*) and 30 g of crystal sugar. First, put Yanwo (*Nidus Collocaliae*) into a bowl. Then, add water and soak Yanwo (*Nidus Collocaliae*) in the bowl until it becomes soft. Secondly, remove all the golden swallow feathers mixed in Yanwo (*Nidus Collocaliae*). Thirdly, wash Yanwo (*Nidus Collocaliae*) again to make it clean with clear water. Fourthly, remove the water and tear it into thin strips and place the strips in the bowl. Fifthly, crush the crystal to pieces and put the pieces into a pot with 250 g of clear water. Dissolve the crystal sugar in boiling water with slow fire. Sixthly, scoop up the floating foam and filter the liquid to remove impurities. Seventhly, pour the liquid into another pot and add Yanwo (*Nidus Collocaliae*) to the liquid. Eighthly, heat the pot until the liquid boils. Finally, fill a clear bowl with the soup for later use. Drink the soup once in the morning and in the evening respectively.

Thick Soup of Yin'er (*Tremella*): 5 g of Yin'er (*Tremella*), an egg, 60 g of crystal sugar and a proper amount of lard. Firstly, soak Yin'er (*Tremella*) in a proper amount of water to make it thoroughly fermented. Secondly, remove the base and wash the drug clean. Thirdly, add a proper amount of water to decoct the drug until the water boils. Fourthly, shift to slow fire to stew Yin'er (*Tremella*) slowly for 2 to 3 hours until it becomes paste. Fifthly, add water to another pot and put the crystal sugar into it. Sixthly, heat the pot until the water boils with slow fire to dissolve the crystal sugar. Seventhly, filter the liquid to remove impurities. Eighthly, take out the egg white and add a bit of clear water to it. Stir the egg white and water evenly and then add the egg white to the pot with crystal sugar water. Ninthly, heat the pot until the water boils and scoop up the floating foam. At this time, pour the water into the pot with

30 g。将燕窝放入碗内，加温水泡至松软，拣净杂入的金丝燕毛，复以清水冲洗，使令洁净。沥去水，细撕如条，置净碗中。将冰糖压碎加入锅中，加清水250 g，文火令沸使冰糖溶解，捞去浮沫并滤除杂质，倾入另锅中，再加入燕窝，加热令沸，盛入净碗备用。每日早晚各服1次。

银耳羹：银耳5 g，鸡蛋1个，冰糖60 g，猪油适量。将银耳以适量温水泡发，发透后，摘除蒂头，洗令洁净，加适量水，武火煮令沸。改用文火慢炖2～3小时，至银耳烂如泥。另器加适量水，放入冰糖，文火令沸使糖溶化，滤除杂质。又取鸡蛋清加少许清水搅匀后加入糖水锅中，加热令沸，捞去浮沫，将此汁倒入银耳锅中。出锅时加入猪油，即得。早晨或睡前服用。

Yin'er (*Tremella*). The Thick Soup of Yin'er (*Tremella*) is finished by adding the lard to the pot with Yin'er (*Tremella*). Drink the soup in the morning and before bed time.

Gruel of Pipaye (*Folium Eriobotryae*): 10 to 15 g of Pipaye (*Folium Eriobotryae*), 50 g of Jingmi (*Semen Oryzae Sativae*) and a proper amount of crystal sugar. First, wrap Pipaye (*Folium Eriobotryae*) in a piece of cloth. Secondly, decoct it to remove dregs and to keep the thick decoction. Or brush off the villi of 30 to 60 g of fresh Pipaye (*Folium Eriobotryae*). Then, cut it into thin slivers and decoct it. Next, remove the dregs and keep the decoction. At this time, add Jingmi (*Semen Oryzae Sativae*) to the decoction to cook gruel. Finally, add the crystal sugar to the gruel when it is down. Again, cook the gruel slightly for later use. Drink the gruel every day in the morning and in the evening.

2.3.3.8 Prescriptions for removing food retention and flatulence, strengthening the spleen and stomach

These prescriptions have the actions of promoting digestion to remove food retention, clearing away heat from the stomach and lowering the adverse flow of the stomach qi, eliminating food retention to get rid of flatulence, strengthening the spleen, drying dampness, etc. They are applicable to the health care and rehabilitation of the diseases of digestive system.

Gruel of Meihua (*Flos Mume Albus*): 5 g of Baimeihua (*Flos Mume Albus*) and 100 g of Jingmi (*Semen Oryzae Sativae*). First, use Jingmi (*Semen Oryzae Sativae*) to cook gruel. Then, add Baimeihua (*Flos Mume Albus*) to the gruel and heat the gruel until it boils for 2 to 3 times. Eat the gruel twice a day on an empty stomach. Three to five days constitute a course of

枇杷叶粥：枇杷叶10～15 g，粳米50 g。冰糖适量。先将枇杷叶用布包起，水煎，去渣取浓汁，或将鲜枇杷叶30～60 g刷尽毛绒，切丝水煎，去渣取汁，加入粳米煮粥，粥将成时加入冰糖，稍煮，供用。每日早晚食用。

8. 导滞除满、健脾和胃类

有消积导滞、清胃降逆、开郁除满、健脾燥湿等作用。适用于消化系统的保健和康复。

梅花粥：白梅花（即绿萼梅）5 g，粳米100 g。先煮粳米将成粥时，加入白梅花煮二三沸即可，每日分2次空腹食用，3～5日为1个疗程。

treatment.

Gruel of Jupi (*Pericarpium Citri Reticulatae*): 15 to 20 g (or 30 g in case of fresh one) of Jupi (*Pericarpium Citri Reticulatae*) and 50 to 100 g of Jingmi (*Semen Oryzae Sativae*). First, decoct Jupi (*Pericarpium Citri Reticulatae*) to keep the decoction and to remove the dregs. Then, add Jingmi (*Semen Oryzae Sativae*) to the decoction to cook gruel. Or dry Jupi (*Pericarpium Citri Reticulatae*) in the sun and grind it into fine powder. Mix 3 to 5 g of the powder with the boiling gruel each time. Finally, cook the gruel again.

Spleen-Benefiting Cake: 30 g of Baizhu (*Rhizoma Atractylodis Macrocephalae*), 6 g of dry ginger, 15 g of Jineijin (*Endothelium Corneum Gigeriae Galli*), 250 g of cooked jujube paste and 500 g of flour. Grind Baizhu (*Rhizoma Atractylodis Macroceph alae*), Jineijin (*Endothelium Corneum Gigeriae Galli*) and dried ginger into powder. Then, add a small amount of water to the cooked jujube paste (Decoct the jujube until it is down. Then, keep the decoction and remove the pit. Finally, crush it to paste). Next, mix the paste with the powder and flour and make them into small cakes. Bake the cakes until they are done. The cakes may be eaten at any time without definite quantity.

2.3.3.9 Prescriptions for moistening bowels to relieve constipation

These prescriptions are applicable to the rehabilitation of patients with constipation.

Fermented Glutinous Rice with Sangshenzi (*Fructus Mori*): 1,000 g of fresh Sangshenzi (*Fructus Mori*) and 500 g of Glutinous rice. Wash the fresh Sangshenzi (*Fructus Mori*) clean and pound it into paste to keep the juice [or decoct 300 g of dry Sangshenzi (*Fructus Mori*) and remove the dregs and keep the decoction]. Then,

橘皮粥：橘皮 15～20 g（鲜者30 g），粳米 50～100 g。先把橘皮煎取药汁去渣，然后加入粳米煮粥。或将橘皮晒干研为细末，每次用 3～5 g，调入已煮沸的稀粥中，再同煮为粥。

益脾饼：白术30 g，干姜6 g，鸡内金15 g，熟枣泥250 g，面粉500 g。白术、鸡内金、干姜生用取粉，熟枣泥（红枣煮熟收汁，将去核枣肉压拌成泥）中加少量水，和入药粉及面粉制小饼，烙熟供用。不拘时、量，可常食。

9. 润燥通便类

多适用于便秘病人的康复。

桑椹子醪：鲜桑椹子1 000 g，元米500 g。鲜桑椹子洗净捣烂取汁（或干桑椹子300 g煎煮去渣取汁），将桑椹子汁与淘净元米共煮米饭，待凉，加适量酒曲，拌匀发酵为

cook rice with the juice or decoction and Glutinous rice. When the rice is cool, add yeast to it and stir the two evenly. After fermentation, the fermented glutinous rice forms. It is used for food.

Gruel of Baiziren (*Semen Biotae*): 15 g of Baiziren (*Semen Biotae*), a proper amount of honey and 100 g of Jingmi (*Semen Oryzae Sativae*). First, remove the peel, shell and impurities of Baiziren (*Semen Biotae*). Then, slightly pound it into paste. Next, use the paste and Jingmi (*Semen Oryzae Sativae*) to cook gruel. When the gruel is to become done, add the honey to the gruel. Finally, decoct the gruel until it boils for one or two times. The gruel is finished now.

Gruel of Roucongrong (*Herba Cistanchis*) and Mutton: 10 to 15 g of Roucongrong (*Herba Cistanchis*), 100 g of fine mutton, 100 g of Jingmi (*Semen Oryzae Sativae*), a bit of fine salt, two segments of scallion stalk, two slices of ginger. First, decoct Roucongrong (*Herba Cistanchis*) in an earthenware pot and keep the decoction and remove the dregs. Then, add mutton and Jingmi (*Semen Oryzae Sativae*) to the decoction and decoct them together. When the decoction boils, add the salt, ginger and scallion stalk. Decoct all the ingredients together again and the gruel is finished.

2.3.3.10 Prescriptions for warming the kidney to induce astringency

These prescriptions are mostly applicable to the rehabilitation of patients with constipation, frequent urination, urinary incontinence, etc.

Gruel of Powder of Qianshi (*Semen Euryales*): 30 to 60 g of powder of Qianshi (*Semen Euryales*) and 100 g of Jingmi (*Semen Oryzae Sativae*). Use the powder of Qianshi (*Semen Euryales*) and clean-washed Jingmi (*Semen Oryzae Sativae*) to cook gruel in the common

酒酿,供服食。

柏子仁粥:柏子仁15 g,蜂蜜适量,粳米100 g。先将柏子仁去尽皮壳杂质,稍捣烂,同粳米煮粥,待粥将成时,兑入蜂蜜,稍煮一二沸即可。

苁蓉羊肉粥:肉苁蓉10～15 g,精羊肉100 g,粳米100 g,细盐少许,葱白2茎,生姜3片。先用沙锅煎苁蓉取汁,去渣,入羊肉、粳米同煮,待煮沸后再加入盐、姜、葱煮为稀粥。

10. 温肾固涩类

多适用于便秘、尿频、尿失禁等病人的康复。

芡实粉粥:芡实粉30～60 g,粳米100 g。取芡实粉与淘洗干净的粳米一同如常法煮粥。早晚食用。

ways. Eat the gruel in the morning and evening.

Gruel of Shanyurou (*Fructus Corni*): 15 to 20 g of Shanyurou (*Fructus Corni*), 100 g of Jingmi (*Semen Oryzae Sativae*) and a proper amount of white sugar. Remove the pit of Shanyurou (*Fructus Corni*) and wash it clean. Use the ingredient and the clean-washed Jingmi (*Semen Oryzae Sativae*) to cook gruel in the common ways. Eat it in the morning and in the evening.

2.3.4 Health care with diet

Ingesting food should be unhurried, moderate, careful in chewing and slow in swallowing. Doing so is beneficial to the digestion and absorption of food, and the protection of the intestine and stomach. When people ingest food, listening to light and lively music is advantageous to improving appetite and enhancing digestive function. People can perform the following nursing activities after ingesting food.

2.3.4.1 Abdominal massage after meals

Massaging the abdomen clockwise for 20 to 30 times continuously is beneficial to abdominal blood circulation, the promotion of gastrointestional digestive functions as well as general health.

2.3.4.2 Taking a walk after meals

"Taking a hundred-step walk after meals can make one live to 99." Taking a walk helps enterogastric peristalsis and promotes digestion and absorption. Besides, taking a walk while massaging the abdomen has better effects.

2.3.4.3 Rinsing the mouth after meals

Rinsing the mouth can make the oral cavity remain clean, teeth firm and prevent diseases such as foul breath and caries.

山萸肉粥：山萸肉 15～20 g，粳米 100 g，白糖适量。山萸肉去核洗净。与淘净的粳米一同如常法煮粥，早、晚食用。

四、饮食保健

进食时应该从容缓和，专心致志，细嚼慢咽。这样有利于食物消化吸收，保护肠胃。进食时，播放轻柔松快的乐曲，有利于增进食欲及加强消化功能。进食之后，为了帮助消化食物，可以作一些必要的护理活动。

1. 食后摩腹

顺时针方向按摩腹部，可连续作二三十次不等。这样有利于腹腔血液循环，促进胃肠消化功能，对全身健康也有好处。

2. 食后散步

"饭后百步走，能活九十九"，散步有利于胃肠蠕动，促进消化吸收。亦可边散步边摩腹，效果更佳。

3. 食后漱口

食后漱口可使口腔保持清洁，牙齿坚固，并能防止口臭、龋齿等疾病。

2.4 Health care methods in sexual life

2.4.1 Sexual life and prolonging life

Sexual function is the human instinct. Only by bringing the instinct into full play can the biological mechanism of mutual causality "between matter and function", which the human body should abide by, achieve balance. On the contrary, failure to bring the functions of genitals into play may result in the disuse of the organs, and cause the disturbances of certain links of the closely-related functions of the organism. As a result, disturbances of vital activities will occur.

Compared with ascetics and people indulging in sensual pleasures, those with normal reproductive activities have marked enhancement of vital activities and obvious extension of life time. However, "Taking food and having sexual life are the human instinct." Sexual life is the human instinct for reproduction while asceticism inhibits this instinct. Nevertheless, indulgence in sensual pleasures may overconsume vital substances. Therefore, both asceticism and indulgence in sensual pleasures go against the basic requirements of health and longevity.

2.4.2 Measures for health care in sexual life

2.4.2.1 Avoiding extreme emotional activities

Healthy sexual life begins with the requirement of peaceful mind and stable emotions. However, excessive impetuosity is not permissible while fright and nervousness are not even more allowable, because all psychic factors

第四节 性生活保健法

一、性生活与延年益寿

性功能是人的本能,只有本能得到充分发扬,则人体必须遵循的"物质-功能"互为因果的生物机制才能得到平衡。反之,如果生殖器官的功能得不到发挥则会造成器官的废用,使环环相扣的机体功能因某一环节的障碍而致生命活动紊乱。

具有正常生殖活动的人,较之禁欲或纵欲的人来说,其生命活动和生命时间都明显地增强和延长。"食、色,性也",合理的性生活是人类生命延续的本能,禁欲即抑制了这种本能,而放纵情欲则会过度地消耗生命物质。因此,禁欲和纵欲都是违反健康长寿的基本要求的。

二、性生活的保健措施

1. 避免情志过激

健康的两性交合,开始时要求心神平静,情志安定,不可过分急躁,更不能惊慌、紧张,因为焦虑、紧张、惊恐或过

like anxiety, nervousness, fright or excessive excitement may exert bad effects on the psychology and physiology during the sexual intercourse and consume human vigor wastefully. If the situation continues long, it may give rise to disturbances of reproductive functions, even disturbances of general functions.

2.4.2.2 Moderating sexual intercourse

The basic viewpoint of TCM life cultivation is "preserving essence and cherishing qi." Sexual overstrain may overburden cerebral cortex, genital gland, and genitals etc. and consume a lot of refined nutritious substances. Genitals in particular are more susceptible to overexcitement and local congestion due to sexual overstrain. If the situation continues long, it will inevitably cause the imbalance between excitement and inhibition. This, in addition to excessive consumption of refined nutritious substances, may give rise to pathological changes of reproductive system or general functional injuries. These injuries are not confined to men, but also involve women.

2.4.3 Taboos on sexual life

2.4.3.1 Forceful sexual intercourse

This refers to frequent intercourse, sexual overstrain, profuse sweat, etc. which should be avoided.

2.4.3.2 Sexual activities after drinking wine

Wine is very hot in nature. It can scorchingly consume essence, blood, fat and marrow of the human body. Besides, it can arouse sexual desire and promote hypersexuality as well. Both "wine" and "sex" consume essence and blood in the same way as a leaking pot with soup is subject to strong fire. This inevitably affects life span and is the root cause of premature ageing. It is true of

度兴奋等精神因素都可能对性交过程中的心理、生理产生不良影响，虚耗人的精神。长期以往，会导致生殖功能乃至全身功能的紊乱。

2. 做到性交有度

中医养生的基本观点是"葆精爱气"。过度性交，对大脑皮质、生殖腺、生殖器官等都会造成过度负担，以致人体精微物质的大量损耗。尤其是生殖器官，更容易因为过度性交而导致高度兴奋，局部充血；长期以往，必然形成兴奋-抑制的不平衡。加上精微物质的过度损耗，就会产生生殖系统病变或全身功能的损害。这些危害并不局限于男子，女性也是同样道理。

三、性生活禁忌

1. 忌强力交合

"强力"指性交频繁过密、劳累过度、汗出过多等情况，应避免。

2. 忌酒后入房

酒性大热，能灼耗人体的精、血、脂、髓，又能煽动性欲之火，促使性欲亢进。"酒"、"色"双耗精血，如同漏锅盛汤遭猛火，必然促人寿命，是早衰的根由。男性如此，女子亦不例外。

men and not exceptional to women, either.

2.4.3.3 Holding urine during sexual activities

Holding urine mainly harms defecation, urination, anterior and posterior genitals. Because retention of urine in urinary bladder makes qi activities of lower energizer obstructed due to sexual intercourse. At this time, sexual activities make meridians obstructed, blood and qi stagnated, with clinical manifestations of difficult urination and defecation, astringing or stabbing pain, swelling and hard underbelly, etc.

2.4.3.4 Sexual intercourse during the menstrual period

During the menstrual period, the ostium of uterus opens, endometria come off, blood vessels rupture and body resistance declines. At this time, sexual intercourse is extremely susceptible to infection, irregular menstruation, metrorrhagia, metrostaxis, leukorrhea, sterility, and accumulation of abdominal masses (including malignant tumor of reproductive system), etc.

2.4.3.5 Sexual intercourse during puerperia

A puerperal woman has not restored her qi and blood, and the ostium of uterus still opens. In this case, sexual coitus may impair meridians, consume essence and blood, bring in pathogenic substances and cause various gynecological diseases. On account of the serious consequences of sexual intercourse during puerperia, the Chinese ancients fixed the date for assuming sexual life after delivery as "One hundred days after the birth, people can assume sexual life."

2.4.3.6 Using drugs to stir up sexual urge

There are many agents for enhancing sexual urge or sexual power with quick effects in traditional Chinese drugs and western agents. But these tonics are only applicable to people with yang deficiency, hypofunctions

3. 忌忍尿入房

忍尿入房主要危害大小便和前后阴。这是因为尿液潴留膀胱，下焦气机因性交而壅滞，此时的交合，使经脉阻塞，血气瘀滞，临床出现大小便困难，尿道涩痛或刺痛，小腹肿硬等症状。

4. 忌经期同房

妇女行经期间，子宫口张开，子宫内膜脱落，血管破裂，抵抗力下降。此时同房，极易造成感染，引起月经不调、崩漏、白带、不孕症、癥瘕积聚（包括生殖系统的恶性肿瘤）等疾病。

5. 忌产褥交合

产后妇女气血未复，子宫口张开，若性交就会损伤经脉，损耗精血，带入致病物质，引起各种妇科病。由于产褥期同房的后果严重，故古人对产后恢复性生活的日期定为"产后满百日，乃可合会。"

6. 忌以药助兴

中西药物中有不少增强性欲或性功能的制剂，壮阳甚速。但这些药物只宜用于身体阳虚，功能低下，肾精不甚

and no severe deficiency of renal essence to remedy defects and balance yin and yang. Moreover, these tonics can be used only momentarily and protracted administration is not advisable. If used as the stimulants for sexual passion, these drugs may harm life and bring about premature death.

2.5 Therapies with sports

The application of physical training with traditional sports activities has the actions of activating meridians and collaterals, promoting qi flow and blood circulation, regulating viscera, eliminating diseases and prolonging life. It possesses unique effects on the restoration of limb functions in particular. The method is applicable to the functional disturbances of limbs such as hemiplegia, flaccidity syndrome, arthralgia syndrome, cervical spondylosis, paraplegia, fracture and injury of the muscle and tendon. In addition, it can promote the metabolism of the organism, bring the compensation of the organism into full play. The method has good accessory therapeutic effects on many chronic diseases as well.

2.5.1 The characteristics and applying principles of enhancing health with sports activities in TCM

2.5.1.1 The main characteristics of traditional Chinese sports activities

2.5.1.1.1 **Being under the guidance of TCM theories** The methods of strengthening health with traditional sports activities are based on TCM theories of yin and yang, viscera, qi and blood, meridians and collaterals, etc. The basic essentials of these sports activities

亏损者，以补偏救弊，平衡阴阳，且只可暂用于一时，不宜久服。如果以其作为情欲刺激剂，就会成为有损健康，促使早夭的毒物。

第五节 运动疗法

运用传统的体育运动方式进行锻炼，有畅达经络、疏通气血、和调脏腑、祛除疾病、益寿延年的功效。尤其对恢复肢体功能有着独特的作用，适用于偏瘫、痿证、痹证、颈椎病、骨折、伤筋等肢体功能障碍性疾病的康复。此外，还能促进机体代偿功能，对病伤和残疾的机体功能障碍，能最大限度地发挥机体的代偿能力。对多种慢性病，也能起到良好的辅助治疗作用。

一、中医运动健身的特点和运用原则

1. 中国传统运动的特点

（1）在中医学理论指导下进行 传统运动健身法，是以中医的阴阳、脏腑、气血、经络等理论为基础，以养精、炼气、调神为运动的基本要点，

include nourishing essence, training qi and regulating the mind. Therefore, people should study TCM theories carefully and apply the theories to the practice of physical training.

2.5.1.1.2 Attaching importance to the harmony and unity of mental concentration, regulating breathing and exercising the body   Mental concentration refers to highly concentrated mind, regulating breathing to regulation of respiration, and exercising the body to training the body, the three of which should be harmonious and cooperative to achieve unity between the body and spirit, interflow of mind and qi, and interaction between the body and qi. Only when the interior and exterior of the body are harmonious, movement and motionlessness are moderate, can the effects of life cultivation and rehabilitation be gained.

2.5.1.2 Applying principles of life cultivation and rehabilitation with sports activities

2.5.1.2.1 Unity of the body and spirit   The main points of life cultivation and rehabilitation with sports activities are the unity of mental concentration, regulating respiration and exercising the body. The relationships among the three are as follows: direct qi with the mind and move the body with qi, the purposes of which are to achieve the harmony between the interior and exterior, general flow of qi and blood, and overall training of the whole organism.

2.5.1.2.2 Being reasonable and moderate   Emphasis should be placed on moderation and orderly and gradual advancement, whereas seeking success impatiently should not be allowed. Otherwise, acting with undue haste may lead to the consequence of more haste, less speed.

2.5.1.2.3 Persevering in one's efforts   "Run-

所以,要认真学习中医理论,并正确运用于运动锻炼。

(2)注重意守、调息和动形的谐调统一 意守指意念专注,调息指呼吸调节,动形指形体运动。三者之间要谐调配合,要达到形、神一致,意、气相随,形、气相感,使形体内外和谐,动、静得宜,方能起到养生、康复的作用。

2. 运动养生、体育康复的运用原则

(1)形神统一 运动养生和体育康复的要领就是意守、调息、动形的统一。三者的关系是:以意领气,以气动形,使内外和谐、气血周流,整个机体可得到全面锻炼。

(2)合理适度 要强调适量的锻炼,循序渐进,不可急于求成。操之过急,否则欲速而不达。

(3)持之以恒 "流水不

ning water is never stale and a door hinge never gets worm-eaten." Only when one perseveres in one's effort can better effects of life cultivation and rehabilitation be achieved. Traditional sports activities train not only the body, but also will and stamina.

2.5.2 Examples of life cultivation and rehabilitation with classical sports activities

2.5.2.1 The five mimic-animal games

It is a classical physical exercise which imitates the motions of the five animals of tigers, deer, bears, monkeys and birds. The exercise has been the method for Chinese people to build up health and to prolong life since the ancient times.

The game of mimic-tiger　It imitates the tiger's image, adopts the tiger's air and its perfect utilization of its paws as well as its motions of shaking the head and wagging the tail, bulging and vibrating the whole body. The game requires concentration of the mind on Mingmen (GV4). It has the functions of strengthening the kidney and waist, enhancing the bone and promoting the production of marrow. The exercise may remove obstruction of governor vessel and eliminate pathogenic wind.

The game of mimic-deer　It imitates the deer's image, adopts the animal's longevity and intelligence as well as its perfect use of the coccyx. The games requires concentration of the mind on the coccyx. It can remove obstruction of meridians and collaterals, promote blood circulation, limber up muscles and joints.

The game of mimic-bear　It imitates the bear's image of being clumsy in bodily movement and great in physical strength, static in exterior and dynamic in interior. The game requires concentration of the mind on Zhonggong (within the navel), and puts emphasis on being dy-

腐,户枢不蠹",只有坚持不懈,才能收到养生、康复效果,传统体育运动不仅是身体的锻炼,也是意志和毅力的锻炼。

二、古典运动养生、康复法举隅

1. 五禽戏

是一种模仿虎、鹿、熊、猿、鸟五种禽兽动作的古典体操,自古至今一直是中国人防病治病、延年益寿的方法。

虎戏:即模仿虎的形象,取其神气、善用爪力和摇首摆尾、鼓荡周身的动作。要求意守命门,有益肾强腰,壮骨生髓的作用,可以通督脉、祛风邪。

鹿戏:即模仿鹿的形象,取其长寿而性灵,善运尾闾。要求意守尾闾,可以通经络、行血脉、舒展筋骨。

熊戏:即模仿熊的形象,熊体笨力大,外静而内动。要求意守中宫(脐内),着重于内动而外静。

namic in the interior and static in exterior.

The game of mimic-monkey It imitates the monkey's image of being alert, dexterous and quick in action, and liable to movement. The game requires concentration of the mind on the navel to seek for physical movement and mental peace.

The game of mimic-bird It is also called the game of mimic-crane which imitates the crane's image of being lithe in flying and unfolding in action. Practicing this games requires concentration of the mind on Qihai (CV6). It can regulate and promote qi flow and blood circulation, dredge meridians and collaterals, limber up the tendons, bones and joints.

The five mimic-animal games not only include bodily movements, but also requires elimination of all stray thoughts, concentration of the mind on Dantian as well as the cooperation of respiration. The games can regulate yin and yang, promote qi flow and blood circulation, strengthen the body resistance to eliminate pathogenic factors. Therefore, it has better actions of nourishing the mind, regulating qi flow and blood circulation, strengthening viscera, dredging meridians and collaterals, limbering up muscles and joints, and facilitating flexible movement of joints. Clinically, the game is commonly applicable to patients with hemiplegia, paraplegia, arthralgia syndrome, flaccidity syndrome, osteoporosis, Parkinson's syndrome, etc. at the stage of recovery.

2.5.2.2　Yijinjing (tendon-exercising technique)

"Yi" means movement and change; "jin", in general sense, refers to the muscle, tendon and bone; "jing" denotes the general law and norm. "Yijinjing" means this technique exercises the muscle, tendon and bone, makes general meridians and collaterals, qi flow and blood

猿戏：即模仿猿的形象，猿机警灵活，好动无定。要求意守脐中，以求形动而神静。

鸟戏：又称鹤戏，即模仿鹤的形象，动作轻翔舒展。练此戏要意守气海，可以调达气血，疏通经络，活动筋骨关节。

五禽戏既有形体动作，又要求排除杂念，意守丹田及呼吸配合，能调理阴阳，流通气血，扶正祛邪，故有较好的养精神、调气血、益脏腑、通经络、活筋骨、利关节的作用，临床则常用于偏瘫、截瘫、痹证、痿证、骨质疏松症、震颤麻痹综合征等患者的康复期。

2. 易筋经

"易"指移动、改变；"筋"，泛指肌肉、筋骨；"经"，指常道、规范。"易筋经"就是活动肌肉、筋骨，使全身经络、气血通畅，从而增进健康、祛病延

circulation unobstructed. As a result, it strengthens health, eliminates diseases and prolongs life. The technique is a traditional method of enhancing health and rehabilitation.

All the movements of Yinjinjing imitate the various ancient postures of physical labor and have evolved from them. For example, the actions of husking grain with a mortar and pestle, carrying grain, putting grain in storage, harvesting crops and storing grain, cherishing grain, etc. all of which are the basic forms based on various movements of physical labor. The specific content includes husking grain with a mortar and pestle, carrying grain on a carrying pole, winnowing impurities from grain, carrying grain on the alternate side of the shoulder, pushing a cart with sacks of grain and piling them up, leading an ox to carry grain, carrying grain on the back, unloading grain with the square-bottomed bamboo basket, enclosing grain for storage with the mat, bending over to protect grain and bending down to pick up grains and bending low to gather crops. The twelve movements are marked by bodily flexion and extension, bending and lifting as well as torsion to achieve the training effect of "limbering up joints". Therefore, this method can remedy the bad postures, promote the growth and development of muscles and skeleton for teenagers; as far as old and weak people are concerned, the method can prevent senile muscular atrophy, promote blood circulation, adjust and strengthen general nutrition and absorption; it is very beneficial to the rehabilitation of patients with chronic diseases as well as delaying ageing. Clinically, the method is commonly applied to patients with hemiplegia, flaccidity syndrome, paraplegia, disuse syndrome, etc. at the stage of recovery.

年的一种传统健身康复法。

易筋经中所设动作都是仿效古代的各种劳动姿势而演化成的。例如：舂谷、载运、进仓、收囤和珍惜谷物等动作，均以劳动的各种动作为基础形态。其具体内容为：捣杆舂粮、扁担挑粮、扬风净粮、换肩扛粮、推袋垛粮、牵牛拉粮、背牵运粮、盘箩卸粮、围芄囤粮、扑地护粮、屈体捡粮、弓身收粮。十二式的活动以形体屈伸、俯仰、扭转为特点，以达到"伸筋拔骨"的锻炼效果。因此，对于青少年来说，这种方法可以纠正身体的不良姿态，促进肌肉、骨骼的生长发育；对于年老体弱者来讲，可以防止老年性肌肉萎缩，促进血液循环，调整和加强全身的营养和吸收，对慢性疾病的恢复，以及延缓衰老都很有益处。临床常用于痿证、废用综合征等病人的康复期。

2.5.2.3 Eight-section brocade

Eight-section brocade consists of eight different movements, hence the name "eight-section". This gymnastic activity strengthens health, prolongs life and eliminates diseases. Its effect is very excellent, just as if a piece of bright and colorful brocade presents itself before people's eyes, hence the name "brocade". Practicing eight-section brocade is not limited by the surroundings and place. Thus, it can be performed at any time and in any place. Besides, the postures are easy to memorize and learn. Meanwhile, its amount of exercise is moderate. The exercise is suitable for both the old and the young. It is not only used for strengthening health, but also for the rehabilitation of many chronic diseases. Accordingly, eight-section brocade has been handed down from ancient times to the present and still has been the popular keep-fit method among the vast number of the Chinese masses.

The content of eight-section brocade has been written in the form of seven-character verse, from which the different effects of different movements on life cultivation can be seen. The verse reads:

Both hands stretch upwards to regulate triple energizer,

bend a bow with alternate hands to shoot at a vulture;

stretch one hand upwards to regulate gastrosplenic functions,

look round to remove seven types of impairment and five kinds of consumptive diseases;

shake the head and move the low back to eliminate the heart fire,

both hands reach for feet to reinforce the kidney and lumbus;

3. 八段锦

八段锦是由八种不同动作组成的运动,故名"八段"。因为这种健身运动可以强身益寿,祛病除疾,其效果甚佳,有如展示给人们一幅绚丽多彩的锦锻,故称为"锦"。由于八段锦不受环境场地限制,随时随地可做,术式简单易记易学,运动量适中,老少皆宜,既可用于强身保健,又可用于多种慢性病的康复。故一直流传至今,仍是广大群众所喜爱的健身方法。

其内容被编为广为流传的七言歌诀,从中可以看出各种动作的不同养生效果:

两手托天理三焦,

左右开弓似射雕;

调理脾胃须单举,

五劳七伤往后瞧;

摇头摆尾去心火,

两手攀足固肾腰;

clench fists with round eyes to enhance physical strength,

hold the neck with interlocked hands and jolt to prevent all diseases.

2.5.2.4 Taijiquan

It is a method of life cultivation and rehabilitation conforming to nature. It requires the close integration of breathing, consciousness and movements to achieve the state of integrating the exterior with interior into one in perfect harmony. The present popular school of Taijiquan is the simplified Taijiquan (24-posture style). The movements vary from simple ones to complicated ones, from easy ones to difficult ones, proceeding in an orderly way and step by step. Accordingly, it is convenient to spread and master. In addition, there are 48-posture Taijiquan, 88-posture Taijiquan, etc., the amount of exercises of which increases in proper order, the movements of which are complicated correspondingly.

The course of Taijiquan is under the guidance of the philosophical theory of Taiji (infinite void). Every stroke and every posture forms the Taiji diagram. The shape of Taijiquan is "Taiji" and the intention of Taijiquan also lies in "Taiji." The movement of Taiji generates yang, while the motionlessness of Taiji generates yin, with both of which stimulate qi and blood of the human body itself to reach the state of "yin is even and well while yang is firm" and to make life brimming with exuberant vigor.

Persevering in practicing Taijiquan can coordinate viscera, promote qi activities, regulate yin and yang and strengthen health. Thus, it has better rehabilitation effect. Clinically, it is commonly applicable to patients with hypertension, hypotension, myocardiac infarction, chronic obstructive pulmonary disease, gastroptosis, chronic hepatitis, etc. at the stage of recovery.

攒拳怒目增气力,

背后七颠百病消。

4. 太极拳

是一种顺应自然的养生、康复方法。它要求呼吸、意识、动作三者紧密结合,达到内外合一,浑然无间的境地。目前比较流行的套路是简化太极拳(二十四式),其动作由简到繁,从易到难,循序渐进,便于普及和掌握。还有四十八式太极拳、八十八式太极拳等,运动量依次增大,动作也相应复杂。

太极拳以"太极"哲理指导拳路,拳路的一招一式又构成了太极图形。拳形为"太极",拳意亦在"太极",以太极之动而生阳,静而生阴,激发人体自身的阴阳气血达到"阴平阳秘"的状态,使生命保持旺盛的活力。

坚持练习太极拳,能协调脏腑,调畅气机,调理阴阳,强壮身体,故有较好的康复医疗作用。临床常用于高血压病、低血压症、心肌梗死、慢性阻塞性肺疾患、胃下垂、慢性肝炎等病人的康复期。

2.6 Therapies with recreation

2.6.1 Musical therapy

Musical therapy is a method to recuperate health and cultivate the mind for the promotion of somatopsychic rehabilitation by asking patients to appreciate music. As early as over two thousand years ago, classics such as *Yue Ji*, or *Records of Music* and *Neijing*, or *Canon of Medicine* carried the account of promoting health with music.

2.6.1.1 Principles of life cultivation and rehabilitation with music

Music exerts effects on the human psychology and physiology through the four major elements of the tune, rhythm, melody, loudness and harmony. Psychologically, music influences people's emotions and behavior by means of artistic appeal. It straightens people out with sentiments to regulate emotional activities. Music with strongly accented rhythms can inspire people; beautiful music with gentle melodies can make people light-hearted, happy and calm; deep and sad music can make people depressed and worried. Physiologically, different scales have different actions as well. Music, the sound wave vibration with given frequency, exerts effects on the human body to make the rhythm of every organ harmonized. Besides, sound exerts effects on the auditory organ and auditory nerve. It further influences the muscle tension, blood circulation and visceral activities. In short, music can regulate emotions, coordinate visceral functions, promote normal qi flow and blood circulation to achieve the purpose of life cultivation and rehabilitation.

2.6.1.2 Commonly-used musical prescriptions

2.6.1.2.1 Prescriptions for expressing emotions and removing worries: Select beautiful songs with

lively rhythms, smooth melodies and happy emotional appeal. For instance, Bubugao (Higher and Higher), Xiyangyang (Jubilance), Don't Worry, Don't Worry! the Golden Water River, and Sea Beach During the Holiday, etc. This type of songs may be applicable to various diseases due to emotional depression.

2.6.1.2.2 **Prescriptions for tranquilizing the mild**: Select songs with slow rhythms, mild and sweet melodies and gentle emotional appeal. For example, The Night of Spring Sea with Flowers and the Moon, the Swallow Flies down the Sandy Beach as well as Calm Lake with the Autumnal Moon, How Wonderful! the South of the Yangtze, etc. This kind of songs has the actions of relieving mental stress, tranquilizing the mind and removing worries. These songs are applicable to various diseases concerning restlessness with anxiety and vexation.

2.6.1.2.3 **Prescriptions for inspiring and arousing people**: Select songs with strongly accented and forceful rhythms, sonorous and arousing melodies, majestic or solemn and stirring tunes. For example, The Yellow River Cantata, March of the Volunteers, etc. This type of songs possesses the actions of arousing emotions, increasing courage and inspiring people. These songs can be applicable to various diseases concerning low-spiritedness, pessimism and disheartenedness.

2.6.1.2.4 **Prescriptions for inhibiting mania and anger**: Select songs with slow rhythms, deep melodies, mournful and sorrowful tunes. For instance, Sea Water, Dirge, Bury Flowers, the Homeless Singing Girl, and the Han Palace Below the Autumnal Moon, etc. This kind of songs has the actions of inhibiting mania and anger, relieving emotional excitement. They are applicable to patients with extreme emotional activities, irascibility, endless laughing and mania.

优美动听一类的曲目，如《步步高》、《喜洋洋》、《莫愁啊，莫愁》、《金水河》、《假日的海滩》等。可用于情志郁结所致的各种病证。

（2）宁心安神　选用节奏缓慢，旋律婉转，情绪柔绵异类的曲目，如《春江花月夜》、《平沙落雁》以及《平湖秋月》、《江南好》等。具有安神宁心，镇静除烦之功效，可用于情志焦躁烦恼有关的各种病证。

（3）振奋激昂　选用节奏鲜明有力，旋律高亢激昂，曲调雄壮或悲壮一类的乐曲。如《黄河大合唱》、《马赛曲》等。具有激昂情绪、增强魄力、振奋勇气之功效，可用于低沉消极、悲观失望有关的各种病证。

（4）抑躁制怒　选用节奏缓慢，旋律低沉，曲调凄切悲凉一类的乐曲，如《江河水》、《哀乐》、《葬花》、《天涯歌女》、《汉宫秋月》等。具有抑制狂躁、愤怒，减轻情绪亢奋之功效。可用于情志偏激易怒以及喜笑不休证、狂躁证者。

2.6.1.2.5 Prescriptions for improving intelligence: Select songs with gay emotions, elegant melodies and quicker rhythms to improve children's and juvenile intelligence. For example, Horse Race, Happy Russell, Fantasia, Spring of Xinjiang, and Cuckoo Walts, etc. Select songs which people were familiar with or loved when they were infants or young to improve mid-aged and old people's intelligence. The songs may vary in people. Guide people to listen and recall something. These songs may delay cerebral ageing of patients, evoke the lost memories and help the rehabilitation of patients with dementia.

Musical therapy can be conducted twice or thrice a day, 30 to 60 minutes each time. The volume should be moderate. The environment should be elegant, peaceful and cozy, free from the interference of noises. If the conditions permit, the effects can be improved with the corresponding cooperation of lights, colors, flowers, etc.

If the conditions permit, patients may be encouraged to adopt active methods such as playing musical instruments, singing and composing musical works.

2.6.2 Singing therapy

Singing therapy is a method to promote life cultivation and rehabilitation by asking patients to sing songs. Singing songs requires concentration of the mind and imagination in order to enter the artistic conception. Meanwhile, regulating bodily postures is needed to direct air and produce sounds. Therefore, singing is the massage beneficial to viscera. Besides moulding sentiments and enhancing health, singing therapy may be applicable to emotional depression and pessimism after being wounded, ill and handicapped as well as various diseases concerning these factors. In addition, it may be applicable to asthma at the stage of recovery. This is because that singing songs can remove the obstruction of air passage, enhance thoracic and diaphragmatic movement, and is thus beneficial to the discharge of sputum and saliva as well as the enhancement of respiratory function. Moreover, singing songs can train and restore the physiological functions of the throat, lips, palates and vocal folds. Accordingly, it is applicable to diseases such as ankyloglossia, stiff tongue, facial paralysis and dysphasia as well as difficulty in raising the palate upwards, etc.

The songs should be selected on the basis of the patient's musical accomplishment, hobbies, and national customs, etc.

2.6.3 Dancing therapy

It is applicable to life cultivation of emotions and emotional disorders such as emotional depression, sorrow, vexation, or hypophrenia, dementia and neurasthenia. Besides, it relaxes muscles and tendons to promote blood circulation. The therapy is applicable to exercising limbs and the rehabilitation of bodily diseases such as flaccidity syndrome, arthralgia syndrome, five types of flaccidity and injury of muscles and tendons at the stage of recovery as well as obesity, osteoporosis and disuse syndrome.

Different dances have different rhythms and movements. Therefore, flexible selection of dances among the local popular dances should be based on the patient's specific conditions.

2.6.4 Drama therapy

There are roles and plots in dramas. Dramas can not only set people roaring with laughter, but also make people grieved and cry; dramas can not only arouse people's feeling, but also make people have a light heart. Accordingly, drama therapy is good at regulating emotional activities and applicable to life cultivation of emotional disorders. Different types and contents of dramas should be selected for the rehabilitation patients with abnormal emotions on the basis of the patient's specific conditions. Light and merry, or lively and inspiring types and contents of dramas should be selected for patients with depression and pessimism such as comedies; peaceful and elegant types and contents of dramas should be selected for patients with dysphoria and emotional excitement such as various orthodox dramas.

2.6.5 Therapies with a musical instrument and chess, practicing paintings and calligraphy

Therapies with a musical instrument and chess are the methods to promote somatopsychic health by asking patients to play a musical instrument and chess. The fine movement and coordination of the fingers are under the control of the brain. Thus playing a musical instrument and chess, practicing painting and calligraphy have positive effects on the prevention of cerebral arteriosclerosis, senile dementia, etc.

2.6.5.1 Playing a musical instrument

Its effects on life cultivation are realized by means of "keeping relaxed and happy" and "exercising fingers to tonify the brain." The single-hearted devotion and the appreciation of peaceful, cheerful and beautiful music during playing a musical instrument make people happy and relaxed. Thus, it has the action of making people have ease of mind and a light heart. Meanwhile, playing a musical instrument can exercise fingers and palms, make them flexible in movements and help finger joints to re-

又可使人心情愉悦,故长于调节情志,用于情志养生;对于情绪异常的康复患者,要针对病人的具体情况,可选择不同的剧种和戏剧内容。凡情绪抑郁、消沉一类的病人,应选择轻松愉快,或热烈激昂的剧种和戏剧内容,如喜剧等;而情绪烦躁、亢奋一类的病人,则应选择恬静优雅的剧种和戏剧内容,如各种正剧。

五、琴棋书画

琴棋疗法是让病人通过弹琴、弈棋,促进身心健康的方法。由于手指的精细动作与协调运动是在大脑的指挥下进行的,因此,琴棋书画对预防脑动脉硬化、老年性痴呆等有积极的作用。

1. 弹琴

其养生作用是通过"怡情悦志"和"运指健脑"两方面实现的。弹琴时的专心致志和恬愉优美的音乐享受,使人心情舒畅,轻松愉快,故有畅娱神情的作用;同时,有练习指掌,使之灵活自如,帮助手指关节恢复活动功能的功效。对于中风后遗症、痿症、痹症、

store active functions. Playing a musical instrument can be used to eliminate finger dysfunctions such as finger spasm and inflexible finger flexion due to sequelae of apoplexy, flaccidity syndrome, arthralgia syndrome, burn, and injury of muscles and tendons, etc.

2.6.5.2 Playing chess

It is a method of life cultivation and rehabilitation to promote intelligence development. When playing chess, people concentrate the mind on the chessboard and get rid of all distracting thoughts. Therefore, playing chess is applicable to people with distractibility and difficulty in concentrating the mind. Besides, playing chess helps to remove depression and have a light heart. It can be applicable to infantile retarded intelligence development and declining intelligence in old people.

Playing chess should be moderate, too. People should not spend too much energy and should not be too particular about the result. The most important aspect is always to while away the time for a light heart and to benefit intelligence.

2.6.5.3 Therapy with painting and calligraphy

Therapy with painting and calligraphy is a method to promote somatopsychic health by asking the patients to watch and practice painting and calligraphy. People should get rid of distracting thoughts before watching and practicing painting and calligraphy. Then, they regulate breathing and direct qi to fingers, wrists, arms and waist to bring all the force of the body onto the pen point or tip of a writing brush. Actually, this already includes regulation of the mind, breathing and bodily movement. Its mechanism lies in the following aspects.

2.6.5.3.1 Regulating emotions
Appreciating and practicing painting and calligraphy can mould temperament, soothe and disperse stagnated qi. Therefore, the

烧伤、伤筋等病证所致手指拘挛、屈指不利等，可通过弹琴以消除手指功能障碍。

2. 弈棋

是一项促进智力发展的养生方法和康复疗法。弈棋时，心神集中，意守棋局，杂念尽消，故适合于注意力分散，精力不易集中者。弈棋还有助于解除郁闷，愉快心情。可用于小儿智力发育迟缓及老人智力衰减。

弈棋亦要注意适度，不能耗神太多，也不能过于计较输赢，而总以遣情益智为要。

3. 书画

书画疗法是让病人通过观看、习练书画，促进身心健康的方法。由于观、作书画之前，要排除杂念，再调节呼吸，运气于指、腕、臂、腰，调动全身之力于笔端，实际上已内蕴调心、调息、调形之义。其养生、康复的机理在于：

（1）调节情志 观赏和习练书画能陶冶性情，舒发郁气，故情绪烦躁、愤怒、抑郁

method is applicable to patients with impetuosity, anger and depression, or patients with disorders of seven emotions. Ancients believed that watching and writing different forms of characters may have different effects on moulding temperament.

(1) Regular script: It has the actions of tranquilizing qi and the mind, removing vexation and impetuosity. Regular script is applicable to diseases due to dysphoria and anger.

(2) Official script: It is imposing and firm, quiet and beautiful, which easily makes people emotionally stable. Official script is also applicable to diseases due to dysphoria and anger. Besides, it is cooperatively used with regular scrip to check activity with tranquility.

(3) Running hand and cursive hand: Both are natural, unrestrained and lively, like floating clouds and flowing water, which can make people in high spirits and have ease of mind. Accordingly, running hand and cursive hand are particularly applicable to patients with depression and pessimism.

2.6.5.3.2 Training the body When practicing painting and calligraphy, people have fine movements of arms, elbows, wrists and fingers. These fine movements can train general tendons, bones and muscles (especially the upper limbs) to regulate and promote qi flow and blood circulation, relax muscles and tendons and activate collaterals. Practicing painting and calligraphy is used to eliminate dysfunctions and restore functions such as spasm or unsmooth flexion of hands, wrists, elbows and arms due to sequelae of apoplexy, flaccidity syndrome, arthralgia syndrome, burn and injury of muscles and tendons.

Practicing painting and calligraphy can also achieve the purposes of arousing inspiration and improving intelligence by focusing on thinking and cleverly applying fin-

者，或七情逆乱者，均可选用。古人认为书写或观赏不同的字体有不同的怡情作用：

楷书：有静气安神，消除烦恼和急躁情绪的作用，适用于烦躁、愤怒致病者。

隶书：凝重稳健，清幽恬静，易使人产生沉稳安定的情绪，亦适用于烦躁、愤怒致病者，并常与楷书配合使用，以静制动。

行书、草书：潇洒活泼，似行云流水，能使人情绪高昂，胸怀舒畅，故对情志抑郁低沉之患者尤为适宜。

（2）锻炼形体 书画之时，臂、肘、腕、指要进行精细活动，能使周身筋骨肌肉（尤其是上肢）得到锻炼而获调畅气血、舒筋活络之效。凡中风后遗证、痿证、痹证、烧伤、伤筋所致手腕肘臂拘挛或屈伸不利者，可习书画以消除障碍，恢复功能。

书画还能通过集中思维、巧运手指而达到激发灵感，增进智力的目的，对弱智儿童、

gers. It may be applicable to the rehabilitation of children with hypophrenia, senile amnesia and dementia, etc. Modern researches also indicate practicing painting has satisfactory effects on rehabilitation of feeble-minded children.

2.7 Life cultivation and rehabilitation with loutrotherapy

Loutrotherapy is a method to eliminate diseases and strengthen health by applying visible or invisible natural physical factors such as water, sunlight, air, mud and sand.

Different bathing forms may relieve exterior syndromes by means of diaphoresis, remove wind and dampness, promote qi flow and blood circulation, relax muscles and tendons, activate collaterals, regulate yin and yang, and inspire enthusiasm, etc. respectively. Bathing forms are numerous, such as hot spring bath, hot water bath, sunbath, seawater bath, sauna, cold water bath, medicated bath, mud bath, sand bath and forestry bath. Because of limited space, this section only introduces the three bathing methods with TCM characteristics.

2.7.1 Medicated bath

Medicated liquid with a certain concentration is used to bathe or soak the whole body. In this way, the active principles of the drugs can exert direct effects on the region of pathological changes to destroy bacteria, kill pain, check itching and relieve inflammation. Meanwhile, by means of skin absorption, the active principles enter blood circulation to reach every tissue and organ of the human body, and to bring the therapeutic effects into full play.

老年健忘、痴呆等可行书画康复疗法。现代研究也表明，绘画对弱智儿童的康复效果颇佳。

第七节 沐浴疗法

沐浴疗法，是利用水、日光、空气、泥沙等有形的或无形的天然物理因素祛病健身的方法。

不同的沐浴方式，可分别起到发汗解表、祛风除湿、行气活血、舒筋活络、调和阴阳、振奋精神等作用。沐浴形式较多，如温泉浴、热水浴、日光浴、海水浴、桑拿浴、冷水浴、药浴、泥浆浴、沙浴、森林浴等，由于篇幅所限，本节仅介绍具有中医特色的三种沐浴法。

一、药浴

用一定浓度的药液，洗浴或浸泡全身，使药物中的有效成分直接作用于病变部位，起杀菌、止痛、止痒、消炎的作用，同时通过皮肤吸收进入血液循环，到达人体各个组织器官，发挥药物的治疗作用。

2.7.1.1 The mechanism of life cultivation and rehabilitation with medicated bath

Medicated bath, like hot spring bath, hot water bath and sauna, can make skin blood vessels dilated and congested, accelerate metabolism and strengthen syringadenous excretion to promote profuse sweating and discharge of metabolite and toxin. Heat can reduce the excitability of nervous system to produce tranquilization and to be beneficial to sleeping, too. The heat of water can reduce muscular tension to relieve muscular pain and spasm as well. Moreover, the drugs in the medicated liquid reach the body directly. Therefore, it can produce a pharmacological action which does not exist in other bathing therapies.

Medicated bath may be applicable to the rehabilitation of hypertension, local soft tissue injury, neurosis, rheumatic arthritis, rhematoid arthritis, lumbago, pain of legs, ischias, sequelae of cerebrovascular accident, obesity, psoriasis, and skin itching, etc.

Before bathing, soak the drug for more than half an hour. Then, decoct the drugs into decoction. Next, mix the decoction with bathing water. The temperature of the water is about 40 to 50℃. The bathing lasts 15 to 20 minutes (soak only the affected part in the case of contagious skin diseases such as tinea manuum and tinea pedis) each time, once a day or once every other day. It is advisable to take the medicated bath after noon or in the evening according to the specific patient's conditions. Each dose can be decocted twice. After bathing, wipe the body drily with a towel. Then, cover the body with a quilt and lie in bed peacefully for a while. However, be cautious not to select the drugs which irritate and corrode the skin; old,

1. 药浴的养生、康复机理

药浴与温泉浴、热水浴、桑拿浴一样,其物理效应可使皮肤血管扩张、充血、新陈代谢加快,汗腺分泌增强,大量排汗,排出代谢产物及毒素。温热又可以降低神经系统的兴奋性,产生镇静作用,有利于睡眠。水的温热作用又可降低肌肉的张力,缓解肌肉疼痛与痉挛。而药浴液中的药物与身体直接接触,所产生的药理作用是其他沐浴疗法所不具备的。

药浴可应用于高血压、局部软组织损伤、神经官能症、风湿性关节炎、类风湿关节炎、腰腿痛、坐骨神经痛、脑血管意外后遗症、肥胖病、银屑病、皮肤瘙痒等疾病的康复。

洗浴前先将药物浸泡半小时以上,煎煮成药汁,再兑入洗澡水中,水温约在40～50℃左右,每次浸浴约15～20分钟(手足癣等传染性皮肤病只浸泡患处),每日1次,或隔日1次,或视病情而定,以午后或晚间进行为宜。每剂药物可煎煮2次。浴后用干毛巾拭干,盖被静卧片刻。但需注意,药物不能选择对皮肤有刺激和腐蚀性的;老、幼、病重者药浴需人护理,避免意外;

very young and seriously sick patients should be nursed to avoid accidents; medicated bath is not advisable in the case of skin injury, excessive starvation, overfeeding, menstrual period and pregnant stage.

2.7.1.2 The commonly-used prescriptions for medicated bath

TCM possesses a large number of prescriptions for medicated bath handed down from the ancient times. Here is a brief introduction only for your reference.

2.7.1.2.1 Prescription for skin itching　90 g of Ganheye (dry *Folium Nelumbinis*), Gaoben (*Rhizoma Ligustici*), Gansong (*Rhizoma Nardostachyos*), Baizhi (*Radix Angelicae Dachuricae*), Weilingxian (*Radix Clematidis*), Cangercao (*Herba Xanthii*), Rendongteng (*Caulis Lonicerae*) and salt respectively.

2.7.1.2.2 Prescription for skin eczema　100 g of fresh Chuanlianpi (*Pericarpium Meliae Toosendan*), 30 g of Qiyeyizhihua (*Cortex Actinodaphnes Obovatae*), Longgu (*Os Draconis*) and Luganshi (*Calamina*) respectively, 25 g of Tufuling (*Rhizoma Smilacis Glabrae*), Kushen (*Radix Sophorae Flavescentis*), Difuzi (*Fructus Kochiae*) and Huzhang (*Rhizoma Polygoni Cuspidati*) respectively, 20 g of Huanglian (*Rhizoma Coptidis*), Huangqin (*Radix Scutellariae*), Huangbai (*Cortex Phellodendri*), Shengdaihuang (*Radix et Rhizoma Rhei*), Baixianpi (*Cortex Dictamni Radicis*), Huajiao (*Pericarpium Zanthoxyli*) and Diyu (*Radix Sanguisorbae*) respectively, 15 g of Chixiaodou (*Semen Phaseoli*), Baiyaojian (*Massa Gallae et Thei Fermentata*), Liujinu (*Herba Artemisiae Anomalae*) and Danpi (*Cortex Moutan Radicis*) respectively, 10 g of Cheqianzi (*Semen Plantaginis*) and Bingpian (*Borneolum Syntheticum*) respectively.

皮肤破损、饥饱过度、月经期、妊娠期不宜药浴。

2. 常用药浴方剂

中医的药浴方剂数量庞大，现简要介绍几则，供参考：

（1）皮肤瘙痒症药浴方
干荷叶、藁本、甘松、白芷、威灵仙、苍耳草、忍冬藤、盐各90 g。

（2）皮肤湿疹药浴方
鲜川楝皮100 g，七叶一枝花、龙骨、炉甘石各30 g，土茯苓、苦参、地肤子、虎杖各25 g，黄连、黄芩、黄柏、生大黄、白鲜皮、花椒、地榆各20 g，赤小豆、百药煎、刘寄奴、丹皮各15 g，车前子、冰片各10 g。

2.7.1.2.3 Prescription for infantile malnutrition
15 g of Kushen (*Radix Sophorae Flavescentis*), Fulingpi (*Epidemis Poriae*), Cangzhu (*Rhizoma Atractylodis*), Sangbaipi (*Cortex Mori Radicis*) and Baifan (*Alumen*) respectively and 15 g of Congbai (*Bulbus Allii Fistulosi*).

2.7.1.2.4 Prescription for sore and scabies due to toxic heat
30 g of Fangfeng (*Radix Ledebouriellae* with the tip removed), Baizhi (*Radix Angelicae Dahuriae*), Xixin (*Herba Asari*), Kushen (*Radix Sophorae Flavescentis*), Wuzhuyu (*Fructus Evodiae*), Kulianzi (*Fructus Meliae Toosendan*), Lilu (*Radix et Rhizoma Veratri*) with the tip removed, Mangcao (*Folium Illicii Lanceolati*) and Mahuanggen (*Radix Ephedriae*) respectively, 15 g of Chuanjiao (*Pericarpium Zanthoxyli*) and 60 g of salt.

2.7.1.2.5 Prescription for tinea manuum and tinea pedis
30 g of Kushen (*Radix Sophorae Flavescentis*), Taoren (*Semen Persicae*), Shechuangzi (*Fructus Cnidii*), Wumei (*Fructus Mume*), Lianqiao (*Fructus Forsythiae*) and Dahuang (*Radix et Rhizoma Rhei*) respectively, 20 g of Gancao (*Radix Glycyrrhizae*) and 40 g of Mangxiao (*Natrii Sulfas*).

2.7.1.2.6 Prescription for arthritis and gout
Equal amount of Laoguancao (*Herba Erodii seu Geranii*), Wujiapi (*Cortex Acnthopancis Radicis*), and Shenjincao (*Herba Lycopodii*), etc. respectively.

2.7.1.2.7 Prescription for strengthening renal yang and sexual function
30 g of Dingxiang (*Flos Caryophylli*), Rougui (*Cortex Cinnamomi*), Zishaohua (*Spongillae Fragillae*), and Shechuangzi (*Fructus Cnidii*) respectively, 60 g of Cangzhu (*Rhizoma Atractylodis*) and Duzhong (*Cortex Eucommiae*) respectively. All the above ingredients are ground into coarse powder. 30 g

（3）小儿发育不良药浴方　苦参、茯苓皮、苍术、桑白皮、白矾各15 g，葱白5 g。

（4）热毒疮疖药浴方　防风、白芷、细辛、苦参、吴茱萸、苦楝子、藜芦、莽草、麻黄根各30 g，川椒15 g，盐60 g。

（5）治疗手足癣　苦参、桃仁、蛇床子、乌梅、连翘、大黄各30 g，甘草20 g，芒硝40 g。

（6）关节炎、痛风药浴方　老鹳草、五加皮、伸筋草各等分。

（7）补壮元阳、治疗性功能减退方　丁香、肉桂、紫梢花、蛇床子各30 g，苍术、杜仲各60 g。上为粗末。每用30 g，加水煎煮，沐浴时薰洗脐、腹部。

of the powder is decocted each time for use. Fumigate and wash the navel, abdomen and Dantian with the decoction.

2.7.2 Mud bath

Unique natural hot mineral mud forms in the central zone of the hot spring in some places with the hot spring due to prolonged moistening of spring water. The temperature of the mud remains 42 to 60℃ and the mud contains a large amount of colloidal substances, salts, gases, etc. Applying such hot mineral mud to bury and clean the body generally or locally can stimulate and regulate the nerves and body fluid of the organism. This has anti-inflammatory, pain-checking and cosmetic actions, etc.

There are natural or artificial mud bath rooms in places with rich geothermal resources. Bathers soak themselves in the mud of the bathing pool for 3 to 5 minutes or about 10 minutes. Then, they go to the sandy beach to lie down. When the mud on the body dries up in the sun and peels off one lump after another, wash the body clean with clear water. Mud bath has specific therapeutic effects on skin diseases and rheumatic arthritis. For healthy people, it also removes fatigue after they are soaked in the mud pool for a period of time.

There existed a kind of mud therapy in the ancient China. However, it was not the hot mud produced by terrestrial heat, but the cold mud dug from the well called "well mud". Medical books in the Tang Dynasty carried this method, such as *Qianjin Yaofang*, or *Valuable Prescriptions* and *Zhenlei Bencao*, or *Classified Materia Medica for Emergency*. It was used to cure diseases such as threatened abortion due to fetal heat at pregnant stage as well as headache due to wind and heat. This

二、泥浆浴

某些有温泉的地方，由于受矿泉的长期滋润，在泉水的中心地带形成了特有的天然热矿泥，其温度在42～65℃之间，并有大量的胶体物质、盐类和气体等。用这样的热矿泥进行全身或局部埋浴、擦浴，能刺激和调节机体的神经和体液，具有消炎、止痛和美容等作用。

在地热资源比较丰富的地方，会有天然的或人工建造的泥浆浴室。浴者先在浴池的泥巴中浸泡三五分钟或者十来分钟，然后到沙滩上躺下，待身上的泥浆晒干后一块块自然剥落，再用清水洗净身体。泥浆浴对治疗皮肤病和风湿关节炎有特效，健康的人在泥浆池内泡上一段时间，也有消除疲劳的益处。

中国古代还有一种泥浴疗法，但不是用地热产生的热泥浆，而是用井底挖出的冷泥浆，称之为"井底泥"。唐代的《千金要方》、《证类本草》等医书中都记载了这种方法，认为治疗妊娠胎热导致的胎动不安，以及风热头痛等疾病。这种方法，实际上就是现代所说

method, in fact, is the so-called humic acidic natrium bath. Besides well mud, the mud in marshland also has the same effects.

Humic acid is the substance produced by putrefied organic substances. It has the actions of regulating the endocrine of the organism, inhibiting various harmful enzymes, accelerating blood circulation, promoting metabolism and increasing the immunity of the human body.

Mud bath has better therapeutic effects on rheumatoid arthritis, arthralgia of limbs, skin purpura, soft tissue injury of the organism, ulcer of digestive tract, certain obstetrical and gynecological diseases as well as hypertension. It has the therapeutic actions of relieving swelling and restoring physical strength especially in the people with sprain due to competitions or training.

2.7.3 Sand bath

Sand bath is the method to achieve the therapeutic effects by means of heat transmission into the body with sand directly contacting the body as the medium. It has very good therapeutic effects on rheumatic arthritis and diseases of motor system.

The mechanism of sand bath mainly lies in the comprehensive therapeutic effects of magnetic therapy (the sand contains magnetic substances), physical therapy (dryness, high temperature and infrared radiation), massage, sunbath, etc. Sand bath can remove obstruction of meridians, relax muscles, tendons and bones, eliminate intractable diseases, promote blood circulation and enhance metabolism.

The method of taking a sand bath is burying the whole body except the head, or part of the body in the hot solarized sand. With the scorching sun overhead and the burning sand under the body, patients perspire all over

的腐植酸钠浴,除了井底泥以外,沼泽地里的泥浆也有同样作用。

腐植酸是有机物腐败后生成的物质,具有调节机体内分泌、抑制各种有害酶、加速人体的血液循环、促进新陈代谢、提高人体免疫力的功能。

泥浆浴对治疗类风湿关节炎、四肢关节疼痛、皮肤紫斑、机体软组织损伤、消化道溃疡、某些妇产科疾病、高血压均有较好的疗效。尤其对因比赛或训练而扭伤者,有消除肿胀、恢复体力的疗效。

三、沙浴

沙浴,就是以沙为媒介,与身体接触,向体内传热,以达到治疗目的的方法。沙浴治疗风湿性关节炎、运动系统疾病有非常好的疗效。

沙浴的机理,主要是通过磁疗(沙子中含有的磁性物质)、理疗(干燥高温和红外辐射)、推拿按摩、日光浴等综合疗效。可通经脉、舒筋骨、祛痼疾,促进血液循环,增强新陈代谢之功效。

沙浴的方法,是将除头以外的整个身体、或身体的局部埋入太阳晒热的沙子之中。上有烈日,下有烫沙,上下夹

the body and the heat is almost unendurable. Sand bath just makes use of such thermal effect to cure diseases. In general, taking sand bath once or twice can eliminate the diseases for patients with rheumatic arthritis, ischias, disturbances of nervous system, etc. It also has therapeutic effects on diseases such as chronic diseases of digestive tract and dysfunctions of autonomic nerve.

Sand bath lasts about 10 to 15 minutes each time in accordance with the air temperature and the sand temperature. Ten days constitute one course of treatment.

攻,使患者大汗淋漓,热不可耐。沙疗正是通过这种热效应来治疗疾病。风湿性关节炎、坐骨神经痛、神经系统障碍等患者,往往一二次沙疗就能拔除病根。对于慢性消化道疾病、自主神经功能紊乱等疾病也有治疗作用。

根据气温、沙子的温度,每次沙浴时间10～15分钟,10天为1个疗程。

3 Techniques of TCM Life Cultivation and Rehabilitation

3.1 Acupuncture therapy

3.1.1 Body acupuncture

Body acupuncture therapy, a TCM therapy, is a method to promote the patient's somatopsychic rehabilitation by needling the acupoints properly selected according to the courses of meridians and collaterals with various needles. Body acupuncture therapy is extensively applied in clinic and plays an important role in health preservation, health care and rehabilitation of TCM. Now, the commonly-used methods are selectively and briefly introduced as follows.

3.1.1.1 Filiform needle therapy

The filiform needle is the most commonly-used instrument in acupuncture. The therapy has the actions of regulating visceral functions, qi flow and blood circulation, relieving pain, sedation, etc. It may be applicable to the disablement due to diseases and maim such as paralysis, convulsion, deafness and dumbness, various diseases during the convalescence such as palpitation due to fright, insomnia, cough with dyspnea, thoracic obstruction, headache and thoracic fullness, various ageing diseases such as dementia, tremor and obesity.

The application of the filiform needle therapy should be strictly handled to avoid the contraindications. For

第三章 养生康复的中医技术

第一节 针灸疗法

一、体针

体针疗法,是按经络循行途径,选择适当穴位,用各种针具施行刺激,以促使患者身心康复的中医疗法。体针疗法临床应用十分广泛,在中医养生保健和康复医疗中占有重要的位置。现择其常用方法概述如下:

1. 毫针法

毫针是针刺治疗中最常用的工具,具有调整脏腑功能,调节气血运行、镇痛、镇静等作用。可用于诸如瘫证、痉证、聋哑等病残伤残;惊悸、不寐、咳喘、胸痹、头痛、痞满等病后诸证以及痴呆、震颤、肥胖等老衰诸证。

施用毫针刺法,必须严格掌握针刺的禁忌证,如过于疲

example, needling is not advisable for patients with over-fatigue and starvation; strong stimulation is not advisable for patients with weak constitution; needling is not advisable in the case of skin infection and ulceration.

3.1.1.2 Therapy with the warming needle

The body of the needle is warmed in certain ways on the basis of therapy with the filiform needle in this therapy. It has the actions of activating yang to dispel cold, promoting qi flow and activating blood circulation.

There are many methods to heat the body of the needle. Generally, the ignited argyi wool and moxa roll or alcoholic cotton ball are used to lean against the handle of the needle, the duration and the temperature of which may be determined by the state of diseases. Therapy with the warming needle is mainly applicable to diseases due to asthenic cold or cold and dampness such as arthralgia due to cold and dampness, cold and pain of the waist and knees, pain due to asthenic cold of middle energizer. When using the warming needle, pay attention to the application and disposal of the fire source to prevent the injury.

3.1.1.3 Therapy with the three-edged needle

This therapy has strong stimulation because it has to stab and wound the skin to bleed a bit. The commonly-used methods include spot pricking, clumpy pricking, and pricking, etc. Therapy with the three-edged needle has the functions of promoting blood circulation to remove blood stasis, inducing resuscitation and purging heat, etc. The method can be used for all the diseases with relatively obvious obstruction of meridians due to internal obstruction of blood stasis in TCM rehabilitation. It is commonly applicable to intractable Bi-syndrome, aphasia from apoplexy, numbness of limbs, intractable neurodermatitis, baldness and psoriasis.

劳、饥饿者不宜进针；体弱者不宜强刺激；皮肤有感染、溃疡处不宜进针等。

2. 温针法

温针法是在毫针治疗的基础上，采取一定的方式，使针体温热，具有通阳散寒，行气活血的作用。

加热体针的方法较多，通常是用点燃艾绒、艾条或酒精棉球紧靠针柄，时间的长短及温度的高低可视病情而定。温针法主要适用于虚寒或寒湿性的病证，如寒湿痹痛、腰膝冷痛、中焦虚寒疼痛等。使用温针，应注意火源的应用处理，以防造成损伤。

3. 三棱针法

三棱针法，因为需刺破皮肤，使之少量出血，故刺激性较强。常用方法有点刺法、散刺法、挑刺法等。三棱针法具有活血祛瘀、疏经通络、开窍泄热等作用，在中医康复医疗中，凡是具有较为明显的瘀血内阻，经脉不通的病证都可使用本法。常用于顽固性痹证、中风失语、肢体麻木、顽癣、脱发、银屑病等病证。

The application of the three-edged needle requires aseptic manipulation. Besides, the action should be swift and the location shallow while profuse hemorrhage is not advisable. Do not injure the large arteries. Meanwhile, the patient should cooperate closely with the doctor to prevent fainting during acupuncture. This method is not advisable for patients with deficiency of qi and blood as well as frequent spontaneous hemorrhage or endless bleeding after injuries.

3.1.1.4 Electro-acupuncture therapy

Electro-acupuncture therapy, a method to promote rehabilitation, uses the electric stimulator to output a small amount of electric current approaching the bioelectricity of the human body which acts on the human body by means of the filiform needle inserted into the acupoint.

The indications of electrotherapy are basically the same as those of therapy with the filiform needle. It possesses better therapeutic effects on various painful diseases, paralysis, Bi-syndrome and abdominal mass, the dysfunctions of organs such as the heart, stomach, intestine, gallbladder and urinary bladder as well as the injuries of joints, muscles and ligaments, etc.

Before using the electric stimulator, check whether it functions well or not; for the electric stimulator with the maximum output voltage over 40V, its maximum output current should be limited within 1 mA in order to avoid getting an electric shock; the electric current should be increased gradually and sudden increase is not allowed; for the patients with heart diseases, avoid the electric current passing through the heart; small amount of electric current is advisable on the regions near to the bulb and spinal cord; for pregnant women, it should be used with caution.

使用三棱针，须无菌操作，且动作要快，部位要浅，出血不宜过多，勿刺伤大动脉；患者应与医生密切配合，防止晕针；气虚血弱及常有自发性出血或损伤后出血不止者，不宜使用本法。

4. 电针法

电针法，是用电针仪输出接近人体生物电的微量电流，通过刺入穴位的毫针作用于人体，使疾病得以康复的一种方法。

电针的适应证与毫针刺法基本相同，对于各种痛证、瘫证、痹证、痞证；心、胃、肠、胆、膀胱等器官的功能失调以及关节、肌肉、韧带损伤等，均有较好的疗效。

在使用电针仪前必须检查其性能是否良好；电针器最大输出电压在40伏以上者，最大输出电流应控制在1毫安之内，避免发生触电事故；电流量的调节应从小到大，切勿突然增加；有心脏病者，应避免电流回路通过心脏；近延髓、脊髓部位电流输出量宜小；孕妇慎用。

3.1.1.5 Hydro-acupuncture therapy

It is also called "acupoint injection". The therapy, a method to promote rehabilitation, uses the injection of drug into acupoints, tender points or sensitive points to regulate the functions of the corresponding viscera and tissues for the improvement of the pathological state by means of needling stimulation and the pharmacological actions of the drugs.

The proper syringe and syringe needle should be selected according to the differences of the location of the acupoints and the amount of the drug during the application of hydro-acupuncture therapy. For example, the syringe needle with size of 5 to 6.5 is selected for ordinary acupoints, while the syringe needle with the size of 9 is selected for deep acupoints, etc. During the injection, let the patient assume the comfortable posture. After the routine sterilization, insert the syringe needle with the liquid medicine quickly according to the angle and direction of inserting the filiform needle. Then, insert the needle deeper gradually. After the arrival of the needling sensation, if there is no blood in the syringe after it is drawn, push the liquid medicine into the acupoint.

The commonly-used drugs: The injections of traditional Chinese medicines include injection of Danggui (*Radix Angelicae Sinensis*), injection of Honghua (*Flos Carthami*), injection of Chuanxiong (*Rhizoma Ligustici Chuanxiong*), injection of Danshen (*Radix Salviae Miltiorrhizae*), compound injection of Danggui (*Radix Angelicae Sinensis*), compound injection of Danshen (*Radix Salviae Miltiorrhizae*), compound injection of Huangqi (*Radix Astragali Hedysari*) and compound injection of Yuxingcao (*Herba Houttuyniae*); the commonly-used injection of antibiotics of modern medicine includes injection of streptomycin, injection of kanamycin, injec-

5. 水针法

又称"穴位注射法"。是将药物注入穴位、压痛点或反应点，通过针刺的刺激和药物的药理作用，调整相应脏腑组织的功能，改善病理状态以促使疾病康复的一种方法。

水针法的运用，当根据腧穴部位及药量的不同，选择合适的注射器和针头，如一般穴位用 5～6 1/2 号针头，深部穴位用 9 号针头等。注射时，让病人取舒适的体位，常规消毒后，将抽好药液的针头按毫针刺法的角度和方向快速刺入，然后缓慢进针，"得气"后，回抽无血，即可将药液注入。

常用药物：中药注射液，如当归、红花、川芎、丹参、复方当归、复方丹参、黄芪、鱼腥草等，西药注射液如链霉素、卡那霉素、普鲁卡因青霉素、争光霉素、氯霉素注射液等抗生素；维生素类，如维生素 B_1、B_6、B_{12}、复合维生素 B、维生素 K_3、C、E 等注射液。其他类如 0.25%～2% 盐酸普鲁卡因、25% 硫酸镁、阿托品、地塞米松、醋酸可的松、维丁胶性钙、

tion of penicillin with procaine, injection of bleomycin, and injection of levomycetin, etc.; the drugs also include the injection of vitamins such as injection of vitamin B_1, injection of vitamin B_6, injection of vitamin B_{12}, injection of vitamin B complex, injection of vitamin K_3, injection of vitamin C and injection of vitamin E. Other types of drugs include injection of 0.25 to 2% procaine hydrochloride, injection of 25% magnesium sulfate, injection of atropine, injection of dexamethasone, injection of cortisone acetate, injection of Schaudinn scolloid calcium, injection of reserpine, injection of adrenosemsalicylate, and injection of 50% glucose, etc.

The dosage of acupoint injection is determined by the injection site, the property and concentration of the drug. Higher dose is applied on the site with thick muscle, generally 2 to 5 ml for one acupoint each time; smaller dose on the site with less muscle, usually 0.1 to 0.5 ml for one acupoint each time.

Hydro-acupuncture therapy may be applicable to various diseases such as every type of tissue damage, arthropathy, neuralgia, headache, insomnia, epilepsy, asthma, hypertension, cholelithiasis, hysteroptosis and allergic rhinitis.

Points for attention: ① Have a good command of the properties, pharmacological actions, doses, expiry date, incompatibilities, side effects, allergic reactions of the medicine to be used. The skin tests should be done before the medicines which may produce allergic reactions are used such as penicillin; the drugs with strong side effects and irritability should be applied with caution. ② Avoid inserting the needle on the nerve trunks or puncture the part shallowly if the injection is to be done on the main nerve trunks in case the bad consequence should occur.

③ It is not advisable to inject the drug into blood vessels, articular cavities and cavities of spinal cord. Besides, hydro-acupuncture therapy is not advisable on the lower abdomen, waist, Sanyinjiao (SP6), Hegu (LI4), etc. in pregnant women.

3.1.1.6 Skin needle therapy

Skin needle is also called "plum-blossom needle" and "seven-star needle". It is a specially-made needle used to percuss the skin along meridians and collaterals or acupoints. Skin needle therapy, a needling method, applies such percussion to dredge meridians and collaterals and regulate visceral functions for the purpose of curing diseases.

The intensity of percussing acupuncture is divided into weak stimulation, moderate stimulation and strong stimulation. Weak stimulation refers to the appearance of flush on the percussed site and freedom from pain in the patient. It is applicable to the old, the weak, women and children as well as the parts of the head and face with shallow and thin muscles; strong stimulation means that blood oozes on the percussed site and that the patient feels painful. It is applicable to the patients with strong physique and with sthenia syndromes as well as on the parts of limbs with rich and thick muscles; moderate stimulation, weaker than the strong one but stronger than the weak one, denotes that flush appears on the percussed site but no oozing of blood occurs, while the patient feels slightly painful. It is applicable to common chronic diseases.

The commonly-used methods of skin needle therapy include percussing along the meridian, percussing the acupoint, local percussing, etc. All these methods have better rehabilitation effects on insomnia, asthma, palpitation, headache, backache, lumbago, facial paralysis, skin numbness, neurodermitis or chronic eczema, alopecia

管,不能注入关节腔与脊髓腔。孕妇的下腹、腰部及三阴交、合谷等处,不宜用水针。

6. 皮肤针

皮肤针又称"梅花针"、"七星针"。它是用特制的针具,沿经络或腧穴叩打皮肤,借以疏通经络,调节脏腑功能,从而达到治病目的的一种方法。

叩刺的强度有弱、中、强之分。弱刺激,是叩刺部位略见潮红,病人无疼痛感,适于老弱妇儿、虚证患者及头面肌肉浅薄处;强刺激,是叩刺部位隐隐出血,病人有疼痛感,适于年壮体强、实证患者及四肢肌肉丰厚处;中等刺激,用力介于强弱之间,是叩刺部位潮红,但无渗血,病人稍有疼痛感,适于一般慢性病证。

皮肤针常用方法有循经叩刺、穴位叩刺、局部叩刺等,对失眠、哮喘、心悸、头痛、脊背痛、腰痛、面瘫、皮肤麻木、顽癣、斑秃、痿证等均有较好的康复作用。

areata, and flaccidity syndrome, etc.

Before using the skin needle therapy, the instruments should be carefully examined; aseptic manipulations are required; the therapy is not advisable to the patients with the ulcer or injury of local skin.

3.1.1.7 Intradermal needle therapy

Intradermal needle therapy is also called needle-embedding therapy, of which the specially-made needle is inserted into the inside of the skin and retained for a certain period of time after the fixation. The therapy just makes use of such weak and persistent stimulation to promote the rehabilitation of diseases.

The duration of retaining the intradermal needle is determined by the specific state of disease. It usually lasts for 1 to 3 days, or for 6 to 7 days in long duration. During embedding the needle, press the site with the hand several times every day to strengthen the stimulation and therapeutic effects.

Intradermal needle therapy is mostly applicable to intractable diseases such as insomnia, asthma, hypertension, palpitation, headache, gastralgia, dysmenorrhea and bed wetting.

Pay attention to the sterilization when using intradermal needle therapy. Avoid water on the needle-embedded site in case infection should occur. In addition, it is not advisable to embed the needle on the part with skin ulcer as well as the parts which often move such as joints, the chest and abdomen. Withdraw the needle in case of discomfort after embedding the needle. Then, change to another site to embed the needle again.

3.1.2 Ear acupuncture

Ear acupuncture therapy, a method to promote rehabilitation, applies the methods such as acupuncture, needle-embedding therapy and electrotherapy to puncture the corresponding acupoints of the specific sites of the auricle according to certain acupoint selection principles.

The auricle is like an inverted fetus with the corresponding sites of the internal organs, limbs and other tissues and organs of the fetus on it. The location and nomenclature of auricular acupoints mostly correspond with such a distribution and have certain regularity.

The auricular acupoint (also called positive point, sensitive spot, tenderness point, and good conducting point, etc.) has double value in diagnosis and treatment. The commonly-used methods of ear acupuncture therapy include needle-embedding therapy, seed-pressing method, needling method with the filiform needle, electrotherapy, warming needle therapy, etc. Ear acupuncture therapy is commonly applicable to various painful diseases as well as many dysfunctional diseases in TCM life cultivation and rehabilitation such as hemicrania, trigeminal neuralgia, toothache, ischias, hypertension, insomnia, aphasia, numbness of limbs, indigestion, gallstone, chronic tracheitis, chronic enteritis, chronic pelvic inflammation, impotence and menopausal syndrome.

Strict measures should be taken for antisepsis during ear acupuncture therapy. Needling is contraindicated on the site with frostbite or inflammation. Immediate treatment is required in case of infection. Besides, needling is contraindicated in pregnant women with a history of habitual abortion; patients with sprain or disturbance of limb movement should move the affected part to improve the rehabilitation effects when the feeling of congestion and fever appears on the auricle after the insertion of the needle.

用针刺、埋针、电针等方法刺激相应穴位，使疾病得以康复的一种方法。

耳郭犹如一个倒置的胎儿，各内脏、肢体及其他组织器官，在耳郭上一般都有相应的部位，而耳郭穴位的定位及其名称，则多与这一分布相适应，具有一定的规律性。

耳穴（又称"阳性反应点"、"敏感点"、"压痛点"、"良导点"等）具有诊断和治疗的双重价值。耳针常用方法有埋针法、压籽法、毫针刺法、电针法、温针法等等。在中医康复医疗中，常用于治疗各种疼痛性病证以及多种功能紊乱性疾病，如偏头痛、三叉神经痛、牙痛、坐骨神经痛、高血压病、失眠、失语、肢体麻木、消化不良、胆结石、慢性气管炎、慢性肠炎、慢性盆腔炎、阳痿、绝经期综合征等。

耳针疗法，消毒措施应严密，炎症或冻伤部位禁针，有感染迹象应及时处理；有习惯性流产的孕妇禁用；扭伤及肢体活动障碍的病人，进针后待耳郭有充血发热感，应适当活动患部，以提高康复疗效。

3.1.3 Scalp acupuncture

Scalp acupuncture therapy is a method to treat diseases or promote the somatopsychic rehabilitation of the patient by needling the specific areas of the scalp.

The specific stimulation areas of the scalp are established on the basis of the location theory of corticocerebral functions. The antero-posterior midline of the scalp and the eyebrow-occiput line, the two standard lines, should be firstly established in order to delimit the stimulation areas of the scalp acupuncture precisely. On the basis of this, specific stimulation areas can be determined respectively. The division of the stimulation areas of the scalp acupuncture may be determined with the help of flexible rule in general. The location may be determined by the experience with the mastery of the skill. Finger measurement may be applicable to patients of different age groups and different scalp types. Generally, the middle finger of an adult measures 2 to 2.5 cm. The division of stimulation areas of scalp acupuncture is very strict. Each stimulation area accurately corresponds to the indications it controls. Therefore, all the areas and their corresponding indications should be mastered and correctly used in TCM life cultivation and rehabilitation.

In scalp acupuncture therapy, the stimulation area opposite to the diseased limb is mostly selected for the disease of the unilateral limb in the stimulation area selection; the bilateral stimulation areas are selected for diseases of bilateral limbs; the bilateral stimulation areas are selected for visceral diseases, and diseases of which the right and left cannot be easily differentiated. In addition, other stimulation areas may be cooperatively selected in accordance with the accompanying symptoms besides the

三、头针

头针疗法,是在头部的特定区域进行针刺,以治疗疾病或促使患者身心康复的一种方法。

头针刺激的特定区域,是在大脑皮质功能定位理论的基础上确定的。为准确地划定头针刺激区,首先必须确定头部前后正中线和眉枕线两条标准定位线,在此基础上,才可分别确定出具体的刺激区域。头针刺激区的划分,一般需用软尺测量,熟练后可凭经验定位,对不同年龄、头型的病人,也可采用手指同身寸测量法,一般成人中指一寸约为2～2.5 cm。头针刺激区,划分确定较为严格,各刺激区临床主治病证针对性较强,在中医康复医疗中,必须一一掌握,正确运用。

头针疗法,在刺激区的选择方面,对单侧肢体病证,多选用病肢对侧刺激区;双侧肢体病变,选用双侧刺激区;内脏疾病及不易区分左右的病证,选择双侧刺激区。另外,除可选用与疾病相关的刺激区外,还可根据兼症配合选用其他刺激区,如下肢瘫痪,除

selection of the stimulation area corresponding to the disease. For example, the foot motor sensory area may be cooperatively selected for paralysis of lower limbs besides the selection of the motor area of lower limbs. Quick speed and a wide range are advisable to twirl the needle in scalp acupuncture (200 times per minute). When twirling and retaining the needle, let or help the patient move the limbs and enhance training. This helps to improve the therapeutic effects.

Scalp acupuncture therapy is applicable to the rehabilitation of cerebrogenic diseases such as hemiplegia, aphasia, facial distortion, tinnitus, numbness, vertigo and chorea; it also has better therapeutic effects on cardiovascular diseases, diseases of digestive system as well as many types of neuralgia and enuresis.

The head with hair is susceptible to infection, accordingly strict sterilization should be done during scalp acupuncture therapy; the therapy is not advisable for the patients with apoplexy; it is not applicable to the patients with accompanying high fever and heart failure, either. In addition, the stimulation of scalp acupuncture is more severe, so needling fainting should be particularly prevented. The scalp with rich blood vessels is subject to hemorrhage. When withdrawing the needle, press the punctured site with the cotton ball.

3.1.4 Moxibustion for health care

The moxibustion for health care mainly makes use of the heat of the ignited argyi wool to give the certain parts of the body the febrile stimulation. The stimulation exerts the effect by means of meridians, collaterals and acupoints to enhance health and prolong life.

选下肢运动区外,还可配足运感区等。头针捻针的速度宜快(每分钟200次左右),捻转幅度宜大。捻针及留针时,让患者(或帮助患者)活动肢体,加强锻炼,有助于提高疗效。

头针法主要适用于脑源性疾患康复,如半身不遂、失语、口眼歪斜、耳鸣、麻木、眩晕、舞蹈病等;此外,头针对治疗心血管疾病、消化系统疾病以及多种神经痛、遗尿等也有较好的疗效。

头部因长有头发,容易感染,故行头针应严格消毒。中风患者在急性期不宜使用;伴有高热、心力衰竭者,也不宜使用。此外,头针刺激量较大,尤应防止晕针,头皮血管丰富,容易出血,起针时要用棉球按压。

四、保健灸

保健灸,主要是借艾绒点燃后的热力,给人体一定部位以温热性刺激,通过经络腧穴的作用,以达到保健强身、益寿延年的目的。

3.1.4.1 Commonly-used moxibustion types for health care

Moxa is mostly used in moxibustion. Moxa is a pungent, warm-and hot-natured drug. After igniting the moxa, place it on the acupoint. The heat is persistent and penetrating. When the feeling of heat penetrates into the deep muscle, it can achieve the purposes of preventing and treating diseases by warming and dredging meridians and collaterals, promoting qi flow and blood circulation, strengthening primordial qi, the spleen and the stomach. Moxibustion is mainly divided into three types of moxibustion with moxa cones, moxibustion with moxa sticks and moxibustion with the warming needle according to different uses of moxibustion. The moxibustion methods can be classified into three kinds of direct moxibustion, indirect moxibustion, suspended moxibustion (Please refer to *Chinese Acupuncture and Moxibustion* of this series of books.

3.1.4.2 Moxibustion methods for health care

The acupoints are well selected according to the physique and the requirement of health preservation and rehabilitation. The ignited moxa stick or moxa cone is aimed at the acupoint to produce a feeling of mild heat, the degree of which is determined by a warm and cozy feeling as well as endurability.

Moxibustion usually lasts for 3 to 5 minutes, the longest one being ten to fifteen minutes. Short moxibustion is advisable to strengthen health and prevent diseases while long moxibustion may be used for treatment and rehabilitation; short moxibustion is advisable in the two seasons of spring and summer while long moxibustion is advisable in autumn and winter; short moxibustion is advisable on limbs and the chest while long moxibustion is advisable on the abdomen and back; short moxibustion is advis-

（一）灸法的种类

灸法一般多用艾灸。艾为辛温、阳热之药，点燃后，置于施灸穴位上，热持久而深入，温热感直透肌肉深层，从而达到温通经脉、行气活血、培补元气、健脾益胃、防病治病的目的。根据艾灸的不同用途，艾灸主要分为艾炷灸和艾条灸、温针灸三种，从灸的方法上分，又可分为直接灸、间接灸和悬灸三种（参见本丛书《中国针灸》）。

（二）保健灸的方法

根据体质及所需的养生、康复要求选好穴位，将点燃的艾条或艾炷对准穴位，使局部感到有温和的热力，以感觉温热舒适，并能耐受为度。

艾灸一般3～5分钟，最长至10～15分钟。健身、预防灸，时间宜短，治疗、康复，施灸时间可长；春、夏两季施灸时间宜短，秋、冬宜长；四肢、胸部时间宜短，腹、背部位宜长；老人、妇女、儿童施灸时间宜短，青壮年则时间可长。

able in old people, women and children while long moxibustion may be used in young people and people in their thirties to fifties.

The order for moxibustion is as follows: Moxibustion is generally applied to the upper part first, and then to the lower part; treat the back first, the abdomen second; the head first and the four extremities second.

Time was measured with the help of the size of the moxa cones and the number of the moxa cones in the ancient moxibustion. The moxa cone is made into the cone-shaped units of measurement by hand which are divided into three types of big cone, medium-sized cone and small cone. The big cone is like a broad bean, the medium-sized cone a soybean and the small cone a wheat grain. Every moxa cone burnt is called one zhuang (a moxa cone). The moxa cones are accordingly selected according to the site used for moxibustion and the state of physique. For instance, small number (roughly 3 to 5 moxa cones) is advisable on the distal ends of limbs while big moxa cones and more number (about 5 to 15 moxa cones) are advisable on the trunk and the proximal ends of limbs; more number of moxa cones is advisable for young people and people in their thirties to fifties while small number of moxa cones is advisable for old people and children.

Besides, pay attention to the contraindications of moxibustion, namely, moxibustion is contraindicated for sthenic heat syndromes, fever due to yin deficiency as well as on the abdomen and lumbosacral portion of pregnant women.

3.1.4.3 Commonly-used moxibustion points for health care

3.1.4.3.1 Zusanli (ST36)

Zusanli (ST36) is the H3-Sea acupoint of the stomach meridian. It has the actions of strengthening the spleen, regulating the stomach, promoting digestion and absorption, improving appetite, etc. and can prevent and treat diseases of enterogastric tract. Besides, it also tonifies renal essence, strengthens the tendons and bones, and has very good therapeutic effects on the prevention and treatment of dizziness, tinnitus, lassitude in the waist and knees, seminal emission and premature ejaculation due to deficiency of renal essence as well as ischias, etc. Modern studies show that moxibustion at Zusanli (ST36) can increase immunity of the organism, regulate gastrointestinal functions, and adjust favorably blood system, respiratory system and circulatory system, etc. The commonly-used moxibustion methods include suspended moxibustion with moxa sticks and scarring moxibustion with moxa cones.

3.1.4.3.2 Shenque (CV 8)

Shenque (CV 8) warms and strengthens the kidney yang, enhances the spleen and stomach in transportation. It is the important acupoint to warm yang and prevent collapse, and has the warming and strengthening effects on pain and cold of the abdomen, diarrhea, cool limbs, etc. due to insufficiency of yang and qi in old and weak people. The commonly-used moxibustion methods include moxibustion with ginger and moxibustion with salt.

3.1.4.3.3 Guanyuan (CV 4)

Guanyuan (CV 4), also called Dantian, is the place where the primordial qi of the whole body accumulates. It can warm the kidney, consolidate body resistance, supplement qi, recuperate depleted yang, regulate and dredge governor vessel (GV) and conception vessel (CV) and regulate qi flow and blood circulation. The acupoint is the important acupoint to preserve health and strengthen physique. It is also the commonly-used acupoint for the moxibustion for health care in old people. Prolonged

收,增进饮食等功能,能防治肠胃道疾病。此外尚能补益肾精、强健筋骨,对于肾精不足所致的头晕耳鸣、腰膝酸软、遗精早泄以及坐骨神经痛等均有很好的防治效果。现代研究表明,艾灸足三里能提高机体免疫力,调节胃肠功能,对血液、呼吸、循环等系统均有良性调整作用。常用灸法,如艾条悬起灸、艾炷瘢痕灸。

2. 神阙

功能温补元阳,健运脾胃,是温阳固脱的重要穴位,对于年老体弱、阳气不足、腹中冷痛、泄泻、四肢发凉等均有温补作用。常用灸法如隔姜灸、隔盐灸。

3. 关元

关元又称"丹田",为一身元气之所在。能温肾固本,补气回阳,通调冲任,理气和血,为全身养生保健、强壮体质的重要穴位,也是老年保健灸的常用穴位。长期艾灸本穴,可使真元之气充足,对于阳气不足,身体虚弱,怕冷乏力以及腹泻、阳痿、早泄等均有防治

moxibustion of this acupoint can make the primordial qi and kidney qi sufficient, and prevent and treat weakness, aversion to cold and fatigue due to deficiency of yang and qi as well as diarrhea, impotence, premature ejaculation, etc. The commonly-used moxibustion methods include moxibustion with ginger, moxibustion with the cake of Fuzi (*Radix Aconiti Praeparata*) and moxa roll moxibustion. The moxibustion is not advisable for pregnant women.

3.1.4.3.4 Qihai (CV 6)

Qihai (CV 6), also called Shangdantian, pertains to conception vessel below the navel. The acupoint, the sea of all types of qi, is the important acupoint to invigorate primordial qi, regulate qi activities generally and preserve health for health care. Prolonged moxibustion of this acupoint can supplement primordial qi and regulate qi activities. It cures diarrhea, impotence, seminal emission, irregular menstruation, etc. due to deficiency of renal qi and primordial qi, disorder of qi activities of lower energizer. The commonly-used moxibustion methods include moxa roll moxibustion, moxibustion with the moxa cone, moxibustion with ginger, moxibustion with the cake of Fuzi (*Radix Aconiti Praeparata*), etc.

3.1.4.3.5 Dazhui (GV 14)

Dazhui (GV 14), also called the sea of yang meridians, is the crossing acupoint of the three yang meridians of the hand and foot and governor vessel. It generally governs all types of yang qi of the body and is the important acupoint to invigorate yang qi and strengthen and preserve health. The acupoint can prevent various consumptive diseases, common cold, etc.; it can refresh the brain, relieve mental stress, improve intelligence and regulate cerebral functions, too. Modern researches discover that Dazhui (GV 14) effectively relieves inflammation,

作用。常用灸法，如隔姜灸、隔附子饼灸、艾条灸。孕妇不宜采用。

4. 气海

气海又名"上丹田"，属任脉，位于脐下，为诸气之海，是大补元气，总调气机，养生保健的重要穴位。常灸此穴，能培补元气，调理气机，对于真元之气不足，下焦气机失调所致的腹泻、阳痿、遗精、月经不调等均有调理作用。常用艾条灸、艾炷灸、隔姜灸、隔附子饼灸等灸法。

5. 大椎

大椎为手足三阳经和督脉的交会穴，又称"阳脉之海"，总督一身之阳气，为振奋阳气，强壮保健的重要穴位。能防治各种虚损和感冒等病证；还可清脑宁神，增强智力，调节大脑功能。现代研究发现，大椎有良好的消炎、退热、解痉、消除黄疸，预防流脑、流感，增强白细胞的作用。常用

abates fever, relieves spasm, eliminates jaundice, prevents epidemic encephalitis and influenza as well as increase white blood cells. The commonly-used moxibustion methods include moxa roll moxibustion and direct moxibustion with the moxa cone.

3.1.4.3.6 Fengmen (GB 12)

Fengmen (GB 12) has the actions of dispelling wind to relieve the exterior syndrome, dispersing the lung qi, clearing away heat, purging fire, etc. The acupoint can prevent and treat diseases of respiratory system such as common cold. It has good therapeutic effects on the prevention and treatment of furuncle, boils and swelling and subcutaneous ulcer, rhinitis, etc. The commonly-used moxibustion methods include moxa roll moxibustion, moxibustion with ginger and moxibustion with garlic.

3.1.4.3.7 Shenzhu (GV 12)

Shenzhu (GV 12) means the prop of the whole body. It is the important moxibustion point of health care for children. The point can activate yang, regulate and restore qi to treat injury and all pediatric diseases. Besides, Shenzhu (GV 12) can tonify the brain, relieve mental distress, promote cerebral development to improve intelligence, disperse the lung qi, increase resistance of the organism against diseases and prevent diseases of respiratory system. The commonly-used moxibustion methods include moxa roll moxibustion, moxibustion with moxa cone and moxibustion with ginger.

3.1.4.3.8 Gaohuang (BL 43)

Gaohuang (BL 43), one of the acupoints of health preservation and health care in the ancient times, can restore health from consumptive diseases, disperse the lung qi, activate yang, prevent common cold and tuberculosis as well as strengthen physique. The commonly-used moxibustion methods include moxa roll moxibustion, moxibus-

灸法,如艾条灸、艾炷直接灸。

6. 风门

风门有疏风解表、宣通肺气、清热泻火等作用,能防治感冒等呼吸系统疾病,对防治疔疮疖肿、痈疽、鼻炎等也有良效。常用灸法,如艾条灸、隔姜灸、隔蒜灸。

7. 身柱

身柱含有全身支柱的意思,是小儿保健灸的重要穴位。能通阳理气,补益虚损,通治小儿科百病。身柱还能健脑宁神,促进大脑发育,增进智力,宣通肺气,提高机体的抗病能力,防止呼吸系统疾病的发生。常用灸法,如艾条灸、艾炷灸、隔姜灸。

8. 膏肓

是古代常用的养生保健穴之一。能补益虚损,宣肺通阳,预防感冒、结核,增强体质。常用灸法为艾条灸、艾炷灸、隔姜灸。

tion with the moxa cone and moxibustion with ginger.

3.1.4.3.9　Yongquan (KI 1)

Yongquan(KI 1), the first acupoints of kidney meridian, can tonify renal essence and qi, strengthen the functional activities of viscera, enhance health and delay ageing. As one of the commonly-used acupoints of health care for old people, it is also one of the main acupoints for emergency treatment simultaneously. It has the actions of promoting resuscitation, refreshing the brain, elevating blood pressure for shock, prostration syndrome, drop of blood pressure, heatstroke, etc. It has specific therapeutic effects on nausea and vomiting as well. The commonly-used moxibustion methods include moxibustion with ginger and direct moxibustion with the moxa cone.

3.1.4.3.10　Quchi (LI 11)

The ancients believed that Quchi(LI 11) is "an ocular moxibustion point" which can make eyes sharp, improve sight and has better therapeutic effects on ocular diseases such as palpebral inflammation and conjunctivitis. Quchi (LI 11) is also the He-Sea acupoint of the large intestine meridian. It can regulate enterogastric functions, prevent and treat intestinal diseases such as diarrhea and constipation. In addition, it also has the actions of unblocking away heat, dispelling wind, unblocking and activating meridians and collaterals, etc. as well as certain therapeutic effects on various types of inflammatory fever, common cold and arthritis of upper limbs. The commonly-used moxibustion methods include moxa roll moxibustion, direct moxibustion with the moxa cone and moxibustion with ginger.

3.1.4.3.11　Zhongwan (CV 12)

Zhongwan(CV 12) is located on the abdomen and is the Front-Mu acupoint of the stomach. It can regulate gastrointestinal functions, promote digestion and absorption,

9. 涌泉

涌泉是肾经的第一个穴位，能滋补肾之精气，增强脏腑功能活动，强身抗衰，为老年人保健常用穴位之一。同时也是急救的主要穴位，对于休克虚脱、血压下降、中暑等均有开窍醒脑、复苏升压的作用，对恶心呕吐亦有特效。常用灸法为隔姜灸、艾炷直接灸。

10. 曲池

古人认为曲池是"目灸"穴，可使眼睛明亮，视力提高，对眼睑炎、结膜炎等眼疾疗效较好。曲池又为大肠经的合穴，能调节肠胃功能，防治腹泻、便秘等肠腑疾患。此外，还有清热祛风、通经活络等作用，对于各种炎性发热、感冒及上肢关节炎有一定的疗效。常用灸法，如艾条灸、艾炷直接灸、隔姜灸。

11. 中脘

中脘位于胃脘部，为胃的募穴，能调理胃肠功能，促进消化吸收，对胃脘不适，食欲

thus has health care functions for discomforts of stomach, poor appetite, gastrointestinal hypofunctions, etc. The commonly-used moxibustion methods include direct moxibustion with the moxa cone, moxa roll moxibustion, moxibustion with ginger, etc.

3.1.4.3.12　Pishu (BL 20)

Pishu (BL 20), the Back-Shu acupoint of the spleen, can strengthen the spleen and stomach in transportation, nourish qi and blood and promote digestion. It well regulates digestive system and blood system. The commonly-used moxibustion methods include moxa roll moxibustion, direct moxibustion with the moxa cone and moxibustion with ginger.

3.1.4.3.13　Shenshu (BL 23)

Shenshu (BL 23), the Back-Shu acupoint of the kidney, can tonify renal essence, warm and activate the kidney yang, strengthen health and the waist and delay ageing. It is the commonly-used acupoint for health care and has better therapeutic effects on diseases of genitourinary system such as impotence and seminal emission. The commonly-used moxibustion methods include moxa roll moxibustion, moxibustion with the warming needle, direct moxibustion with the moxa cone and moxibustion with ginger.

3.1.4.3.14　Sanyinjiao (SP 6)

Sanyinjiao (SP 6), the acupoint of the spleen meridians and the crossing acupoint of the three yin meridians of the foot, can strengthen the spleen, regulate the stomach, eliminate dampness, regulate splenogastric functions and enhance digestion. It is one of the commonly-used health care acupoints for diseases of digestive system. Moreover, it links with the three yin meridians of the foot. Therefore, it can tonify the liver, kidney, qi and blood, unblock and activate meridians. The acupoint has

不振，胃肠功能低下等有保健作用。常用灸法，如艾炷直接灸、艾条灸、隔姜灸等。

12. 脾俞

脾俞为脾的腧穴，能健运脾胃，补养气血，促进消化，对消化系统和血液系统有很好的调整作用。常用灸法，如艾条灸、艾炷直接灸、隔姜灸。

13. 肾俞

肾俞为肾的俞穴。能补益肾精，温通元阳，强身壮腰，延缓衰老，是常用的保健穴位，对于阳痿、遗精等泌尿生殖系统的疾病有较好的疗效。常用灸法，如艾条灸、温针灸法、艾炷直接灸、隔姜灸。

14. 三阴交

三阴交是脾经和足三阴经的会穴，能健脾和胃化湿，调节脾胃功能，增强消化，是消化系统疾病常用的保健穴位之一。而且它与足三阴经相通，因此能调补肝肾气血，舒通经脉，对妇科疾病、泌尿生殖系统疾病等均有良效。常用灸法，如艾条灸、艾炷灸。

good therapeutic effects on gynecological diseases, diseases of genitourinary system, etc. The commonly-used moxibustion methods include moxa roll moxibustion and moxibustion with the moxa cone.

3.1.4.3.15 Yanglingquan (GB 34)

Yanglingquan (GB 34), the influential acupoint of tendons, is a commonly-used health care acupoint. It is also the He-Sea acupoint of gallbladder meridian and can regulate and improve the functions of the liver and gallbladder and promote the excretion of bile to help digestion and absorption. The acupoint has very good therapeutic effects on diseases of system of the liver and gallbladder. Besides, it is also the specific acupoint to regulate the stomach and inhibit gastric acid. The acupoint has better therapeutic effects for patients with nausea and acid regurgitation. The commonly-used moxibustion methods include moxa roll moxibustion and direct moxibustion with the moxa cone.

3.1.4.3.16 Mingmen (GV 4)

Mingmen (GV 4), the gate of life, is the important acupoint to nourish the kidney, strengthen yang and preserve health. It has very good therapeutic effects on seminal emission, impotence, premature ejaculation, leukorrhea, diarrhea, cold limbs, cold of abdomen, etc. due to qi deficiency of the kidney and insufficiency of the kidney yang. The commonly-used moxibustion methods include moxa roll moxibustion, direct moxibustion with the moxa cone, moxibustion with ginger and moxibustion with the cake of Fuzi (*Radix Aconiti Praeparata*).

3.1.4.3.17 Hegu (LI 4)

Hegu (LI 4), an important acupoint to prevent and treat diseases of the head, face and five sense organs, has good therapeutic effects on many diseases of five sense organs. It also has a very good action of relieving pain and is

15. 阳陵泉

阳陵泉为筋会,是强壮筋骨、舒通经脉的常用保健穴,又为胆经的合穴,可调节和改善肝胆功能,促进胆汁的排泄,有利于消化吸收,对肝胆系统疾病有良好的效果。还是和胃制酸的特效穴,对恶心、口中泛酸者有较好的作用。常用灸法,如艾条灸、艾炷直接灸。

16. 命门

命门是"生命之门",是滋肾壮阳,养生保健的重要穴位,对于肾气不足,肾阳虚衰引起的遗精、阳痿、早泄、带下、泄泻、肢冷腹寒等有很好的疗效。常用灸法,如艾条灸、艾炷直接灸、隔姜灸、隔附子饼灸。

17. 合谷

合谷是防治头面五官疾病的重要穴位,对五官科许多病证均有良效。还有良好的镇痛作用,是治疗各种痛证的首

the first acupoint selection to treat various painful diseases. Besides, it can expel wind to relieve the exterior syndrome, disperse the lung qi and prevent common cold. The commonly-used moxibustion methods include moxa roll moxibustion, direct moxibustion with the moxa cone, moxibustion with ginger and moxibustion with garlic.

3.1.4.4 Commonly-used moxibustion methods for health care

3.1.4.4.1 Moxibustion methods of regulating the spleen and kidney

Acupoint selection: Zusanli (ST 36), Pishu (BL 20), Weishu (BL 21), Zhongwan (CV 12) and Tianshu (ST 25). The commonly-used moxibustion methods include moxa roll moxibustion and moxibustion with ginger. One to two acupoints are selected each time for alternate use.

3.1.4.4.2 Moxibustion methods of preventing common cold

Acupoint selection: Fengmen (BL 12), Feishu (BL 13), Dazhui (GV 14), Hegu (LI 4), Zusanli (ST 36) and Danzhong (CV 17). The commonly-used moxibustion methods include moxa roll moxibustion, moxibustion with the mild moxibustion instrument, direct moxibustion with the moxa cone, crude herb moxibustion and electrothermal moxibustion.

3.1.4.4.3 Moxibustion methods of nourishing the heart to calm the mind

Acupoint selection: Neiguan (PC 6), Xinshu (BL 15), Shenmen (HT 7), Zusanli (ST 36), Danzhong (CV 17) and Juque (CV 14). The commonly-used moxibustion methods include suspended moxibustion with the moxa stick, direct moxibustion with the moxa cone, moxibustion with the mild moxibustion instrument and moxa cone moxibustion with ginger.

选穴位；并能祛风解表,宣通肺气,防治感冒。灸法,如艾条灸、艾炷直接灸、隔姜灸、隔蒜灸。

（四）常用保健灸法

1. 调和脾胃灸法

取穴：足三里、脾俞、胃俞、中脘、天枢。常用灸法,如艾条灸、隔姜灸。每次选1~2个穴位,交替进行。

2. 预防感冒灸法

取穴：风门、肺俞、大椎、合谷、足三里、膻中。常用灸法为艾条灸、温灸器灸、艾炷直接灸、天灸、电热灸。

3. 养心安神灸法

取穴：内关、心俞、神门、足三里、膻中、巨阙。常用灸法,如艾条悬起灸、艾炷直接灸、温灸器灸、艾炷隔姜灸。

3.1.4.4.4 Moxibustion methods of regulating emotions

Acupoint selection: Yanglingquan (GB 34), Zhangmen (LR 13), Qimen (LR 14), Ganshu (BL 18), Sanyinjiao (SP 6), Zhigou (TE 6) and Danzhong (CV 17). The commonly-used moxibustion methods include moxa roll moxibustion and direct moxibustion with the moxa cone.

3.1.4.4.5 Moxibustion methods of tonifying the brain to benefit intelligence

Acupoint selection: Baihui (GV 20), Taiyang (EX-HN 5), Fengchi (GB 20), Fengfu (GV 16) and Dazhui (GV 14); the adjunct acupoints of Hegu (LI 4) and Zusanli (ST 36). The moxibustion methods include moxa roll moxibustion, direct moxibustion with the moxa cone and electrothermal moxibustion.

3.1.4.4.6 Moxibustion methods of tonifying the kidney and strengthening the body

Acupoint selection: Shenshu (BL 23), Taixi (KI 3), Mingmen (GV 4), Guanyuan (CV 4), Yongquan (KI 1), Sanyinjiao (SP 6), Gaohuang (BL 43) and Guanyuanshu (BL 26). The moxibustion methods include moxa roll moxibustion, direct moxibustion with the moxa cone, moxibustion with ginger, moxibustion with salt and moxibustion with Fuzi (Radix Aconiti Praeparata) cake.

3.1.4.4.7 Moxibustion methods of infantile health care

Shenzhu (GV 12) and Tianshu (ST 25) are selected to strengthen the body and preserve health; Zhongwan (CV 12), Pishu (BL 20), Shenque (CV 8) and Tianshu (ST 25) are selected to strengthen the spleen and regulate the stomach; Fengmen (BL 12), Feishu (BL13), Shenzhu (GV 12), Dazhui (GV 14) and Gaohuang (BL 43) are selected to tonify the lung and supplement qi; Dazhui (GV 14), Shenzhu (GV 12) and Gaohuang (BL

4. 调畅情志灸法

取穴：阳陵泉、章门、期门、肝俞、三阴交、支沟、膻中。灸法为艾条灸、艾炷直接灸。

5. 健脑益智灸法

取穴：百会、太阳、风池、风府、大椎，配穴合谷、足三里。灸法为艾条灸、艾炷直接灸和电热灸。

6. 补肾强身灸法

取穴：肾俞、太溪、命门、关元、涌泉、三阴交、膏肓、关元俞。灸法为艾条灸、艾炷直接灸、隔姜灸、隔盐灸、隔附子饼灸。

7. 小儿保健灸法

强身保健取身柱、天枢穴，健脾和胃取中脘、脾俞、神阙、天枢穴，补肺益气取风门、肺俞、身柱、大椎、膏肓穴，健脑益智取大椎、身柱、膏肓穴。灸法如艾条灸、艾炷直接灸、隔姜灸、隔蒜灸、葱白灸。

43) are selected to tonify the brain and benefit intelligence. The moxibustion methods include moxa roll moxibustion, direct moxibustion with the moxa cone, moxibustion with ginger, moxibustion with garlic and moxibustion with scallion stalk.

3.1.4.4.8 Moxibustion methods of health care for young people

Acupoint selection: Guanyuan (GV 4), Shenshu (BL 23) and Sanyinjiao (SP 6). For the patients with weak physique and susceptibility to common cold, Fengmen (BL 12) and Feishu (BL 13) are added. The moxibustion methods include moxa roll moxibustion, direct moxibustion with the moxa cone, moxibustion with the mild moxibustion instrument and moxibustion with garlic.

3.1.4.4.9 Moxibustion methods of health care for middle-aged and old people

Acupoint selection: Zusanli (ST 36), Qihai (CV 6), Sanyinjiao (SP 6), Shenshu (BL 23) and Guanyuan (GV 4). The moxibustion methods include moxa roll moxibustion, moxibustion with the mild moxibustion instrument and moxa cone moxibustion with ginger.

3.2 Massage therapy

Massage (called "an mo" in ancient times) is a rehabilitation method in which different manipulations are applied on the certain parts of the patient's body to dredge meridians and regulate qi and blood for the promotion of somatopsychic health.

3.2.1 The applying principles of massage

3.2.1.1 Proceeding in a proper order

In general, apply the manipulation of massage from the upper to the lower, from the internal to the external, from the proximal to the distal, from the shoulder to the wrist in the case of massaging upper limbs, from the shoulder to the waist in the case of massaging the back and from the midline to the two sides in the case of parting-pushing, etc.

3.2.1.2 Combination of high speed with low speed

When applying the manipulation or changing the manipulation during the treatment, follow the manipulation speed principle of being "low-high-low". For example, apply the pulling and shaking manipulations slowly at the beginning for the patients with inflammation around the shoulder joints. When the soft tissues around the shoulder joints get relaxed, accelerate the manipulation gradually. Then, the manipulation slows down again till the end.

3.2.1.3 Alternation of the forceful manipulation and mild manipulation

When applying one manipulation or different manipulations, the forceful one is "gang" (forceful) while the mild and swift one is "rou" (mild). The alternation of the forceful manipulation and mild manipulation means that the principle of being "mild-forceful-mild" should be followed in all the selection of many manipulations and the application of one manipulation when massage is used in treatment. For example, swift and mild kneading and pushing manipulations should be applied at the beginning and in the end while forceful kneading, pressing and pulling manipulations are used amidst the process of curing the injury of femoral adductor muscle. The force shifts from mild one to heavy one, then from heavy one to mild one.

As for the commonly-used massage methods and their application, please refer to *Chinese Tuina* (*Massage*) of this series of book.

远,如上肢应由肩至腕;背部应由肩背至腰部;分推法应由中线推向两侧等。

2. 快慢结合

在施以推拿手法或在治疗过程中变换手法时,操作速度应遵循"慢—快—慢"的原则。如对肩关节周围炎患者,在进行牵抖时,开始速度应慢,待肩关节周围软组织基本松弛后,再逐渐加快,然后再减慢速度至结束。

3. 刚柔相济

同一种手法或不同手法之间,强劲有力者为"刚",柔和轻快者为"柔"。刚柔相济,即要求在施行推拿治疗时,多种手法的选择及同一种手法的运用顺序上,均应按"柔—刚—柔"的原则进行。如对股内收肌损伤,开始和结束应用轻快柔和的揉、推法,中间用强有力的揉、按、推法。力量由轻到重,然后再由重到轻。

推拿常用手法及其应用,参见本丛书《中国推拿》。

3.2.2 Manipulations of self-massage and their application

The manipulations of self massage refer to the fact that the patient himself massages a certain part of the body surface with certain manipulations to strengthen the body, eliminate diseases and prolong life. Almost all parts of the body can be used for self massage except the back due to its inconvenience.

3.2.2.1 Massage of the head and face

3.2.2.1.1 Kneading-pressing Jingming (BL 1)
Press the two sides of Jingming (BL 1) respectively with the tips of the thumb and index finger for 20 times to 30 times. It is applicable to blurred vision, near-sightedness and many other diseases.

3.2.2.1.2 kneading-pressing Yintang (EX-HN 3)
knead and press Yintang (EX-HN 3) with the whorled surface of the thumb for 20 to 30 times. It is applicable to headache, vertigo, etc.

3.2.2.1.3 Pushing the forehead on either side
Close up two to five fingers of both hands and place these fingers on Yintang (EX-HN 3). Push outwards along the two eyebrows respectively to reach Taiyang (EX-HN 5) for three to five times. Then, push vertically and upwards along Yintang (EX-HN 5) and gradually push outwards on either side to reach the hairline. Afterwards, push downwards gradually on either side to reach the two eyebrows. It is applicable to headache, head distension, vertigo, insomnia, etc.

3.2.2.1.4 Kneading-pressing Baihui (GV 20)
Knead Baihui (GV 20) forwards with the middle finger or the palmar side of the index finger from gently to forcefully step by step for 20 to 30 times. It is applicable to visceroptosis, proctoptosis, vertigo, headache, tinnitus, in-

二、自我推拿手法及其运用

自我推拿法，是患者本人运用某些简单的手法，在体表一定部位进行推拿，以强身健体、祛病延年的一种方法。除背部稍有不便外，几乎全身都可进行自我推拿。

1. 头面部

（1）揉按睛明穴 以拇、食两指尖分别按两侧睛明穴20～30次。用于治疗视物模糊、近视以及其他多种眼疾。

（2）揉按印堂穴 以拇指罗纹面揉按印堂穴20～30次，可用于治疗头痛、眩晕等病证。

（3）分推前额 两手二至五指并拢附于印堂穴，沿两眉毛向外分推到太阳穴3～5次，然后沿着印堂穴垂直向上逐次升高向外分推，直至前发际下，之后再逐次向下分推，到两眉处。用于头痛、头胀、眩晕、失眠等。

（4）揉按百会穴 用中指或食指指腹由轻渐重向前揉百会穴20～30次。用于内脏下垂、脱肛、眩晕、头痛、耳鸣、失眠等病证。

somnia, etc.

3.2.2.2 Massage of upper limbs

3.2.2.2.1 Rubbing the shoulder Press and knead Jianyu (LI 15) forcefully with the whorled surface of one middle finger until soreness and distension occur. It is applicable to periarthritis of shoulder, rheumatalgia, and paralysis of upper limbs, etc.

3.2.2.2.2 Pressing-kneading around the elbow joint Alternately press and knead Quchi (LI 11), Shousanli (LI 10), Chize (LU 5), Quze (PC 3), etc. with the whorled surface of one thumb until local soreness and distension occur. It is applicable to bronchial asthma, dry and sore throat, pain of the elbow and arm, numbness, etc.

3.2.2.2.3 Pressing-kneading Hegu (LI 4) Press the contralateral Hegu (LI 4) with one thumb and press the corresponding site of the palm surface with the index finger from gently to forcefully for 20 to 30 times. It is applicable to headache, toothache, sore throat, ocular pain, facial paralysis, abdominalgia, diarrhea, constipation as well as pain of upper limbs, numbness, spasm of the finger, etc.

3.2.2.3 Massage of lower limbs

3.2.2.3.1 Digitally pressing Huantiao (GB 30) Digitally press the homolateral Huantiao (GB 30) with the first finger joint of the thumb or the thumb tip for 20 to 60 times. It is applicable to rheumatic arthralgia, sciatica, paralysis of lower limbs, etc.

3.2.2.3.2 Pressing-kneading Zusanli (ST 36) Press the homolateral Zusanli (ST 36) with the thumb, with the other four fingers keeping close to the back of the leg. Press and knead Zusanli (ST 36) outwards for 20 to 40 times. It is applicable to gastralgia, vomiting, abdominal distension, dysphagia, diarrhea, insomnia, dizziness,

2. 上肢

（1）擦肩 以一手中指罗纹面用力按揉肩髃，酸胀为宜。用于肩周炎、肩臂风湿痛、上肢瘫痪等。

（2）按揉肘关节周围 以一手拇指罗纹面，在曲池、手三里、尺泽、曲泽等穴位处交替按揉，以局部出现酸胀为宜。用于支气管哮喘、咽喉干痛、腹痛肠鸣、肘臂痛、麻痹不仁等。

（3）按揉合谷穴 一手拇指按于对侧合谷穴，食指按于掌面相对部位，由轻至重揉按 20～30 次，可用于头痛、牙痛、咽痛、目痛、面神经麻痹、腹痛腹泻、便秘以及上肢疼痛、麻木、手指痉挛等。

3. 下肢

（1）点按环跳穴 以拇指第一指关节，或用拇指尖点按同侧环跳穴 20～60 次。用于风湿痹痛、坐骨神经痛、下肢瘫痪等。

（2）按揉足三里穴 以拇指按同侧足三里穴，其余四指附于小腿后，向外按揉 20～40 次。用于胃痛、呕吐、腹胀、噎膈、泄泻、失眠、头晕、下肢萎软无力、瘫痪等。

flaccidity of lower limbs, paralysis, etc.

3.2.2.3.3 Rubbing Yongquan (KI 1) Keep one minor thenar eminance close to Yongquan (KI 1) of the sole and rub the acupoint rapidly and forcefully until the site is hot. Rub the two feet alternately. The method is applicable to pain of vertex, vertigo, sore throat, aphasia, insomnia, and pain of the sole, etc.

3.2.2.4 Massage of the waist

Pressing and kneading Yaoyan (EX-B7): Clench the fists tightly and press Yaoyan (EX-B 7) with the metacarpophalangeal articulations of the thumb to rotate, press and knead forcefully until local soreness and distension occur. It is applicable to aching pain of the waist, inflexible movement, diarrhea, etc.

3.2.2.5 Massage of the chest and abdomen

3.2.2.5.1 Scrubbing the chest Keep the major thenar eminance or the palm close to Zhongwan (CV 12) and scrub it forcefully. Its application is the same as the above one.

3.2.2.5.2 Kneading Zhongwan (CV 12) Keep the major thenar eminance or the palm close to Zhongwan (CV 12) and knead it forcefully and clockwise for about two to five minutes. It is applicable to epigastric discomfort, indigestion, abdominalgia, diarrhea, etc.

3.3 Therapies with traditional Chinese drugs

Rehabilitation with traditional Chinese drugs is a method to promote the somatopsychic health of patients by regulating them with selected drugs according to their different states of diseases under the guidance of TCM theories such as the concept of the organism as a whole, the concept of differentiating syndrome to decide treatment as

（3）擦涌泉穴　用一手小鱼际紧贴足心涌泉穴，快速用力擦，以发热为度，两足交替。用于头顶痛、眩晕、咽喉痛、失音、失眠、足心痛等。

4. 腰部

按揉腰眼　两手握拳，用拇指指掌关节紧按腰眼，旋转用力按揉，以局部出现酸胀为宜。用于腰酸腰痛、活动不灵、腹泻等。

5. 胸腹部

（1）擦胸　以手大鱼际或手掌紧贴中脘穴，用力揉和。应用同上。

（2）揉中脘穴　以一手大鱼际或手掌紧贴中脘穴，用力揉和，作顺时针方向旋转揉动，约2～5分钟，用于胃脘不适、消化不良、腹痛腹泻等。

第三节　中药疗法

药物康复法，是以中医整体观、辨证观以及中药方剂理论为指导，针对患者疾病的不同，有选择地运用药物进行调整，从而促使患者身心康复的一种方法。药物养生、康复法

well as the theory of traditional Chinese drugs and prescriptions. Life cultivation and rehabilitation with traditional Chinese drugs can be divided into two main types: oral medication and external treatment.

3.3.1 Therapies with oral medications

The characteristics of the application of oral medication in TCM life cultivation and rehabilitation are as follows.

3.3.1.1 Curing deficiency and removing stagnation

Curing deficiency and removing phlegm stagnation and blood stasis are the two major therapeutic methods of rehabilitation with oral medication. The differences among qi, blood, yin and yang should be differentiated in curing deficiency. For the patients with qi deficiency, Sijunzi Decoction (Decoction of Four Noble Drugs), Buzhong Yiqi Decoction (Decoction for Strengthening the Middle Energizer and Supplementing Qi), etc. may be selected and modified according to the symptoms; for the patients with blood deficiency, Siwu Decoction (Decoction of Four Ingredients), Guipi Decoction (Decoction for Invigorating the Spleen and Nourishing the Heart), etc. are accordingly modified; for the patients with deficiency of both qi and blood, qi and blood should be both tonified, and Bazhen Decoction (Decoction of Eight Precious Ingredients), prescriptions such as Renshen Yangrong Pill (Ginseng Pill for Nourishing the Face) and the like may be selected; for the patients with deficiency of body fluids, Maimendong Decoction (Ophiopogon Decoction), and Yangyin Qingfei Decoction (Decoction for Nourishing Yin and Clearing away Heat from the Lung), etc. are accordingly selected; for the patients with yin deficiency, prescriptions such as Liuwei Dihuang Bolus (Six-Ingredient

可分内服法和外治法两大类。

一、内服法

中药内服法在中医养生、康复医疗中的运用特点如下。

1. 补虚疏郁

补虚损、祛痰瘀是药物内服养生、康复法的两大治法。补虚损,当辨别气血阴阳的不同。气虚者,可选四君子汤、补中益气汤等随证加减;血虚者,可在四物汤、归脾汤等基础上增损;若气血皆虚,则应气血双补,选方如八珍汤、人参养荣丸之类;津液亏虚者,可酌情选用麦门冬汤、养阴清肺汤等;阴虚者,可用六味地黄丸、大补阴丸等方剂化裁;阳虚者,则可选用金匮肾气丸、右归丸之类。疏郁滞,除了应辨别痰阻、血瘀的不同,分别给予处理之外,还应注意痰瘀的相互夹杂为患,不失时机地作相应的治疗。另外,不论是补虚损还是疏郁滞,分析判断疾病所处的部位,掌握"虚"、"郁"的脏腑经络所属,也极为重要。只有在明确病因、病性、病位的基础上,才有

Bolus with Rehmanni) and Dabuyin Bolus (Bolus for Replenishing Yin) may be selected and modified; for the patients with yang deficiency, Jingui Shenqi Bolus (Bolus for Tonifying the kidney Qi), Yougui Bolus (Bolus for Strengthening the Kidney Yang) and the like may be selected. The patients with obstruction should be differently treated based on differentiating the differences between phlegm stagnation and blood stasis. Besides, timely and corresponding treatment should be given to the patients by paying attention to the pathogenic phlegm stagnation intermingled with blood stasis. Moreover, it is of vital importance to analyze and determine the location of the disease, determine the viscera, meridians and collaterals which deficiency and stagnation pertain to no matter whether the doctor is to cure deficiency or to remove stagnation. Only when the cause, nature and location of the disease are determined can satisfactory therapeutic effects be achieved. The indications of rehabilitation are marked by long course and slow development of disease. Therefore, it is generally hard to gain quick therapeutic effects. Moreover, prolonged administration of decoction of drugs makes the patients bored and it is also inconvenient in many aspects. Accordingly, rehabilitation with oral medication should be various in the selection of dosage forms. For instance, pill, powder, plaster, oral liquid, etc. all can be accordingly selected.

3.3.1.2 Combination of treatment with recuperation

The nourishment in the principle of combination of treatment with recuperation in rehabilitation with oral medication has two senses: the first one means that during the treatment, attention should always be paid to curing deficiency and protecting healthy qi; the second one denotes that importance should be attached to the recuperation in daily life as well. TCM pays full attention to the important roles which pathogenic factors play in the occurrence and development of diseases. Meanwhile, it emphasizes even more the leading role of healthy qi in the struggle between the organism and diseases. Basically speaking, all the rehabilitation measures in TCM are to strengthen healthy qi, the self regulatory ability, adaptive capacity and resistance against diseases of the organism. Therefore, the principle of combination of treatment with recuperation should be always followed during rehabilitation. For patients with weakness due to prolonged diseases, it is natural to supplement qi mainly in the presence of deficiency of qi, blood and body fluids. Pathogenic factors should be eliminated for the patients with marked phlegm stagnation and blood stasis, or for the patients with additional new diseases besides the old ones, while healthy qi should be strengthened at the same time. In this case, the patients should not ignore the weakness of the body only to eradicate pathogenic factors rashly. It is not enough to aim at treatment with oral medication only in TCM rehabilitation. In order to achieve good rehabilitation effects, it is also of vital importance for the doctors to ask the patients to pay attention to their recuperation in daily life. The formation of numerous TCM rehabilitation indications is closely related to the daily life habits. It is difficult to recover from diseases if attention is not paid to the correction of unfavorable life habits for the organism and the elimination of harmful factors while the dependence is only on treatment with oral medication.

3.3.1.3 Following the therapeutic methods and prescriptions

The indications of TCM rehabilitation have the characteristic of longer course of disease in most cases. Besides, there are no great changes in the pathogenesis

气在疾病发生和发展过程中的重要作用的同时,更加强调正气在机体与疾病抗争过程中的主导作用。从根本上看,中医养生、康复医疗的一切措施,就是以扶养正气,增强机体的自我调节能力、适应能力和抗病能力为目的的,所以,面对久病体虚的康复适应证患者,在用药过程中,必须始终遵循治养结合的原则。对于气血津液亏虚者,自然要以补益为主;对于痰阻血瘀较明显,或在原有病患基础上又有新感者,也应在扶邪的同时,注意顾护正气,切不可置素体亏虚于不顾,只图祛邪,妄加攻伐。在中医康复医疗中,仅仅着眼于药物治疗是不够的,为了获得好的康复效果,让患者注意在日常生活中进行调养也十分重要。众多中医康复适应证的形成,与日常生活习惯密切相关,如果不注意调整于机体不利的生活习惯,消除有害因素,只依赖于药物治疗,疾病就难以得到康复。

3. 守法守方

中医康复适应证,多有病程较长的特点,而且在较长时间内,其病机变化不大,基本

while the basic types of syndromes are relatively stable. Thus, the principle of no changes in syndromes, no changes in therapeutic methods should be generally followed as long as the syndrome differentiation is precise during rehabilitation with oral medication. The therapeutic methods and prescriptions should be followed and the drug actions patiently waited for. If the therapeutic methods and prescriptions are changed as soon as no therapeutic effects can be seen, the therapeutic steps will be disturbed, and more sufferings and burdens will be added to the patients. The therapeutic methods should be meticulously established and prescriptions carefully selected. Meanwhile, both the patients and doctors should wait patiently without the desire for quick success. In these circumstances, good therapeutic effects can be achieved in the patients with rehabilitation indications. This has been proved correct by practice. Nevertheless, no satisfactory therapeutic effects can be mostly achieved in the patients with frequent changes in the prescriptions. In addition, careful observation is needed to synthesize the local and general pathological changes. On the one hand, attention should be paid to the discovery and analysis of the ordinary improvement of local symptoms to enhance the confidence in treatment. On the other hand, it is necessary to prepare mentally for the protracted and complex nature of the diseases. The doctors should not be satisfied with the remission of local symptoms to ignore the analysis and judgment of the whole development of the disease.

3.3.2 Life cultivation and rehabilitation with external therapy

3.3.2.1 Fumigating and steaming therapy

This means steaming the patient's body with the steam produced by boiling certain traditional Chinese

证型相对稳定。所以,在施行药物内服进行康复治疗时,只要辨证准确,遣方用药得当,一般应遵循证不变,法亦不变的原则,守法守方,耐心等待药效的发挥,切不可一见疗效不显,就变法更方,不仅打乱了治疗的步骤,而且给患者带来不必要的痛苦和负担。实践证明,对于康复适应证患者,只要精心立法选方,静守缓图,多能取得好的效果,而朝三暮四,随手更方者,疗效多不理想。另外,还必须细心观察,综合分析局部和整体的病理变化,既要注意发现和分析一般性的局部症状的改善,增强治疗的信心;又要对疾病的长期性和复杂性做到心里有数,不能因满足于局部症状的缓解而忽视对整个病势趋向的分析判断。

二、外治法

1. 熏蒸法

利用中药加水煎煮沸腾后产生的蒸气,熏蒸病人肌

drugs so as to promote his recovery from a disease. This therapy can not only be performed on a specially-made therapeutic bed, but also in a self-designed vessel according to the differences of the specific state of disease, location of disease, conditions, etc. In general, put the prepared traditional Chinese drugs into a gauze bag and bind it up at first. Then, place the bag into the vessel with the drugs and add a proper amount of water to the vessel. Next, decoct the drugs until the water boils for about 20 minutes. At this time, the drugs can be applied, once or twice a day, 30 minutes a time. It is proper that the steam has enough warm sensation but does not give rise to scald and burn.

The prescriptions may be accordingly selected for fumigating therapy according to the difference of syndromes. For example, the prescriptions for promoting blood circulation to remove blood stasis may be selected for the patients with meridional blood stasis; the prescriptions for warming meridians to dispel cold, removing dampness and stagnation may be selected for the patients with cold, dampness and stagnation, etc. The theory of selecting the prescription according to syndrome differentiation is identical to that of rehabilitation with oral medication. In sum, fumigating and steaming therapy with both the actions of heat and the effects of drugs has the functions of dredging sweat pores, removing toxic substances, checking itching, regulating qi and blood, removing blood stasis, relieving swelling, warming meridians to dispel cold, removing arthralgia, checking pain, etc. It can be applicable to the rehabilitation of various intractable skin diseases, rheumatic arthritis, headache, flaccidity syndrome, paralysis as well as traumatic pain of tendons, bones and muscles, etc.

Attention should be paid to the fact that the site

肤，以促使病体康复的方法，称为"熏蒸法"。其既可在特制的治疗床上进行，也可根据具体病情、病位、条件等的不同，自行设计器皿。一般先将配制的中药装入纱布袋内扎好，放入贮药器皿中，加适量水煎煮至沸，20分钟左右后即可开始使用。每日1～2次，每次30分钟。以既有较强的温热感而又不至烫伤、烧伤为度。

熏蒸法所用方药，可根据病证的不同酌情选用。如经脉瘀滞者，可选具有活血化瘀功效的方剂；寒湿痹阻者，可选温经散寒，除湿通痹类方剂等。其辨证立法，依法处方之理，与药物内服法相同。总之，熏蒸法通过温热和药气两方面的作用，具有疏通毛窍、解毒止痒、调畅气血、化瘀消肿、温经散寒、除痹止痛等功效，可用于各种皮肤顽疾、风湿痹痛、头痛、痿证、瘫证以及外伤性筋骨肌肉酸痛等病证的康复治疗。

使用熏蒸法时需注意：熏

(general or local) used for fumigating and steaming therapy should be determined according to the state of disease and should not be invariable. The therapy is contraindicated in the patients with hemorrhage or the tendency to bleed, suppuration with carbuncle and swelling, as well as skin ulceration. The method should be used with caution in pregnant women and during the menstrual period.

3.3.2.2 Washing-soaking therapy

Washing-soaking therapy is a method to promote the rehabilitation of the affected organism by bathing and soaking the body generally or locally with the decoction of traditional Chinese drugs. When applying this method, wrap the drugs in a piece of gauze first. Then, add eight to ten times of clear water and soak the drugs for fifteen to twenty minutes. Decoct the drugs for about 20 minutes after the water boils. Filter the decoction and pour the decoction into a sink, a tub or another vessel. At this time, fumigate and steam the affected part first. When the decoction is warm and cannot scald the skin, soak or dip the affected part in the decoction to bath the body generally or locally with a towel, once or twice a day. One dose of the drugs may be applied for two or three times.

Many prescriptions may be used for washing-soaking therapy. These prescriptions should be accordingly selected according to the differences of diseases. The general washing-soaking therapy can clean the skin directly, kill parasites and check itching. Besides, with the help of the medicinal property and heat, the therapy can dispel wind, remove dampness, warm meridians to expel cold, and promote qi flow and blood circulation, etc. It is commonly applicable to general or local skin itching, hemorrhoid, hysteroptosis, baldness, sequalae of poliomyelitis at the early stage as well as paralysis, flaccidity syndrome, infantile malnutrition and various traumatic diseases. Pay

蒸部位（全身或局部），必须根据病情决定，不可千篇一律。正在出血或有出血倾向者、痈肿化脓、皮肤溃烂者禁用。孕妇、月经期间慎用。

2. 洗浸法

用中草药煎水洗浴，浸泡全身或局部，以促使患病机体病康复的方法，称为洗浸法。用时先将药物用纱布包好，加清水8～10倍，浸泡15～20分钟，煮沸后再煮20分钟左右，过滤药液，倒入池、盆或其他器皿中，先熏蒸患部，待温不致烫伤皮肤后，再浸泡或用毛巾蘸药水洗浴全身或局部。每日1～2次，每剂药可用2～3次。

可作洗浸用的方药很多，应根据病证的不同酌情选用。一般洗浸法可直接清洁皮肤，杀虫止痒，借助药性和温热作用，还可驱风除湿、温经散寒、行气活血等，常用于治疗全身或局部的皮肤瘙痒、痔疮、子宫脱垂、脱发、小儿麻痹后遗症早期以及瘫证、痿证、疳证和外伤诸证。

使用洗浸法时应注意：注意避风寒，勿过度疲劳。洗浸

attention to avoiding wind, cold and overfatigue when applying washing-soaking therapy. The patients should have bed rest soon after the washing-soaking therapy. The therapy is contraindicated in all the patients with skin hemorrhage and women during menstrual periods. The washing-soaking therapy should be stopped if adverse reactions occur such as dizziness, palpitation and retching during the washing-soaking process.

3.3.2.3 Plastering therapy

Plastering therapy is a method to promote the recovery from a disease by applying prepared herbal medicines on the affected part or acupoints directly. Pound the fresh selected herbs into paste, or grind the dry herbs into fine powder. Then, add a proper amount of water, or vinegar, or honey, or sesame oil, or egg white, or vaseline, etc. to the powder to make the powder into paste. Afterwards, apply the paste on the affected part or certain acupoints. Replace the paste with fresh one once every one to three days.

Plastering therapy is widely applied because many fresh herbs and the commonly-used decoction, bolus, etc. in clinic can be mostly pounded into paste or made into paste. The therapy is applicable to aphasia, asthma, insomnia, vertigo, headache, abdominalgia, tympanites, Bi-syndrome, flaccidity syndrome as well as dysmenorrhea, infantile malnutrition, fracture, and soft tissue injury, etc. during rehabilitation according to the different selection of drugs.

Pay attention to the fact that plastering therapy is contraindicated in the patients with local ulceration. Pay attention to the observation of local pathological changes at all times to prevent infection. Apply the method with caution on the abdomen and lumbosacral portion of a preg-

后应立即卧床休息。凡皮肤出血、妇女月经期间禁用洗浸法。洗浸过程中若出现头晕、心慌、干呕等不良反应,应暂停洗浸。

3. 敷贴法

用加工过的中草药直接敷贴于患部或穴位,借以促使疾病康复的方法,称为"敷贴法"。使用时,将所选鲜药捣烂成泥,或将干药研成细末,加适量水或醋、蜜、麻油、鸡蛋清、凡士林等调和成膏状,直接敷于患处或某个穴位,一般每隔1~3天换药1次。

不少鲜药及一般临床上常用的汤剂、丸剂等,大多可以捣烂成泥或制成膏状作敷贴用,所以敷贴法的运用范围较为广泛,根据选方用药不同,在康复医疗中,一般可用于失音、咳喘、失眠、眩晕、头痛、腹痛、鼓胀、痹证、痿证以及痛经、小儿疳证、骨折、软组织损伤等病证。

使用敷贴法时应注意:局部破溃者慎用。随时注意观察局部病变情况,防止感染。孕妇腹部及腰骶部慎用。

nant woman.

3.3.2.4 Plastering-ironing therapy

Plastering-ironing therapy is a method to promote the rehabilitation of the body by applying the heated medicinal herbs on the affected part or certain acupoints directly or by ironing externally with the cloth bag containing the drugs. The specific usage is as follows: Apply the heated medicinal herbs on the affected part or certain acupoints directly and then bind up the part or acupoints with a piece of cloth. Heat the site with certain methods (like ironing with an iron). Besides, two cloth bags with hot steamed or hot parched drugs may be alternately applied on the affected part or certain acupoints. Replace the cold one with the hot one. The bag is moved upwards and downwards, from the left to the right. The therapy is generally applied once or twice a day, 30 minutes or so each time.

With the help of the heat and medicinal potency, plastering-ironing therapy has the actions of warming meridians to dispel cold, promoting qi flow to remove stagnation, activating blood circulation, dredging collaterals, etc. With different formulas and medicines, the therapy is commonly applicable to diseases such as various types of Bisyndrome due to wind, cold and dampness, headache, hypochondriac pain, epigastralgia and abdominalgia with cold, impotence, sterility due to uterine cold, unsmooth urination and proctoptosis due to prolonged diarrhea.

Pay attention to these points during applying plastering-ironing therapy: it is contraindicated in the patients with skin injury, on the underbelly or lumbosacral portion of a pregnant woman; the temperature should be proper to prevent scald.

4. 熨贴法

用中草药加热后直接敷于患部或穴位,或以布袋盛装外熨以促进病体的方法,称为"熨贴法",其用法是:直接将加热后的药敷于患部或穴位,用布包扎。若冷则设法(如用热熨斗)加热。也可用两个布袋盛蒸热或炒热的药物,一袋熨摩患部或穴位,并上下左右移动,冷则另换一袋,交替使用,一般每日1~2次,每次30分钟左右。

熨贴法借热力和药力的作用,具有温经散寒、行气导滞、活血通络等功效。根据选用方药不同,常用于治疗各种风寒湿痹痛、头痛、胁痛、脘腹冷痛、阳痿、宫寒不孕、小便不畅、久泻脱肛等疾病。

使用熨贴法时应注意:皮肤破损者禁用。孕妇小腹及腰骶部禁用。注意温度适宜,防止烫伤。

3.3.3 Drugs and prescriptions for promoting longevity

Drugs and prescriptions for promoting longevity refer to the drugs or prescriptions that have the actions of eliminating diseases and strengthening the body. These drugs and prescriptions can be categorized into four types of invigorating qi, tonifying blood, nourishing yin and strengthening yang according to their specific actions.

3.3.3.1 Qi-invigorating drugs

3.3.3.1.1 Renshen (*Radix Ginseng*)

It is sweet, slightly bitter and warm-natured, and has the function of replenishing primordial qi and promoting body fluid production to quench thirst. It is especially applicable to the old people with qi deficiency and the patients with prostration syndrome due to chronic diseases. Renshen Yiwei Decoction (Ginseng Decoction), also called Dushen Decoction (Ginseng-Only Decoction), has the actions of supplementing qi to prevent prostration syndrome. Prolonged administration of the decoction in old people with weak physique may strengthen the body, delay ageing and prolong life. If cut into slices and made into sucking tablets, the drug can tonify the body and increase the resistance of the organism against diseases if it is sucked or drunk as tea. Modern researches have proved that Renshen (*Radix Ginseng*) can regulate the function of reticuloendothelial system, and the active constituent it contains has anti-ageing action.

3.3.3.1.2 Huangqi (*Radix Astragalis seu Hedysari*)

It is sweet and slightly warm-natured and has the functions of invigorating qi, elevating yang, supplementing qi and consolidating superficial resistance, etc. Prolonged administration can strengthen the bone and

三、长寿药物

长寿药物,是指有病祛病,无病强身,融祛病、强身于一体的药物或方剂。按其具体的作用,分为补气、补血、补阴、补阳四类。

(一)补气类

1. 人参

味甘微苦,性温,有大补元气、生津止渴作用,对老年气虚、久病虚脱者尤为适宜。人参一味煎汤,名"独参汤",具有益气固脱之功效,年老体弱者,长服此汤,可强壮身体,抗衰延年。人参切成饮片,每日嚼化或泡茶饮用,可补益身体,增强机体的抗病能力。现代研究证明,人参可调节网状内皮系统功能,其所含活性成分具有抗衰老作用。

2. 黄芪

味甘性微温,具有补气升阳、益卫固表等功效。久服可壮骨强身,用于气虚证候。现代研究表明,黄芪可增强机体

body. It is applicable to symptoms due to qi deficiency. Modern studies have indicated that Huangqi (*Radix Astragalis seu Hedysari*) can enhance resistance of the organism against diseases, regulate blood pressure and immune function, has the corticoid functions and improve blood circulation of coronary artery and heart functions. It also has the ability to prolong the life of certain primary cells and certain diploid cell strains.

3.3.3.1.3　Fuling (*Poria*)

It is sweet and tasteless and neutral-natured, and can benefit the heart and spleen, promote diuresis, remove dampness. The drug cannot only strengthen body resistance against diseases, but also eliminate pathogenic factors. It is the fine commonly-used tonic and drug for prolonging life. The so-called Fuling (*Poria*) Gruel is cooked with 12 g of fine Fuling (*Poria*) powder and 100 g of Jingmi (*Semen Oryzae Sativae*). Drinking the gruel regularly has the preventive action of senile edema, obesity and tumor to a certain degree. The Fuling (*Poria*) Cake handed down so far from the Qing Dynasty is the fine food to tonify the body, eliminate diseases and prolong life. Modern researches have proved that the active principle of Fuling (*Poria*) is mainly pachman. It strengthens the human immunity and has certain antitumor actions.

3.3.3.1.4　Huaishanyao (*Rhizoma Dioscoreae*)

It is sweet, neutral-natured and has the actions of strengthening the spleen, tonifying the lung, reinforcing the kidney to benefit renal essence. Modern studies have indicated that the drug is rich in nutrients and contains amylase, choline, phlegm, glucoprotein, free amino acid, fat, carbohydrate, and vitamin C, etc. It is both the drug and food with good tonification. For instance, Huaishanyao (*Rhizoma Dioscoreae*) Gruel is cooked with 50 g of dry slices of Huaishanyao (*Rhizoma Dioscoreae*), or

抵抗力,调整血压,调节免疫功能,有类皮质激素样作用,可改善冠状动脉血液循环和心脏功能。并有延长某些原代细胞和某些二倍体细胞株寿命的能力。

3. 茯苓

味甘淡,性平,可益心脾,利水湿。既能扶正,又可祛邪,为平补之佳平,是常用的延年益寿药物。如将白茯苓磨成细粉,取12 g,与粳米100 g煮粥,名为"茯苓粥",常吃此粥,对老年性浮肿、肥胖症以及肿瘤有一定的预防作用。再如流传至今的清代宫廷名品茯苓饼,是滋补祛病延年的佳品。研究证明,茯苓的有效成分主要是茯苓多糖,能增强人体免疫功能,并有一定的抗癌作用。

4. 怀山药

味甘,性平,具有健脾补肺、固肾益精作用。现代研究表明,本品营养丰富,内含淀粉酶、胆碱、黏液质、糖蛋白和自由氨基酸、脂肪、糖类、维生素C等,是滋补作用较强的药食两用之品。如怀山药粥,用干怀山药片50 g,或鲜怀山药100 g,粳米400 g,同煮粥。每

100 g of fresh Huaishanyao (*Rhizoma Dioscoreae*) and 400 g of Jingmi (*Semen Oryzae Sativae*). Eating the warm gruel in the morning and evening every day can strengthen the spleen, supplement qi, stop diarrhea and dysentery, and is also applicable to senile diabetes, chronic nephritis, etc.

3.3.3.1.5　Yiyiren (Semen Coicis)

It is sweet, tasteless, cool-natured and has the actions of strengthening the spleen, tonifying the lung, eliminating dampness, etc. The pharmacological tests have discovered that the drug can inhibit the growth of cancer cells. The gruel cooked with Yiyiren (*Semen Coicis*) alone, or the rice or gruel cooked with Yiyiren (*Semen Coicis*) and Jingmi (*Semen Oryzae Sativae*) is very beneficial to middle-aged and old people if they eat or drink regularly.

3.3.3.2　Blood-tonifying drugs

3.3.3.2.1　Shudihuang (Radix Rehmanniae Praeparata)

It is sweet, slightly warm-natured and has the actions of tonifying blood and nourishing yin. Modern researches believe that the drug has very good cordial, diuretic and hypoglycemic actions. For example, decoct 1 500 g of Shudihuang (*Radix Rehmanniae Praeparata*) in three different times and then filter the decoction. Next, mix the decoctions of the three times together. Afterwards, add a proper amount of white honey to the mixed decoction and keep it airtight for later use. Take it orally with warm boiled water, 10 g each time, twice a day. The decoction has the actions of tonifying blood, nourishing yin, strengthening the kidney and replenishing marrow for the people with deficiency of renal essence and blood.

日早晚温热服食，可健脾益气，止泻痢，对老年性糖尿病、慢性肾炎等病，均有益处。

5. 薏苡仁

味甘、淡，性凉。具有健脾、补肺、除湿等功效。药理试验发现，本品能抑制癌细胞生长。单用薏苡仁煮粥，或与粳米同用煮饭或煮粥，中老年人经常服用，很有益处。

（二）补血类

1. 熟地黄

味甘，性微温。具有补血滋阴之功。现代研究认为，本品有很好的强心、利尿、降血糖作用。如用熟地黄 1 500 g，熬 3 次，每次过滤去渣滓，合并滤液，加白蜜适量，装瓶密封备用。每次服 10 g，日服 2 次，用白开水送下。对于肾之精血不足者，可起到养血滋阴、益肾添髓的作用。

3.3.3.2.2 Heshouwu (*Radix Polygoni Multiflori*)

It is bitter, sweet, puckery, warm-natured and has the actions of tonifying the liver and kidney, arresting spontaneous seminal emission. Modern studies have indicated that the drug contains anthraquinones, lecithin, starch, coarse fat, etc., of which lecithin can promote the growth and development of central nervous system. The drug can also lower blood fat, remit atherosclerosis and has cordial action. The drug has the action of prolonging life if decocted alone in water or in spirit or decocted into paste, or used in a prescription with other ingredients.

3.3.3.2.3 Guiyuanrou (*Arillus Longan*)

It is sweet, warm-natured and has the actions of tonifying the heart and spleen, supplementing qi and nourishing blood. The gruel cooked with 15 g of Guiyuanrou (*Arillus Longan*), 4 Chinese dates and 100 g of Jingmi (*Semen Oryzae Sativae*) has better therapeutic effects on palpitation, insomnia, listlessness, hypodynamia due to asthenia of both the heart and spleen, etc.

3.3.3.2.4 Ejiao (*Colla Corii Asini*)

It is sweet, neutral-natured and has the actions of tonifying blood, nourishing yin, checking hemorrhage, and preventing abortion, etc. Modern researches believe that the drug contains collagen, multiple amino acid, calcium, sulfur, etc. which can accelerate the production of red blood cells and hemoglobin, promote blood coagulation, tonify blood and stop bleeding. The drug is applicable to various types of blood deficiency. It is generally melted by boiling water or hot yellow rice wine, or by stewing the vessel containing it in water, 5 g each time.

3.3.3.2.5 Ziheche (*Placenta Hominis*)

It is sweet, salty, slightly warm-natured and has the actions of nourishing blood, tonifying qi, benefiting

2. 何首乌

味苦、甘、涩,性温,具有补益肝肾、涩精止遗的功效。研究表明,本品含有蒽醌类、卵磷脂、淀粉、粗脂肪等成分,其中卵磷脂可促进中枢神经系统的生长发育。本品尚能降低血脂,缓解动脉粥样硬化的形成,有强心作用。单用水煎或酒煎、熬膏,或与其他益寿药物配伍使用,均有益寿延年之功。

3. 桂圆肉

味甘,性温,具用补心脾、益气血之功。如用桂圆肉15 g,大枣4枚,粳米100 g,一起煮粥,每日早晚食用。对于心脾两虚引起的心悸、失眠、神疲乏力等有较好的补养作用。

4. 阿胶

味甘,性平,具有补血滋阴、止血安胎等作用。近代研究认为,本品含有胶原、多种氨基酸、钙、硫等成分,可以加速红细胞和血红蛋白生成,促进血液凝固,能补血止血,用于各种血虚证。一般用开水或热黄酒烊化,或隔水炖化,每次5 g。

5. 紫河车

味甘、咸,性微温,具用养血补气益精等功效。实验研

essence, etc. Experimental studies and clinical practice have proved that Ziheche (*Placenta Hominis*) has sex-hormonoid actions, can promote the development of the mammary gland and uterus, and enhance the human body resistance against diseases. The drug may be taken orally alone and may be taken with other ingredients in a prescription as well. When taken alone, the drug may be stewed for eating or ground into powder for oral administration. The stewing method: Select a fresh human placenta and remove the blood vessels. Then, wash and clean it. Afterwards, stew it until it is down. Or wash it clean. Then, stove it to be ground into fine powder. Take the powder by infusing it in warm boiled water, 6 g each time.

3.3.3.3 Yin-nourishing drugs

3.3.3.3.1 Gouqizi (*Fructus Lycii*)

It is sweet, neutral-natured and has the actions of nourishing the kidney, moistening the lung, calming the liver and improving sight. Modern studies have indicated that Gouqizi (*Fructus Lycii*) contains betaine, carotin, thiamine, ovoflavin, nicotinic acid, vitamin C, calcium, phosphorus, and iron, etc. It has the actions of inhibiting the fat deposit in liver cells, preventing fatty liver and promoting cell regeneration. The drug can effectively prevent and treat light-headedness, pain and flaccidity of the waist and knees, and blurred vision due to deficiency of the kidney yin in old people, and treat diabetes.

3.3.3.3.2 Yuzhu (*Rhizoma Polygonati Odorati*)

It is sweet, neutral-natured and has the actions of nourishing yin, moistening the lung, removing dysphoria and quenching thirst. Prolonged administration is advisable for the people with yin deficiency. Modern studies

究及临床实践证明，紫河车有性激素样作用，可促进乳腺和子宫的发育，能增强人体的抵抗能力。本品可单味服用，也可配方服用，单味服用可炖食，亦可研末服。炖食：用新鲜胎盘一个，挑去血络，漂洗干净后，炖熟。或洗净后，烘干，研为细末，每次6g，温水冲服。

（三）补阴类

1. 枸杞子

味甘，性平，具有滋肾润肺、平肝明目之功效。研究表明，枸杞子含有甜菜碱、胡萝卜素、硫胺、核黄素、烟酸、抗坏血酸、钙、磷、铁等成分，具有抑制脂肪在肝细胞内沉积，防止脂肪肝，促进肝细胞新生的作用。本品泡茶饮服，或与粳米煮粥常食，能有效地防治中老年人因肝肾阴虚所致的头晕目眩，腰膝酸软，视物昏花，并用于糖尿病的治疗。

2. 玉竹

味甘，性平，具有养阴润肺、除烦止渴作用。适用于阴虚之人常服。研究表明，本品有降血糖及强心作用，对于糖

have indicated that the drug has the action of lowering blood sugar, having cordial function and certain therapeutic effects on the patients with diabetes and palpitation.

3.3.3.3.3 Huangjing (*Rhizoma Polygonati*)

It is sweet, neutral-natured and has the actions of strengthening the spleen and stomach, moistening the heart and lung, replenishing essence and marrow. It is applicable to tiredness, hypodynamia, dry mouth, and scanty body fluid, etc. due to yin deficiency or deficiency of both qi and yin. Modern researches believe that Huangjing (*Rhizoma Polygonati*) has the actions of lowering blood pressure, preventing atherosclerosis and fatty liver, etc.

3.3.3.3.4 Sangshenzi (*Fructus Mori*)

It is sweet, cold-natured and has the actions of tonifying the liver and kidney, improving hearing and sight. It is generally made into paste for oral administration. Modern clinical practice has proved that Sangshenzi (*Fructus Mori*) has better therapeutic effects on anemia, neurasthenia, diabetes and hypertension due to yin deficiency.

3.3.3.3.5 Nüzhenzi (*Fructus Ligustri Lucidi*)

It is sweet, slightly bitter, neutral-natured and has the actions of tonifying the liver and kidney, nourishing yin, and improving sight, etc. Modern studies have proved the drug has cordial and diuretic actions and can also treat hectic fever of tuberculosis of lymph nodes and pulmonary tuberculosis, etc.

3.3.3.4 Yang-strengthening drugs

3.3.3.4.1 Tusizi (*Semen Cuscutae*)

It is sweet, pungent, slightly warm-natured and has the actions of replenishing essence and marrow, strengthening the tendon and bone, supplementing qi and strength, etc. Prolonged administration of the drug can

尿病、心悸患者，有一定的作用。

3. 黄精

味甘，性平，具有益脾胃、润心肺、填精髓之作用。用于阴虚或气阴两虚所致的身倦乏力，口干津少等。现代研究认为，黄精具有降血压、防止动脉粥样硬化及脂肪肝等功效。

4. 桑椹子

味甘，性寒。具有补益肝肾、聪耳明目之功效。一般制成膏剂服用。现代临床证实，桑椹子对于贫血、神经衰弱、糖尿病及阴虚型高血压有较好的疗效。

5. 女贞子

味甘、微苦，性平，具有补益肝肾、滋阴明目等作用。研究表明本品有强心、利尿作用，还可治颈淋巴结核及肺结核所致的潮热等症。

（四）补阳类

1. 菟丝子

味甘、辛，性微温，具有补肝肾、益精髓、壮筋骨、益气力等功效。常服久服，可延年益寿。

prolong life.

3.3.3.4.2 Lurong(*Cornu Cervi Pantotrichum*)

It is sweet, salty, warm-natured and has the actions of strengthening the kidney yang, replenishing essence and blood and strengthening the tendon and bone. It may be infused in water or stewed for oral administration. The powder of Lurong(*Cornu Cervi Pantotrichum*) is used for infusion, 1.5 g or so each time. 3 g of Lurong(*Cornu Cervi Pantotrichum*) is put into a cup with water and stewed with the cup for oral administration. It is contraindicated in the patients with excessive fire due to yin deficiency, pulmonary heat and hyperactive yang of the liver.

3.3.3.4.3 Roucongrong(*Herba Cistanchis*)

It is sweet, salty, warm-natured and has the actions of tonifying the kidney, strengthening the kidney yang, loosening the bowel to relieve constipation. 10 g of the drug or so may be decocted for oral administration or used to cook gruel with Jingmi(*Semen Oryzae Sativae*) for eating. Modern researches believe that the drug contains orobanchin, microalkaloid, glycosides and substances of organic acid. It has hormonoid action and the actions of lowering blood pressure, strengthening the body, and the resistance of organism against diseases and possesses cordial effect, etc.

3.3.3.4.4 Duzhong(*Cortex Eucommiae*)

It is sweet, warm-natured and has the actions of tonifying the liver and kidney, strengthening the tendon and bone. Animal experiments have proved that Duzhong (*Cortex Eucommiae*) contains Gutta-percha, resin, etc. and that the drug has the actions of tranquilization and lowering blood pressure.

2. 鹿茸

味甘、咸,性温,具有补肾阳、益精血、强筋骨作用。可单味冲服,亦可炖服。冲服时,用鹿茸末,每次服1.5g左右。炖服是把3g鹿茸放杯内加水,隔水炖服。阴虚火旺及肺热、肝阳上亢者忌服。

3. 肉苁蓉

味甘、咸,性温,具有补肾助阳、润肠通便之功效。本品可用10g左右,加水煎服或与粳米煮粥食用。近代研究认为,本品含有列当素、微量生物碱、苷类、有机酸类物质。具有激素样作用,还有降压、强心、强壮、增强机体抵抗力等作用。

4. 杜仲

味甘,性温,具有补肝肾、强筋骨作用。动物实验证明,杜仲含有杜仲胶、树脂等,有镇静和降低血压作用。

3.4 Nursing of TCM Rehabilitation

Nursing of TCM rehabilitation helps the patient restore his physiological functions, viability and social adaptive capacity and promotes his somatopsychic health by means of the specialized nursing measures which make use of various nursing techniques accompanied by rehabilitation measures and traditional rehabilitation training methods. The main targets of rehabilitation nursing are the patients with various types of morbid disablement such as mental and physical disablement, various types of maim, senile diseases, and chronic diseases, etc. It is very hard to achieve therapeutic effects with one or several methods. Therefore, many rehabilitation techniques and methods are comprehensively adopted to nurse the patients.

3.4.1 Nursing with the concept of wholism

Nursing with the concept of wholism means that during the rehabilitation nursing period, nursing staff should understand thoroughly the mutual relationships among various viscera and tissues of the human body and consider the roles which the seasonal climatic changes, social environment, etc. play in the rehabilitation of diseases, and that only in this way can the somatopsychic health be restored to the greatest extent in the patient so that he will return to society as soon as possible.

3.4.1.1 Nursing in conformity to seasonal changes

Man lives in nature and is closely related to nature. Seasonal changes with summer going and winter coming during a year, etc. all can unavoidably influence the ascension and descension of yin and yang, circulation of qi and blood and visceral asthenia and sthenia of the human body. Rehabilitation nursing should conform to the natural law to arrange reasonable nursing. For example, in summer, the rehabilitation ward should be well-ventilated, cooled and the cold color light and curtain installed to achieve the cool and comfortable feeling; in winter, attention should be paid to the prevention of cold and heat preservation, and the ward should be equipped with the warm color light and curtain; in spring, yang qi rises and ask the patient to have more outdoor activities; in the scorching summer, it is advisable for people to have activities in the shade of trees and indoors to avoid profuse perspiration and prevent sunstroke due to consumption of qi and yin; in autumn and winter, yang qi contracts internally and yin and essence are in storage interiorly. Therefore, large amount of exercise is not advisable to prevent the consumption of essence and qi.

3.4.1.2 Adaptation to social environment

As an element of society, man's various activities are influenced by the social environment. Especially, the occurrence, development, even rehabilitation of certain emotional disorders are closely related to the social environmental factors. Good environmental factors and cheerful emotions may promote the patient's recovery as soon as possible; poor environmental atmosphere is not beneficial to rehabilitation, even may aggravate diseases. The rehabilitation nursing staff should be familiar with the patient's interpersonal relationships such as marriage, love, family and friends as well as the social status, working conditions, likes and dislikes, etc. They should make the patient mentally prepared and straight him out intentionally so as to restore the normal psychology of the patient with the psychological disorder or disturbance as soon as possible.

流通及脏腑的虚实。康复护理工作必须顺应自然规律,进行合理地护理。如康复病室夏季要通风降温,配用冷色调灯光、窗帘,给人以凉爽舒适的感觉;冬季则应注意防寒保暖,用暖色灯光、暖色调窗帘。春日阳气升发,让病人多做户外活动;夏季炎热,宜在树荫下或室内活动,避免大汗淋漓,防止气阴耗伤,发生中暑;秋冬季节阳气内收,阴精内藏,运动量不宜过大,以防精气耗散。

2. 适应环境

人作为社会的一分子,其种种活动要受到社会环境的影响。特别是某些情志疾病的发生和发展,乃至康复过程,与社会环境因素有着密切的关联。良好的环境因素和舒畅的情志,会促使病人早日康复;而不良的环境氛围,则不利病体的康复,甚至可能使病情恶化。康复护理者必须熟悉病人的婚恋、家庭、朋友等人际关系,以及社会地位、工作条件、喜好厌恶等,做细致的思想工作,进行针对性的疏导,使心理疾病患者或有心理障碍的病人,及早恢复正

3.4.1.3 Attaching equal importance to internal and external factors

The human body is an indispensable organic whole. Man's viscera, limbs and skeleton are physiologically related to and pathologically influence one another. Accordingly, the rehabilitation nursing staff should familiarize themselves with the internal relationships among viscera and tissues, observe the patient's condition closely, discover the developing tendency of the disease at all times so that the reliable material can be provided for the doctor to work out or revise the rehabilitation measures.

3.4.2 Differentiating syndrome to decide nursing

Differentiating syndrome to decide treatment is one of the basic TCM principles. This principle should be observed during the rehabilitation nursing. One disease may be divided into several syndromes according to its clinical manifestations. Different therapeutic methods and nursing measures should be adopted for different syndromes of one disease. For example, the patients with qi deficiency should be nursed mainly by calm mind and a good rest to avoid overstrain; preserving yin and body fluids should be taken into account in the patients with yin deficiency; strengthening yang and qi should be taken into consideration in the patients with yang deficiency to prevent attack by cold; the patients with qi stagnation should be mainly nursed by regulating emotions, etc. In addition, each person varies from others in the congenital inheritance, postnatal living conditions and surroundings and personal hobbies. Moreover, everybody is different from others in the age, sex, behavior and habits. These individual variations should be specifically dealt with during the rehabili-

常心理。

3. 内外兼顾

人体是一个不可分割的整体。人的五脏六腑、四肢百骸生理上互相联系,在病理上互相影响。因此,康复护理人员必须熟悉脏腑组织的内在联系,密切观察病情,随时发现疾病的发展趋势,为康复医生制订或修正康复措施提供可靠的资料。

二、辨证护理

辨证施治是中医学的基本原则之一,在康复护理时也应时时遵循这一原则。同一病证,据其临床表现可分为若干证型,证型不同,就应采取不同的治疗方法和护理措施。例如,气虚者的护理应以清心静养为主,切忌过度劳累;阴虚者应注意顾护阴液;阳虚者应温补阳气,避免受寒;气郁者的护理应以调畅情志为主等。此外,每个人先天禀赋各异,后天的生活条件和环境不同,兴趣爱好有别,还有年龄、性别、行为习惯、病情轻重也各不相同,这些个体的差异,要求康复护理时必须具体对待。

tation nursing.

3.4.3 Comprehensive nursing

3.4.3.1 The combination of general nursing with special nursing

Special nursing should be given to the patient at the stage of recovery according to the patient's condition in special cases besides the routine nursing. For instance, the key link of preventing the complications such as bed sore should be seized in the patients with hemiplegia, paraplegia and prolonged bed rest. For these patients, nursing in urination, defecation and affected limbs should be even more careful. The methods such as acupuncture, massage, ear acupuncture and hot medicated compress may be adopted in nursing to keep smooth defecation. The affected limbs should keep locally warm and often applied with safflower oil and massaged while injection should be avoided on the affected limbs as much as possible. As for the diseases of respiratory system, close attention should be paid to the state of asthma. Generally, critical symptoms easily occur in the early morning such as polypnea, profuse accumulation of sputum and saliva and difficulty in supination due to gasp. Therefore, the nursing staff should help the patient to expectorate the sticky sputum by turning him over, patting his back and wiping his chest, and with finger-press method and acupuncture in time. Mental recreation and work nursing should be simultaneously arranged besides the routine nursing for the patients with mental defect.

3.4.3.2 The integration of various nursing methods

Comprehensive nursing is mostly adopted in rehabilitation nursing due to the specific characteristics in the rehabilitation patients. For example, various nursing

三、综合护理

1. 一般护理与特殊护理相结合

康复期患者除常规护理外，对于特殊情况还应结合病情进行特殊护理。如偏瘫、截瘫、长期卧床的患者应抓住预防褥疮等并发症这一重要环节。对这类病人，二便和患肢的护理更要仔细。可用针刺、按摩、耳针、热熨等方法进行护理，保持大便通畅。患肢要注意局部保暖，经常用红花酒等外搽按摩，尽量避免在患肢注射。呼吸系统的疾病，除常规护理外，要密切注意咳喘情况，一般凌晨容易出现呼吸急促、痰涎壅盛、喘息难卧等危重病候，要及时给患者翻身、拍背、抹胸、指压、针刺，帮助咳出粘痰。对于智力残疾者，在常规护理的同时，要合理安排好精神娱乐及作业护理。

2. 多种护理方法相结合

因为康复对象的特殊性，康复护理多采用综合护理，如饮食护理、心理护理、运动健

methods may be commonly adopted like diet nursing, psychological nursing, strengthening health with sports and functional training; the patients with aphasia and paralysis suffer physically and most of them have mental and emotional disturbances at the same time because of the lack of communication with the outside world due to prolonged bed rest. Thus, the nursing staff should not only turn them over, bathe them, replace their underclothes with the new ones and do other such kinds of routine nursing regularly, but also cooperate with functional training and massage of the affected limbs as well as attach importance to psychological nursing. The comprehensive application of various rehabilitation techniques and methods can promote the rehabilitation process.

3.4.3.3 The combination of self-nursing and family nursing with hospital nursing

Self-nursing mainly includes careful prevention of exogenous pathogenic factors, cultivation of temperament, regulation of diet, physical training with sports, etc. It attaches importance to self nursing and recuperation, and benefits the rehabilitation of the diseased body.

The nursing staff are mainly the patient's family members in terms of family nursing. They should take care of the patient's daily life and diet arrangement, and communicate emotionally with the patient. All these are of prime importance for the rehabilitation of the patient's somatopsychic health.

Hospital nursing is mainly undertaken by rehabilitation nurses. Rehabilitation nurses should receive certain specialized training and have a good command of certain special skills such as various functional training methods and massage. Rehabilitation nurses are responsible for the specific implementation of rehabilitation methods, provide the preventive measures of various complications and

身、功能训练等多种护理方法常可配合进行。如失语、瘫痪者在身体痛苦的同时,因长期卧床,缺乏与外界的交流,大多有精神情志方面的障碍,所以在既要经常给他们翻身、擦澡、更换内衣,做一些常规护理外,还要配合功能训练,按摩患肢,并要重视心理护理。多种康复技术和方法综合运用,可促进康复进程。

3. 自我护理、家庭护理与医院护理相结合

自我护理,主要包括谨避外邪、怡情养性、饮食调摄、运动锻炼等内容,注重自我护理和调养,有利于病体的康复。

家庭护理方面,护理人员主要是病人的家属,他们要照顾康复对象的日常起居,饮食安排,经常与之交流感情等,这些对于病患者身心的康复也极为重要。

医院护理,主要由康复护士担任。康复护士须经过一定的专业训练,掌握一定的特殊技能,如各种功能训练方法、按摩等。康复护士负责康复方法的具体实施,提供各种并发症的预防措施,动态反映

dynamically report the changes of the patient's condition and the comprehensive nursing from the operation of nursing techniques and functional training with sports to mental and dietary recuperation, etc. The rehabilitation effects are not only related to the evaluation of the doctors and rehabilitation medicine, but also have close ties with the nursing work.

The organic combination of self nursing and family nursing, with hospital nursing, which cooperate and supplement mutually, is one of the characteristics of the rehabilitation nursing in traditional Chinese medicine. It plays an important role in smoothly carrying out the comprehensive rehabilitation nursing, promoting the patient's recovery and preventing complications.

3.4.4 The nursing methods of attaching equal importance to somatic and psychic health

Rehabilitation involves not only overcoming the patient's physical suffering, but also regulating the psychological state of the rehabilitation patient so as to make him return to society with good somatopsychic health as much as possible. Preserving both physique and mentality and attaching equal importance to somatic and psychic health are one of the creams of life cultivation and rehabilitation theories in TCM. Therefore, people who preserve health should pay attention to the unity of physique and mentality. Only in this way can good health be guaranteed and life prolonged. The injury of physique is mostly accompanied with emotional impairment in most rehabilitation indications; emotional impairment in most cases is accompanied by the injury of physique. In other words, the injury of physique involves mentality while the impairment of mentality involves physique. Accordingly, the thought

病情变化，从护理技术操作、功能运动训练，到精神饮食调养等各方面进行综合护理。康复效果不但与康复医生的康复评价、康复医疗有关，而且与护理工作也有着密切的关系。

将自我护理、家庭护理与医院护理有机地结合起来，相互配合与补充，是中医康复护理的特色之一，对于顺利开展综合康复护理，促进病人康复，预防并发症，均有重要的作用。

四、心身并重的护理法

医疗康复不仅要解决患者躯体的痛苦，而且要调整康复对象的心理状况，使其尽可能身心俱健地重返社会。形神共养、心身并重是中医养生、康复理论的精华之一。因此，养生康复必须注意形神的统一，才能保证身体健康，获得延年益寿。在大多数康复适应证中，伴随形体之损，多有神志之伤；神志之伤者，亦多有形体之损，就是形损必及于神，神伤必及于形，因而，形神并重的指导思想，也贯穿于整个康复医疗实践之中，对治形为主者，辅以调神；对调神

of attaching equal importance to physique and mentality also permeates in the whole rehabilitation practice. The treatment of physique as the main purpose is assisted by regulating mentality, while the regulation of mentality as main object is supplemented by treating physique. Attach equal importance to physique and mentality, and physique and mentality complement each other so as to effectively promote the patient's somatopsychic health.

为主者,辅以治形,形神并重,相得益彰,从而有效地促使患者身心的康复。

4 Forbidden Points for Life Cultivation and Rehabilitation

4.1 Abstinence from smoking and drinking

4.1.1 Smoking is harmful to health

Smoking is absolutely harmful. Tobacco contains nicotine, ammonia and cyanide. When burnt, tobacco generates carbon monoxide. The acute toxicity of nicotine is not less than ammonium cyanate, and the amount of nicotine generated by twenty cigarettes can make an ox die immediately. The tar in tobacco stimulates the lung greatly, injures the pulmonary tissue and the mucosa of respiratory tract, and weakens the protective function of pulmonary epithelial cells and the phagocytic function of macrophage. This lays the foundation for chronic infection and canceration. Tobacco tar contains carcinogenic substances, mainly some chemical compounds of polycyclic aromatic hydrocarbon. This type of substances is generated when tobacco is burnt. In addition, the substances the tobacco contains such as amine nitrite are also carcinogenic substances. The carbon monoxide inspired enters blood to replace oxygen and hinders the function of blood to transport oxygen. Moreover, the high-concentration carbon monoxide may also injure cardiovascular system and markedly increases the incidences of myocardial infarction and atherosclerosis. The ammonia generated by smoking can stimulate oral

第四章　养生康复禁忌

第一节　戒烟酒

一、吸烟有害健康

吸烟有百害而无一利。烟草里含有尼古丁、氨、氰化物,燃烧时产生一氧化碳。尼古丁的急性毒性不亚于氰氢酸,20支烟的尼古丁可使一头牛立即死亡。烟草中的烟焦油对肺的刺激性很大,使肺组织和呼吸道黏膜损伤,并降低肺上皮细胞的保护功能和巨噬细胞的吞噬功能,为慢性感染和癌变提供了基础。烟油中含有致癌物质,主要是一些多环芳烃化合物。这类物质在烟草燃烧时生成。此外,所含的亚硝氨等亦是致癌物质。吸烟时吸进去的一氧化碳进入血液,取代了氧气的位置,妨碍了血液输运氧气的功能。并且高浓度的一氧化碳还会损害心血管系统,使心肌梗死和动脉粥样硬化发病显著增

cavity, throat, pulmonary and gastric mucosae, cause poor appetite, unsmooth respiration, even gingival atrophy, gingival bleeding and odontoseisis in severe cases. It can be seen from the above that smoking may influence the functional activities of every system of the human body and is a factor to promote the occurrence of diseases. Meanwhile, smoking is one of the major causes why many diseases are too intractable to be cured.

Smoking is not only harmful to the smoker, but also to the non-smokers around. It has been determined that in the smog exhaled by the smoker, the concentration of tobacco tar and nicotine is two times as much as that of the smog inhaled by the smoker. Consequently, smoking does not only harm the smoker's health, but also causes "public nuisance". Accordingly, please do not smoke or give up smoking as soon as possible for the sake of your and others' health.

One should stress the methods besides his personal determination and willpower when quitting smoking. For instance, the smoker can smoke less and less in order to give up smoking gradually. In addition, he can place himself in the non-smoking environment. In this case, it can make the smoker feel ashamed and fearful and counteract his desire for smoking. Take some methods for another example. Make the smoker feel slightly uncomfortable, even disgusted during or after smoking with certain methods. Then, he can take advantage of it to quit smoking. For instance, add Renshenlu (*Rhizoma Ginseng*), the mild-natured and atoxic emetic, to the cigarette to make him nauseated. Besides, successful abstention from smoking has been reported, too. For example, puncture the depression between Lieque and Yangxi with the filiform

加。吸烟时产生的氨,能刺激口腔、咽喉、肺和胃黏膜,引起食欲不振、呼吸不畅,严重者口腔牙龈萎缩、出血、牙齿松动。可见,吸烟可影响到人体各系统的功能活动,是疾病发生的一个促进因素,同时也是许多病证经久不愈难以康复的主要原因之一。

吸烟不仅对吸烟者自身有害,还对吸烟者周围的人有害。据测定,在吸烟者吐出的烟气里,烟油和尼古丁的浓度是吸烟者吸进去的烟气里含量的2倍。因此,吸烟不仅危害本人健康,而且还造成"公害",所以,为了自己和他人的健康,劝君不要吸烟或尽早戒烟。

戒烟时,除了个人的决心和毅力外,还要讲究方法。如吸烟由多到少,逐步戒除,并尽可能将自己置身于禁止吸烟的环境中,对吸烟感到羞愧、惧怕,可以抵消吸烟的欲望,再如通过某些方法,使吸烟者在吸烟时或吸烟后感到轻微不适,甚或产生厌恶之情,然后得以顺势戒除,如在香烟中加入性缓无毒的催吐药人参芦,使其吸烟后有恶心欲吐之感。此外,以针灸戒烟,也有一些成功的报道,如在列缺穴与阳溪穴之间的凹

needle, 3 mm in depth, and retain the needle for 15 minutes; apply the needle-embedding therapy on Naodian and Xindian of the auricle. When wanting to smoke, press the two acupoints for several times. It is also effective to some degree.

4.1.2 Drinking and health

Since ancient times, spirit has been closely related to human life. Spirit is used as a drug in TCM. TCM believes that spirit as the king of all drugs has the actions of dredging meridians, activating collaterals, promoting the circulation of qi and blood, improving appetite, removing fatigue, making people happy and relaxed with brisk sensation if it is moderately drunk. The main constituent of spirit is ethyl alcohol. Drinking spirit causes excitation, dilates blood vessels and accelerates blood circulation. Therefore, it can excite nerves and relieve fatigue. The stimulation of spirit on taste sense and olfaction can reflectively increase respiratory capacity and excretion of digestive juice. Accordingly, drinking a small amount of spirit before meals can strengthen the stomach and improve appetite; drinking a small quantity of spirit before bed time can relieve fatigue due to muscular tension and promote sleeping; drinking a bit of spirit at daytime can excite nerves and make people work energetically. Studies in recent years have discovered that drinking a little spirit can prevent myocardial infarction and cerebral thrombosis, reduce the incidence of cardiocerebrovascular diseases.

A great number of ancient and modern, Chinese and foreign data have indicated that drinking a small amount of spirit is beneficial to the human body while overdrinking spirit and addiction to it may be harmful and give rise to various diseases or aggravate diseases. Prolonged stimulation

陷处,用毫针刺入3 mm,留针15分钟;在耳郭上取心点或脑点埋针,想吸烟时按压数次,也有一定的效果。

二、饮酒与健康

自古以来,酒与人类生活有着密切的联系,在中医学中,酒被当作一种药物来使用。认为酒为百药之长,适量少饮,有通经活络,促进气血运行,增进食欲,消除疲劳,使人轻快的作用。酒中主要成分是乙醇,饮后有兴奋作用,可使血管扩张,血液循环加快,故能兴奋神经,解除疲劳。酒对味觉、嗅觉的刺激,可反射性地增加呼吸量和消化液分泌。所以,饭前饮少量酒,可健胃,增进食欲;晚上睡前小啜,可消除肌肉紧张所致的疲劳,有助于睡眠;白天少量饮酒可兴奋神经,使工作精力充沛。近年来研究发现,喝少量的酒能预防心肌梗死和脑血栓形成,减低心脑血管病人的死亡率。

古今中外大量资料表明,少量饮酒对人体有益,但若饮酒过多,嗜酒成瘾,则会变利为害,导致多种疾病的产生或加重原有的疾患。因为胃长

of spirit on the stomach may cause chronic gastritis and malnutrition; prolonged drinking spirit on an empty stomach may result in fatty liver and cirrhosis due to the decomposition of spirit within the liver; drinking spirit may induce cardiac lipoidal change, reduce myocardiac elasticity and cardiac contractility, promote angiosclerosis and cerebrovascular accident in the patients with chronic alcoholism; overdrinking spirit may aggravate primary diseases and is not beneficial to the recovery from diseases and longevity in some patients with chronic hepatic diseases, chronic bronchitis, bronchial asthma, pulmonary emphysema and chronic gastritis.

4.2 Abstinence from food preference

Food preference refers to the addiction to a particular food or condiment that exceeds the endurance of the organism and consequently brings harm to the organism.

"People regard food as Heaven." Food is of prime importance for human existence and provides essential nutrients for the growth, development and various physiological activities of the human body to maintain the normal human vital activities. Foods are various and the nutrients are different from one another. On the other hand, the nutrients constituting the human body and maintaining the metabolism of the human body are very various. These nutrients should be obtained from numerous foods while one type or several types of foods cannot possibly contain all these nutrients. Besides, there exists the requirement of a reasonable proportion among various nutrients essential to the human body. If the content of a certain substance is excessive or scanty in the human body, this may influence the absorption and actions of other substances. Accordingly, scientific feeding and reasonable proportions should be advocated in diet in order to make the nutrients in various foods supplement mutually. The advocation of eating various foods, alternative dietary methods and complete diet has the great guiding significance for TCM life cultivation and rehabilitation.

Foods mainly include five flavors: sour, bitter, sweet, pungent and salty as well as four natures of cold, hot, warm and cool. Foods of different natures and flavors vary from one another in their actions. So, food preference inevitably gives rise to diseases or is not beneficial to the treatment of and recovery from diseases if it lasts long. For instance, the patients with yin deficiency or diseases due to yin deficiency should select sweet and moist-natured foods or sweet and cool-natured food to nourish yin and clear away heat. If they eat or addict to warm-natured tonic foods, this not only makes it difficult to restore the balance among qi, blood, yin and yang, but also promotes the internal generation of heat to further consume yin and essence and aggravate the original state of diseases; on the contrary, the patients with yang deficiency or diseases due to yang deficiency should select sweet, warm-natured and tonic food while addiction to cold-and cool-natured foods unavoidably makes yang deficient and cold even more severe, and the diseases worsened. The same is true of flavor preference. For example, overeating pungent foods may cause fire to consume yin; overeating sweet foods may stagnate the functional activities of qi; overeating salty foods may injure the bone

求,若机体内某一种物质的含量太多或太少,都有可能影响到其他物质的吸收及其作用的发挥。因此,饮食应该提倡科学进食、合理搭配,使各种食物中的营养成分彼此取长补短,相互补充。提倡杂食和轮流交替的饮食方法和全面膳食的思想,对中医养生保健和康复医疗具有重要的指导意义。

食物主要有酸、苦、甘、辛、咸五味,有寒、热、温、凉四性,不同性味的食物,其功能各异,因此在食物选择时,既要结合体质特点,又要考虑病证的性质,不能过于偏嗜某种食物,否则,偏嗜成性,久则必致疾病发生,或不利于疾病的治疗和康复。如素体阴虚或阴虚病证者,应选用甘润或甘凉的食物以养阴清热,若进食或偏嗜温补之品,不仅难以恢复气血阴阳之间的平衡,而且还会因滋补之物助生内热,更加损耗阴精,加重原有病情;相反,若素体阳虚或阳虚病证者,应选用甘温补益之品,偏嗜寒凉之物,势必使阳虚阴寒更甚,病变加深。同样,嗜好五味,如过食辛辣可动火伤阴,过食甘味壅滞气机,过咸伤肾耗气,过于苦燥伤耗胃津,过食酸敛则令肝气郁滞、

and consume qi; overeating bitter foods may dry and consume gastric fluid; overeating sour and astringent foods may make the liver qi stagnated and the spleen qi consumed, etc. Therefore, TCM has been advocating "the balance of the five flavors" since ancient times. Only by balancing the five flavors can the human body take in nutrients in an all-round way and health be enhanced. This is beneficial to the treatment of diseases and the rehabilitation of the body.

4.3 Abstinence from overstrain

Overstrain includes physical overstrain, mental overstrain and sexual overstrain. Strain and rest are relative: strain involves rest; strain combines with relaxation properly. Only when strain integrates with rest, can good health and freedom from diseases or the rehabilitation of the diseased body be guaranteed.

4.3.1 Abstinence from mental overstrain

Mental overstrain refers to excessive mental labor and mental overfatigue. Over-exertion in daily study and work as well as ignorance of proper rest is the main cause of mental overstrain. Besides, mental overstrain may result from the prolonged anxieties due to lack of correct understanding of certain things or phenomena in daily life, inability to meet the desire, failure to solve a problem despite much thought, or poor adaptive capacity to various outside stimulations. It has been clinically proved that long-term mental stress and excessive mental labor are not beneficial to the rehabilitation of diseases such as coronary heart disease, hypertension, cerebrovascular accident, cancer and ulcer. In addition, the exacerbation or deterioration of these diseases is closely related to heavy mental labor and constant overanxiety.

Abstinence from mental overstrain should avoid excessive mental labor during the process of work and study at first. Especially during the rehabilitation and recuperation, people should give up the original work and study to get the brain fully relaxed. Secondly, deal with all the patients correctly. Some patients cannot endure the cruel blow when faced with the lifelong or very harmful diseases such as traumatic paraplegia and cancer. In these cases, they feel unfair and are in the mental state of prolonged anxiety and suffering. As a result, the disease worsens. Medical and nursing staff should straighten out these patients actively and offer psychological treatment to them purposefully. Thirdly, people should approach various unhappy happenings in life correctly. Consider every thing from a long-term point of view, be free from avarice and wild fancy and do not be preoccupied with the personal gains and losses. Finally, people should reasonably arrange various recreational activities to use the brain. These activities should not affect the normal rest. Moreover, people should not be preoccupied with the losing and winning.

4.3.2 Abstinence from physical overstrain

"Running water is never stale and a door-hinge never gets worm-eaten." Physical labor and moderate physical training promote the circulation of qi and blood, improve appetite, enhance physique and are the essential conditions of human existence and preserving good health. However, overlong physical labor or physical training, overburden and ignorance of proper rest may exceed the

为不利，而且这些疾病的加重或恶化，与繁重的脑力劳动、经常性的焦虑过度有着密切的关系。

戒神劳，一是要避免工作和学习过程中的用脑过度。尤其在康复疗养期间，应抛开原有的工作、学习，让大脑得到充分的休息。二是要正确对待所患的疾病。有些病人面对终身性的或危害性大的疾病，如外伤性截瘫、癌症等，承受不住病残的打击，心理严重失衡，长时间处于焦虑、痛苦的心境中，结果使疾病加重。对这类病人，医护人员要给予积极的开导，有针对性地进行心理治疗。三是要正确对待生活中可能发生的各种不愉快的事情，凡事从长远着想，清心寡欲，不斤斤计较个人得失。另外，要合理安排各种用脑的娱乐活动，既不能因此而影响到休息，更不能过于计较输赢。

二、戒体劳

"流水不腐，户枢不蠹"。劳动及适当的体育锻炼，有助于气血流通，增进食欲，增强体质，是人类生存和保持健康的必要条件。但如果劳动或运动的时间过长，负担过重，不注意应有的休息，超过了机

endurance of the organism. As time passes, these factors may make healthy people break down from constant overwork and the patients' diseases worsened. For instance, though the patients with various maims and chronic diseases are badly in need of participation in the physical labor and physical training in their power, they are susceptible to the exacerbation or deterioration of the diseases due to physical overstrain of physique, for these patients generally have poorer endurance of physical labor and training than healthy people. For example, the patients with coronary heart disease and myocarditis themselves have different degrees of muscular ischemia and muscular hypoxia. If they do not limit the amount and duration of their physical labor or physical training to cause overfatigue, this may induce angina pectoris, heart failure, even give rise to sudden death due to overburden of the heart. Take diabetics for another example. The physical overstrain during the treatment is extremely susceptible to hypoglycemic reaction.

The following points should be paid attention to in order that the patients can not only persevere in physical labor or physical training but also avoid physical overstrain. Firstly, the amount of physical labor or physical training should be strictly followed under the guidance of the doctor. Physical labor or physical training should proceed in an orderly way and step by step, from small amount to large amount. Secondly, the types, time, intensity, etc. of physical labor or training should be scientifically selected under the guidance of the medical and nursing staff. It is the best to combine the scientific nature with interesting nature in selecting the types of physical labor or physical training; it is the best to arrange the time in the early morning or one to two hours after the breakfast; the intensity of physical training is always determined by

体的耐受能力，久而久之，就有可能使无病者积劳成疾，有病者疾病加重。如各种伤残和慢性病患者，虽然极需要参加力所能及的劳动及运动，但这类病人对劳动和运动的耐受能力一般较健康人低，很容易因形体过劳而使病情加重或恶化。如冠心病、心肌炎患者本身就有不同程度的心肌缺血缺氧，如果对劳动或运动的量和时间不加限制，过于疲劳，就会因过多增加心脏的负担，诱发心绞痛、心力衰竭，甚至导致突然死亡。又如糖尿病患者，若在治疗期间形劳过度，极易发生低血糖反应。

为了让患者坚持劳动或运动锻炼而又避免体劳过度，必须注意以下问题：一是对劳动或运动的量，应严格遵照医嘱进行。一般应从小到大，循序渐进，逐步增加；二是对劳动或运动种类的选择和运动时间、强度的确定等方面，应以科学的态度，在医护人员的指导下进行。运动的种类最好能科学性和趣味性结合起来，运动的时间以清晨或早饭后1～2小时之后为好；运动强度总以身体感到温热、微微汗出，运动后感到轻松、舒适、

warmth, mild sweating as well as relaxation, comfort, good appetite and sound sleep after the training. Thirdly, the abnormal sensations during the physical labor or training should be instantly reported to the medical and nursing staff such as headache, dizziness, palpitation, declined appetite and poor sleep so as to be noticed. Regular physical examination is conducted to revise the training plan whenever necessary in accordance with the patient's conditions.

4.3.3 Abstinence from sexual overstrain

Sexual overstrain refers to exhaustion due to intemperance in sexual life. Abstinence from sexual overstrain is not only the important measure to preserve health and prevent diseases, but also the objective requirement at the stage of recovery.

Sexual behavior is the human instinct and the important component part of life. From the viewpoint of medicine, moderate sexual life is the physiological and psychological needs of the human body, while celibacy and asceticism are by no means beneficial to health and longevity. But this does not mean overindulgence in sexual life, but temperance should be exercised. Intemperance in sexual life inevitably consumes renal essence, impairs primordial qi and injures the human health.

For the patient's part, he should set aside his worries and have a good rest due to deficiency of essence and qi to supplement qi and restore health. However, overindulgence in sexual life without temperance consumes his essence even more seriously to result in the development of the disease into an incurable one. For instance, the patients with pulmonary tuberculosis suffer from deficiency of yin and essence. Their yin and essence should be nourished. If indulging in sexual life frequently, they are

食欲及睡眠均好为度；三是对劳动或运动过程中出现的异常感觉，如头痛、头晕、心慌、食欲减退、睡眠不好等，应及时向医护人员汇报，引起充分的注意，定期做健康检查，必要时，根据病情，随时修改锻炼计划。

三、戒房劳

房劳，即性生活过度。戒房劳，既是养生防病的重要措施，也是病后康复的客观要求。

性行为是人类的本能，是生活中的重要组成部分。从医学的观点看，适当的性生活是人体生理和心理的需要，独身或禁欲并不利于健康长寿。但也不可纵欲无度，必须有所节制。房事不节制，必然耗伤肾精，损及元气，给人体健康带来损害。

对于患者来说，由于精气亏损，需要静心休养，以使气血得充，体虚得复。若恣情纵欲，房事不节，则更耗其精，则有可能致使疾病发展到无法挽救的地步。比如肺痨患者，素本阴虚精亏，当滋养阴精，若性生活仍不节制，反复泄其精，极易导致病情恶化。再如

extremely susceptible to the deterioration of the disease. Take the renal disease, hypertension and coronary heart disease for examples. These diseases may be aggravated or deteriorated because of indulgence in sexual life as well. In severe cases, indulgence in sexual life even may cause vital crises such as cerebral bleeding and myocardiac infarction. Accordingly, sexual life should be moderated during the daily health care and rehabilitation. In severe cases, sexual life should be stopped for the time being.

4.4 Abstinence from extreme emotional activities

Normal emotional activities are the protective reactions of the organism to the outside irritating factors and harmless to somatopsychic health. Optimistic emotions and being full of vigor are of great significance in maintaining health, eliminating diseases and prolonging life. Nevertheless, extreme emotional activities may turn out to be pathogenic factors, giving rise to the occurrence or the deterioration of diseases. The commonly-seen emotional pathogenic factors fall into two categories. The first category is the great emotional variations, extreme and violent emotional activities like overjoy, fury, sudden terror and great fear. More often, these emotional activities may cause diseases and injure people such as mental diseases due to sudden psychic trauma and abrupt onset of apoplexy due to great anger impairing the liver. The other category is the less extreme emotional variations with long duration like prolonged melancholy, prolonged grief or overanxiety. If such bad states of the mind last long, people are also very susceptible to diseases like neurasthenia, ulcer, hypertension and cancer. The occurrence and development of these diseases are all related to the chronic mental stimulation to a certain extent.

Attention should be mainly paid to the following aspects during life and clinical practice. First, develop good moral cultivation, treat people magnanimously and handle things without seeking fame and wealth. During daily life and work, people should actively create a happy environment, treat others open-mindedly and kindly; properly handle the relationships between neighbors and colleagues; do not seek for fame and wealth; do not worry about personal gains and losses. Only in this way can emotions be stable, qi and blood harmonious. Secondly, overcome the mental pressure due to diseases. Some patients lose their confidence in treating their diseases and are often depressed. Therefore, they may become agitated and furious just for some trifles. As for these patients, the medical and nursing staff should enlist their trust and then help them establish their confidence in defeating the diseases and root out the bad emotions with scientific reasons and specific examples. Thirdly, the medical and nursing staff should try to seek the patients' cooperation and straighten them out with scientific and proper methods as far as the bad emotions are concerned. The methods to regulate emotions include patient-pleasing method, method of checking one emotion with another, suggestion method, and method of straightening out patients, etc.

在生活及临床实践中,戒恼怒、戒抑郁,应当注意以下几个方面：① 培养良好的道德修养,宽以待人,淡泊以待事。在日常的生活和工作中,要主动地去创造欢乐的环境,要心胸宽阔,与人为善,处理好与邻里、同事的关系,不争名利,不患得失,只有这样,才能使情绪稳定,气血调和。② 消除因疾病带来的精神压力。有些患者因为对自己所患的疾病丧失了治疗的信心,常因此而郁郁不乐,或因一些小事就烦躁发怒,对这些病人,医护人员在取得病人信任的前提下,以科学的道理及具体实例,帮助其树立战胜疾病的信心,去除不良情绪产生的根源。③ 对已产生的不良情绪,医护人员必须设法求得患者的合作,采取科学的、适宜的办法进行疏解开导,调节情志的方法如顺情法、情志相胜法、暗示法、开导法等。

5 Examples of TCM Life Cultivation in Accordance with Individual Differences

Human individuals and different groups of people differ greatly from one another in psychology, physiology as well as susceptibility. Accordingly, only when health is preserved on the basis of the individual condition under the guidance of the thought of syndrome differentiation can the TCM life cultivation techniques be brought into full play to prolong life during the life cultivation.

5.1 Constitutional cultivation

Constitution refers to the relatively stable characteristics in morphology, psychology and physiological functions formed during the growth, development and ageing due to the congenital inheritance and the influences of various postnatal factors. These characteristics usually determine the susceptibility of the organism to certain pathogenic factors and the tendency of pathological changes.

There are many ways to divide constitution, of which the ordinary one divides constitution into two types of normal constitution and poor constitution. Normal constitution refers to strong physical power, lustrous complexion, good appetite, sound sleep, smooth urination and defecation, normal pulse condition, freedom from marked tendency of relative excess or deficiency of yin, yang, qi

第五章　因人制宜的养生实例举隅

人类的个体及不同人群之间有着很大的差异，不同的个体（人群）可有不同的心理和生理特征，对疾病的易感性也不尽相同。因此，养生应因人辨证施养，才能最大限度发挥中医养生技术的功效，达到益寿延年的目的。

第一节　体质养生

体质是指人体禀赋于先天，受后天多种因素影响，在其生长发育和衰老过程中，所形成的形态及心理、生理功能上相对稳定的特征，这种特性往往决定着机体对某些致病因素的易感性和病变过程的倾向性。

中医学对体质进行分类的方法很多，一般分为正常体质、不良体质两大类。凡体力强壮、面色润泽、眠食均佳、二便通调，脉象正常、无明显阴阳气血偏盛偏衰倾向者，为正常体质。反之，有明显的阴

and blood. On the contrary, poor constitution means marked tendency of yin deficiency, yang deficiency, qi deficiency, blood deficiency, phlegm and dampness, excess of yang, blood stasis, etc. The life cultivation in poor constitution is as follows.

5.1.1 Constitution with yin deficiency

Constitutional characteristics: Emaciation, facial flush in the afternoon, dry mouth with scanty saliva, occasional vexation, feverish palms and soles, poor sleep, constipation, dark urine, dislike of spring and summer, preference to cold drink, thready and rapid pulse, red tongue with a little fur.

5.1.1.1 Regulating the mind

The people with yin deficiency are impetuous-natured, and often vexed and irascible. Accordingly, they should enhance self-control, argue less with others to avoid being enraged; they should participate less in the competitive recreational activities. Besides, it is also very important to moderate sexual life.

5.1.1.2 Regulating according to the environment

The people with yin deficiency fear heat but like cool. It is easy for them to spend the cold winter but hard to spend the summer heat. Thus, they should pay attention to the prevention of sunstroke. "Nourishing yin in autumn and winter" is more important for the people with yin deficiency, especially, the dry climate in autumn consumes yin more easily. The living environment should be quiet and it is the best to live in the house facing south.

5.1.1.3 Regulating the diet

The principle is to nourish yin and suppress yang. It is advisable to eat bland foods such as sesame, round-grained nonglutinous rice, honey, milk products, sugarcane, vegetable, fruit, bean curd and fishes. Meanwhile,

虚、阳虚、气虚、血虚、痰湿、阳盛、血瘀等倾向的属于不良体质。以下为不良体质的养生：

一、阴虚体质

体质特点：形体消瘦，午后面色潮红，口干少津，心中时烦，手足心热，少眠，便干，尿黄，不耐长夏，多喜冷饮，脉细数，舌红少苔。

1. 精神调养

阴虚体质之人性情急躁，常常心烦易怒，应加强自我涵养，少与人争，以减少激怒；要少参加争胜负的文娱活动。此外，节制性生活也很重要。

2. 环境调摄

阴虚者畏热喜凉，冬寒易过，夏热难受。因此，夏季应注意避暑。"秋冬养阴"对阴虚体质之人更为重要，特别是秋季气候干燥，更易伤阴。居室环境应安静，最好住坐北朝南的房子。

3. 饮食调养

原则是滋阴潜阳，宜食芝麻、元米、蜂蜜、乳品、甘蔗、蔬菜、水果、豆腐、鱼类等清淡食物，并食用沙参粥、百合粥、枸

it is suitable to drink Gruel of Shashen (*Radix Adenophorae*), Gruel of Baihe (*Bulbus Lilii*), Gruel of Gouqizi (*Fructus Lycii*), Gruel of Sangshen (*Fructus Mori*) and Gruel of Shanyao (*Rhizoma Dioscoreae*). If the conditions permit, these people may eat edible bird's nest, tremella, sea cucumber, mussel, tortoise meat, crab meat, Chinese caterpillar fungus, and old male duck, etc. However, they should eat less pungent and hot-natured things like green Chinese onion, ginger, garlic, chives, macrostem onion and hot pepper.

5.1.1.4　Physical training

The strenuous exercise is not advisable while Taijiquan, eight-section brocade, etc. are more suitable.

5.1.1.5　Life cultivation with drugs

Drugs of nourishing yin, clearing away heat, nourishing the liver and kidney may be selected such as Nüzhenzi (*Fructus Ligustri Lucidi*), Shanzhuyu (*Fructus Corni*), Wuweizi (*Fructus Schisandrae*), Hanliancao (*Herba Ecliptae*), Maimendong (*Radix Ophiopogonis*), Tianmendong (*Radix Asparagi*), Huangjing (*Rhizoma Polygonati*), Yuzhu (*Rhizoma Polygonati Odorati*), Xuanshen (*Radix Scrophulariae*), Gouqizi (*Fructus Lycii*), Sangshenzi (*Fructus Mori*) and Guiban (*Carapax et Plastrum Testudinis*). Constitution with yin deficiency can be further divided into constitution with deficiency of the kidney yin, constitution with deficiency of the liver yin, constitution with deficiency of the lung yin, constitution with deficiency of the heart yin, etc. For instance, in the case of deficiency of the lung yin, Baihe Gujin Decoction (Lily Decoction for Strengthening the Lung) is advisable; in the case of deficiency of the heart yin, Tianwang Buxin Decoction (Cardiotonic Decoction) is advisable; in the case of deficiency of the spleen yin, Shenrou Yangzhen Decoction is advisable; in the case

杞子粥、桑椹子粥、怀山药粥。条件许可者，可食用燕窝、银耳、海参、淡菜、龟肉、蟹肉、冬虫夏草、老雄鸭等。对于葱、姜、蒜、韭、薤、椒等辛辣燥烈之品则应少吃。

4．体育锻炼

不宜过激活动，太极拳、八段锦等较为适合。

5．药物养生

可选用滋阴清热、滋养肝肾之品，如女贞子、山茱萸、五味子、旱莲草、麦门冬、天门冬、黄精、玉竹、玄参、枸杞子、桑椹子、龟版等。常用中药方剂有六味地黄丸、大补阴丸等。阴虚体质又有肾阴虚、肝阴虚、肺阴虚、心阴虚等不同，如肺阴虚，宜服百合固金汤；心阴虚，宜服天王补心丸；脾阴虚，宜服慎柔养真汤；肾阴虚，宜服六味地黄丸；肝阴虚，宜服一贯煎。

of deficiency of the kidney yin, Liuwei Dihuang Pill (Bolus of Six Drugs In cluding Rehmanni) is advisable; in the case of deficiency of the liver yin, Yiguan Decoction (An Ever Effective Decoction for Nourishing the Liver and Kidney) is advisable.

5.1.2　Constitution with yang deficiency

Constitutional characteristics: White and fat physique, or pale complexion, aversion to cold and preference to warmth, cold hands and feet, clear and profuse urine, occasional loose stool, pale lips, frequent spontaneous sweating, deep pulse, hypodynamia, enlarged tongue with pale color.

5.1.2.1　Regulating the mind

The people with deficiency of yang mostly manifest bad emotions. For instance, the people with yang deficiency of the liver are susceptible to fear while the people with yang deficiency of the heart are susceptible to grief. These people should properly regulate their emotions to eliminate or reduce the influences of bad emotions.

5.1.2.2　Regulating according to the environment

The people with yang deficiency have poor ability to adapt themselves to the changes of cold and heat. They feel too cold to endure when it turns slightly cool. Therefore, they should "avoid cold and approach warmth" in winter while they should strengthen yang in spring and summer. These people may take sunbath for 20 to 30 times, 15 to 20 minutes each time in summer. But they can not sleep in the open and should avoid being directly fanned to prevent "wind disorders" like numbness of hands and feet, hemiplegia or facial paralysis.

5.1.2.3　Physical training

These people should persevere in physical training, once or twice a day. They can select the events accord-

二、阳虚体质

体质特点：形体白胖，或面色淡白，平素畏寒喜暖，手足欠温，小便清长，大便时稀，唇淡口和，常自汗出，脉沉乏力，舌淡胖。

1. 精神调养

阳气不足者常表现出情绪不佳，如肝阳虚者善恐、心阳虚者善悲。应妥善调节自己的感情，消除或减少不良情绪的影响。

2. 环境调摄

阳虚者适应寒暑变化之能力差，稍微转凉，即觉冷不可受。因此，冬季要"避寒就温"，春夏之季要培补阳气。可在夏季进行20～30次日光浴，每次15～20分钟。但切不可在室外露宿，睡眠时不要让电扇直吹，以防手足麻木不遂或面瘫等"风痹"病的发生。

3. 体育锻炼

要坚持体育锻炼，每日1～2次。项目酌情选择散步、

ingly such as taking a walk, jogging, Taijiquan, five mimic-animal games, eight-section brocade, ball games and various dance activities. They may take sunbath and air bath as well.

5.1.2.4 Regulating the diet

More foods of strengthening yang should be eaten like mutton, dog meat, venison and chicken. Fuzi (*Radix Aconiti Praeparata*) Gruel or Yangrou Fuzi Soup (Soup of Mutton and Radix Aconiti Praeparata) may be eaten once in every ten dog days of the three ten-day periods of the hot season according to the principle of "nourishing yang in spring and summer".

5.1.2.5 Life cultivation with drugs

The people with yang deficiency may select drugs of strengthening yang to remove cold, warming and tonifying the liver and kidney. The commonly-used ones include Lurong (*Cornu Cervi Pantotrichum*), Haigoushen (*Peni et Testes Callorhini*), Gejie (*Gecko*), Dongchongxiacao (*Cordyceps*), Bajitian (*Radix Morindae Officinalis*), Yinyanghuo (*Herba Epimedii*), Xianmao (*Rhizoma Curculigins*), Roucongrong (*Herba Cistanchis*), Buguzhi (*Fructus Psoraleae*), Hutao (*Semen Juglandis*), Duzhong (*Cortex Eucommiae*), Xuduan (*Radix Dipsaci*), and Tusizi (*Semen Cuscutae*), etc. These people may select the prescriptions of Jinkui Shenqi Pill, Yougui Bolus (Bolus for Reinforcing the Kidney Yang) and Quanlu Pill. In the case of marked yang deficiency of the heart, Guizhi Gancao Decoction (Decoction of Cinnamon Twig and Liquorice) with Rougui (*Cortex Cinnamomi*) may be often taken while in the case of severe yang deficiency of the heart, Renshen (*Radix Ginseng*) may be added; in the case of marked yang deficiency of the spleen, Lizhong Pill (Pill for Regulating Middle Energizer) or Fuzi Lizhong Pill (Pill of Aconite for Regulating

慢跑、太极拳、五禽戏、八段锦、球类活动和各种舞蹈活动等,亦可常作日光浴、空气浴。

4. 饮食调养

多食有壮阳作用的食品,如羊肉、狗肉、鹿肉、鸡肉。根据"春夏养阳"的法则,夏日三伏,每伏可食附子粥或羊肉附子汤1次。

5. 药物养生

选用补阳祛寒、温养脾肾之品,常用药物有鹿茸、海狗肾、蛤蚧、冬虫夏草、巴戟天、淫羊藿、仙茅、肉苁蓉、补骨脂、胡桃、杜仲、续断、菟丝子等。方剂可选用金匮肾气丸、右归丸、全鹿丸。若偏心阳虚者,常服桂枝甘草汤加肉桂,虚甚者可加人参;若偏脾阳虚者,选择理中丸,或附子理中丸;脾肾两虚者可用济生肾气丸。

Middle Energizer) may be selected; in the case of asthenia of both the spleen and kidney, Jisheng Shenqi Pill (Life-Preserving Pill for Strengthening the Kidney Qi) may be selected.

5.1.3 Constitution with qi deficiency

Constitutional characteristics: Emaciation or relatively fat physique, pale complexion, low and timid voice, frequent spontaneous sweating worsened by moving, tiredness, amnesia, pale tongue with whitish fur, feeble and weak pulse.

5.1.3.1 Regulating the diet

The people with qi deficiency may regularly eat round-grained nonglutinous rice, polished glutinous rice, wheat, millet, glutinous millet, barley, Chinese yam, polished long-grained nonglutinous rice, naked oats, potato, jujube, carrot, Xianggu mushroom, bean curb, chicken, goose meat, hare meat, quail, beef, dogmeat, black carp and silver carp. In the case of severe qi deficiency, the prescription of dietary therapy "Renshen Lianrou Soup" (Soup of Ginseng and Lotus Seed) should be selected for tonification.

5.1.3.2 Life cultivation with drugs

It is advisable to take Jinkui Shuyu Pill regularly. In the case of qi deficiency of the spleen, Sijunzi Decoction (Decoction of Four Noble Ingredients) or Shenling Baizhu Powder (Powder of Ginseng, Poria and Bighead Atractylodes) is advisable; in the case of qi deficiency of the lung, Lung-Tonifying Decoction is advisable; in the case of qi deficiency of the kidney, more Shenqi Bolus (Bolus for Strengthening the Kidney Qi) should be taken.

5.1.4 Constitution with blood deficiency

Constitutional characteristics: Pale and lustreless or

三、气虚体质

体质特点：形体消瘦或偏胖，面色㿠白，语声低怯，常自汗出，动则尤甚，体倦健忘，舌淡苔白，脉虚弱。

1. 饮食调养

可常食粳米、元米、小米、黄米、大麦、怀山药、籼米、莜麦、马铃薯、大枣、胡萝卜、香菇、豆腐、鸡肉、鹅肉、兔肉、鹌鹑、牛肉、狗肉、青鱼、鲢鱼。若气虚甚，当选用人参莲肉汤以食疗补养。

2. 药物养生

宜常服金匮薯蓣丸。脾气虚，宜选四君子汤，或参苓白术散；肺气虚，宜选补肺汤；肾气虚，多服肾气丸。

四、血虚体质

体质特点：面色苍白无华

5 Examples of TCM Life Cultivation in Accordance with Individual Differences

sallow complexion, pale lips, failure to endure physical labor, susceptibility to insomnia, pale tongue and thready pulse without force.

5.1.4.1 Regulating the mind

The people with blood deficiency often have low spirits, insomnia, amnesia and distraction. Therefore, they should inspire their enthusiasm. They may appreciate music and dramas, watch humorous Xiaopin (humorous performance), etc.

5.1.4.2 Regulating the diet

The foods of supplementing and tonifying blood may be regularly taken such as mulberry, litchi, pine nut, black edible fungus, spinach, carrot, pork, mutton, cattle liver, sheep liver, soft-shelled turtle, sea cucumber and butterfish.

5.1.4.3 Life cultivation with drugs

People with blood deficiency may often take Danggui Buxue Decoction (Chinese Angelica Decoction for Replenishing Blood), Siwu Decoction (Decoction of Four Ingredients), or Guipi Decoction (Decoction for Invigorating the Spleen and Nourishing the heart). In the case of deficiency of both qi and blood, qi and blood should be both tonified. The selected prescriptions include Bazhen Decoction (Decoction of Eight Precious Ingredients), Shiquan Dabu Decoction (Decoction of Ten Powerful Tonics), or Renshen Yangrong Decoction (Ginseng Nutrition Decoction). The above prescriptions may be also changed into the dosage form of pill for prolonged administration.

5.1.4.4 Regulating daily life

"Prolonged use of eyes consumes blood." Accordingly, overuse of eyes or mental overstrain should be avoided.

5.1.5 Constitution with excessive yang

Constitutional characteristics: Sturdy physique,

或萎黄,唇色淡白,不耐劳作,易失眠,舌质淡,脉细无力。

1. 精神调养

血虚者时常精神不振、失眠、健忘、注意力不集中,故应振奋精神。可以欣赏音乐、戏剧,观赏幽默小品等。

2. 饮食调养

常食有补血养血的作用的桑椹子、荔枝、松子、黑木耳、菠菜、胡萝卜、猪肉、羊肉、牛肝、羊肝、甲鱼、海参、鲳鱼等食物。

3. 药物养生

可常服当归补血汤、四物汤,或归脾汤。若气血两虚,则须气血双补,选八珍汤、十全大补汤或人参养荣汤,亦可改汤为丸长久服用。

4. 起居调摄

"久视伤血",不可过用目力,亦不可劳心过度。

五、阳盛体质

体质特点:形体壮实,面

flushed complexion, loud voice and breathing, preference to cool with aversion to hotness, preference to cold drink, dark and feverish urine and foul stool.

5.1.5.1 Regulating the mind

The people with excessive yang are susceptible to movement and irascibility. Therefore, they should enhance self-cultivation of morality and temper their will-power in daily life and cultivate good personality. They should control themselves consciously and overcome the emotional impulse rationally when encountered with things exasperating.

5.1.5.2 Physical training

Fishing, playing the game of go, etc. are the first events to be selected. In addition, swimming and Taijiquan may be selected according to personal hobbies.

5.1.5.3 Regulating the diet

The people with excessive yang should abstain from pungent, hot-natured and dry-natured foods like hot pepper, ginger and Chinese green onion, eat less warm-natured and yang-natured foods like beef, dog meat, chicken and venison, eat more cool-natured fruits and vegetables such as banana, water melon, persimmon, bitter gourd, tomato and lotus root. They should abstain from excessive drinking.

5.1.5.4 Life cultivation with drugs

Soak Juhua (*Flos Chrysanthemi*) and Kudingcha (*Herba Lactucae Taiwanianae*) in boiling water for oral administration at ordinary times. In the case of constipation, Maziren Pill (Sesame Pill) or Runchang Pill (Bowel-Loosening Pill) may be used; in the case of dry mouth and tongue, Maimendong Decoction (Ophiopogon Decoction) may be used; in the case of vexation and irascibility, Danzhi Xiaoyao Powder (Ease Powder of Moutan Bark and Cape Jasmine Fruit) may be used.

赤声高气粗,喜凉怕热,喜冷饮,小便热赤,大便秽臭为其特点。

1. 精神调养

阳盛之人好动易发怒,故平日要加强道德修养和意志锻炼,培养良好的性格,有意识控制自己,遇到可怒之事,用理性克服情感上的冲动。

2. 体育锻炼

垂钓、围棋等是首选项目。此外,游泳、太极拳,也可根据爱好选择进行。

3. 饮食调理

忌辛辣燥烈食物,如辣椒、姜、葱等,少食牛肉、狗肉、鸡肉、鹿肉等温阳食物。可多食凉性水果、蔬菜,如香蕉、西瓜、柿子、苦瓜、番茄、莲藕。戒酗酒。

4. 药物调养

常用菊花、苦丁茶沸水泡服。大便干燥者,用麻子仁丸,或润肠丸;口干舌燥者,用麦门冬汤;心烦易怒者,宜服丹栀逍遥散。

5.1.6 Constitution with blood stasis

Constitutional characteristics: Dim and sluggish complexion, dark lips and eye sockets, dry skin, purple tongue or with petechiae, thready and unsmooth pulse.

5.1.6.1 Regulating the mind

People with blood stasis should develop optimism. In the case of a cheerful frame of mind, qi and blood flow harmoniously, nutrient qi and defensive qi circulate smoothly. This is beneficial to the improvement of constitution with blood stasis. Conversely, depression and melancholy may aggravate the tendency of blood stasis.

5.1.6.2 Regulating the diet

People with blood stasis may often eat the foods of activating blood circulation to remove blood stasis such as walnut, rape, arrowhead and black soybean. They may often drink a bit of spirit and a proper amount of vinegar. The medicated diet includes Haw Gruel and Peanut Gruel.

5.1.6.3 Life cultivation with drugs

The drugs of promoting blood circulation and tonifying blood may be selected like Dihuang (*Radix Rehmanniae*), Danshen (*Radix Salviae Miltiorrhizae*), Chuanxiong (*Rhizoma Ligustici Chuanxiong*), Danggui (*Radix Angelicae Sinensis*), Wujiapi (*Cortex Acanthopancis Radicis*), Diyu (*Radix Sanguisorbae*), Xuduan (*Radix Dipsaci*) and Chongweizi (*Semen Leonuri*).

5.1.6.4 Physical training

Participating in physical training moderately is beneficial to promoting blood circulation and activating collaterals such as various dances, Taijiquan and eight-section brocade.

5.1.7 Constitution with phlegm and dampness

Constitutional characteristics: Fat physique, muscular

六、血瘀体质

体质特点：面色晦滞，口唇色暗，眼眶暗黑，肌肤干燥，舌紫暗或有瘀点，脉细涩。

1. 精神调养

培养乐观的情绪。精神愉快则气血和畅，营卫流通，有利血瘀体质的改善。反之，苦闷、忧郁则可加重血瘀倾向。

2. 饮食调理

常食桃仁、油菜、慈姑、黑大豆等具有活血祛瘀作用的食物，可经常少量饮酒，适量食醋。药膳可选山楂粥、花生粥。

3. 药物养生

选用地黄、丹参、川芎、当归、五加皮、地榆、续断、茺蔚子等活血养血之品。

4. 体育锻炼

适当运动锻炼，有利于活血通脉，如各种舞蹈、太极拳、八段锦等。

七、痰湿体质

体质特点：形体肥胖，肌

relaxation, addiction to fatty and sweet foods, listlessness with heavy sensation of the body, disinclination to move, lethargy, sticky and greasy sensation in the mouth, or loose stool, soft and slippery pulse, enlarged tongue with slippery and greasy fur.

5.1.7.1　Regulating according to the environment

Avoid living and working in the damp environment.

5.1.7.2　Regulating the diet

Eat less fat, sweet and fine foods, drink less all kinds of spirit and do not overeat. More foods of strengthening the spleen to remove dampness, eliminating phlegm and dampness may be eaten such as radish, water chest nut, laver, jellyfish, onion, loquat, ginkgo, jujube, hyacinth bean, coix seed, red bean, broad bean and cabbage.

5.1.7.3　Physical training

The people with phlegm and dampness mostly are fat, heavy and easily tired. Accordingly, they should persist in physical training. They may select taking a walk, jogging, ball games, Wushu (martial arts), eight-section brocade, five mimic-animal games as well as various dances. The amount of exercise should be gradually increased.

5.1.7.4　Life cultivation with drugs

Phlegm and dampness are closely related to the three zang organs of the lung, spleen and kidney. If the lung fails to disperse and descend, body fluids will not be transported and distributed, giving rise to phlegm generated from the accumulated body fluids. In this case, Erchen Decoction (Decoction of Two Old Drugs) is selected to disperse the lung and resolve phlegm. If the spleen fails to transport, the accumulated dampness will turn into phlegm. On this occasion, Liujunzi Decoction (Decoction

肉松弛,嗜食肥甘,神倦身重,懒动,嗜睡,口中粘腻,或便溏,脉濡而滑,舌体胖,苔滑腻。

1. 环境调摄

避免在潮湿环境中生活和工作。

2. 饮食调理

少食肥甘厚味,酒类也不宜多饮,食勿过饱。可多食白萝卜、荸荠、紫菜、海蜇、洋葱、枇杷、白果、大枣、扁豆、薏苡仁、赤小豆、蚕豆、包菜等具有健脾利湿,化痰祛湿的食物。

3. 体育锻炼

痰湿者多形体肥胖,身重易倦,故应坚持体育锻炼,散步、慢跑、球类、武术、八段锦、五禽戏,以及各种舞蹈,均可选择。活动量应逐渐增强。

4. 药物养生

痰湿与肺脾肾三脏关系最为密切,若因肺失宣降,津失输布,液聚生痰者,选用二陈汤宣肺化痰;若因脾不健运,湿聚成痰者,选用六君子汤或香砂六君子汤健脾化痰;若肾虚不能制水,水泛为痰者,选用金匮肾气丸温阳化痰。

of Six Ingredients) or Xiangsha Liujunzi Decoction (Decoction of Cyperus and Amomum with Six Ingredients) is selected to strengthen the spleen and resolve phlegm. If the asthenic kidney fails to check water, the excessive water will transform into phlegm. Under this circumstances, Jinkui Shenqi Pill is selected to warm yang and resolve phlegm.

5.1.8 Constitution with qi depression

Constitutional characteristics: Emaciation or relatively fat physique, dim or sallow complexion, occasional impetuosity and irascibility, susceptibility to excitement, occasional melancholy, choking sensation and discomfort in chest, occasional inclination to sighing, reddish tongue with pale fur and taut pulse.

5.1.8.1 Regulating the mind

The people with qi stagnation are introverted and liable to melancholy. According to the principle "Joy checks melancholy", they should seek for joy actively, participate in more social activities and collective recreational activities, watch more comedies and dramas, but should not watch tragedies. Besides, they may listen to more light, cheerful and lively music.

5.1.8.2 Physical training

Sports and traveling activities can both exercise the body, promote the circulation of qi and blood. Thus, it is advisable for these people to take part in more such activities.

5.1.8.3 Regulating the diet

They may drink a small quantity of spirit to dredge blood vessels and eat more food of promoting qi flow such as fingered citron, orange, mandarin orange peel, buckwheat, chives, fennel, garlic, ham, Chinese sorghum, sword bean and Chinese toon.

八、气郁体质

体质特点：形体消瘦或偏胖，面色苍暗或萎黄，时或性情急躁易怒，易于激动，时或忧郁寡欢，胸闷不舒，时欲叹息，舌淡红、苔白、脉弦。

1．精神调摄

气郁者性格内向，常抑郁，根据"喜胜忧"的原则，应主动寻求快乐，多参加社会活动，集体文娱活动，常看喜剧、滑稽剧等，不要看悲苦剧目，多听轻松、开朗、明快的音乐。

2．体育锻炼

体育和旅游活动均能运动身体，流通气血，宜多参加。

3．饮食调养

可少量饮酒，以疏通血脉。多食佛手、橙子、柑皮、荞麦、韭菜、茴香菜、大蒜、火腿、高粱、刀豆、香橼等行气食物。

5.1.8.4 Life cultivation with drugs

The drugs of soothing the liver, regulating qi flow and relieving depression are commonly used such as Xiangfu (*Rhizoma Cyperi*), Wuyao (*Radix Linderae*), Chuanlianzi (*Fructus Meliae Toosendan*), Xiaohuixiang (*Fructus Foeniculi*), Qingpi (*Pericarpium Citri Reticulatae Viride*) and Yujin (*Radix Curcumae*). The prescriptions like Yueju Pill (Pill for Relieving Stagnancy) may be selected. The drugs of promoting blood circulation to remove blood stasis may be used to make up a prescription in the case of blood stasis due to qi stagnation.

5.2 Life cultivation in the pregnant women

The health status of the pregnant woman directly influences the development, inheritance as well as the lifelong health and life span of the fetus. Improper health preservation may give rise to retarded growth of the fetus, abortion or susceptibility to diseases in the pregnant woman, abnormal inheritance of the fetus, and more often congenital diseases and prenatal deformities.

5.2.1 Prenatal conditioning

Prenatal conditioning means that the enhancement of mental, moral and dispositional cultivation provides the pregnant woman with a comfortable and happy environment and state of mind to exert a favorable effect on the fetus and promote the fetal intelligence development during the pregestational, gestational and productive periods.

5.2.1.1 Keeping sanguine and open-minded

The pregnant woman should be broad-minded and sanguine, free from selfish ideas, without worrying about personal gains and losses; she should be content with her lot in life, generous to people, pleased to help others, free from jealousy, dignified and easy in words, deeds and behavior. In this way, the fetus can have favorable inheritance and it is helpful to the development of the good fetal disposition and character.

5.2.1.2 Cultivating temperament

The pregnant woman may participate in the local recreational and sports activities to a proper degree, develop interest and hobbies in various fields to enrich her life. Besides, she may mould her temperament by means of playing a musical instrument, playing chess, practicing calligraphy and painting, reciting poems, and traveling, etc.

Excessive emotional tension during the gestational period may cause hypercorticoidism and fetal developmental deformity. Excessive emotional tension or anxiety gives rise to severe fetal movement. After birth, the fetus is often liable to restlessness, rage, irritation and cry. Accordingly, various measures should be taken to regulate the pregnant woman's emotions.

5.2.1.3 Avoiding evil things

TCM holds that frequent contact with beautiful things may beautify the fetus. Therefore, the pregnant woman should avoid bad stimulations like obscene and evil things, violence, killing and ugliness so as not to affect the fetal development.

5.2.1.4 Fetal education

The guidance in the fetal sensory function and action should be instantly performed step by step in a planned way to promote the development of infantile intelligence and behavior during the best developmental period of the function of the fetal sensory system. For example, 13 weeks after the gestation, planned speaking and recitation of poems are kept for the fetus; singing songs and playing

乐,处事无妒忌之心,言行举止端庄大方。这样胎儿禀气纯正,有助于良好气质与性格特征的形成。

2. 怡情养性

可适当地参加文体活动,培养多方面的兴趣和爱好,以丰富自己的生活,通过琴棋书画、诵读诗歌及旅游等途径陶冶情操。

孕期情绪过度紧张,会使肾上腺皮质激素分泌过多,引起胎儿发育畸形。情绪过于紧张或焦虑则胎动剧烈,胎儿出生后也往往多动,容易激怒,好哭闹。所以要采用各种措施调节孕妇情绪。

3. 远避邪恶

中医认为,多接触美好的事物,可使秀气入胎,回避淫邪、行凶、丑陋等不良刺激,以免影响胎儿发育。

4. 胎儿辅导

应在胎儿感觉系统功能发展的最佳期,及时对胎儿进行有计划、有步骤的感觉功能与动作辅导,有助于出生婴儿智力与行为的发展。如:从妊娠的第 13 周开始,坚持有计划地对胎儿说话、诵读诗歌,

tapes may be arranged to let the fetus listen to the melodious and beautiful music or songs. Apart from these, the mother's sounds of talking and laughing with others, the bird's singing, the insect's singing and the murmuring stream in a forest are all the good information to promote the development of the fetal auditognosis and nervous system. Researches have found that if the pregnant woman often listens to lively and sweet music, the fetus will be less restless and grow and develop well; if the pregnant woman is usually exposed to the noisy and deafening rock and roll music, the fetus will be more restless.

Every night before bed time, lying in the bed, the pregnant woman put her hands on her abdomen and strokes the fetus to promote the fetal movement. This can arouse the initiative of fetal movement to let the fetus receive earlier training in standing and walking than the untrained fetus. This method is advisable for regular use and it is more important during the gestational period. But it is contraindicated in the pregnant woman with early uterine contraction.

5.2.2 Regulating the diet

The pregnant woman's diet should be fresh, bland, nutritious, light, and moderate in amount.

First trimester of pregnancy (three months since conception): Small amount of fine diet is advisable due to the slow fetal development as well as the reaction of pregnancy. The pregnant woman may select the food suitable for her taste and slightly sour orectic food, fresh vegetables and fruits being the best ones. However, the fishy, pungent and irritative foods should be contraindicated to avoid aggravating the vomiting of pregnancy.

Second trimester of pregnancy (four to seven months

in pregnancy): The fetus grows fast. Ingestion of food rich in protein, calcium and phosphorus is advisable for the pregnant woman. Paddy, beans, meat, fish and eggs contain rich proteins. Calcium exists in yolk, milk, dried small shrimps, animal skeletons and green leafy vegetables; phosphorus in soybean, chicken and mutton. Eating these foods can promote tissue growth, strengthen the bone, benefit marrow, tonify the brain to promote the fetal development.

Third trimester of pregnancy (eight to ten months in pregnancy): The fetal growth and development accelerate. This is the crucial period for the cerebral development. Thus, more nutrients should be stored. The pregnant woman should eat more fine proteins, pay attention to a proper proportion of animal protein and vegetable protein, eat less salt and basic food to prevent edema. The pregnant woman should avoid irritative foods like hot pepper, sensitized foods like crab meat, and river deer and hare. It is advisable for her to give up smoking, drinking spirit and strong tea in case abortion, premature labor, dead fetus, monster and congenital diseases should occur.

5.2.3　Living a normal daily life

After conception, exogenous pathogenic factors easily invade the pregnant woman, giving rise to various fetal diseases, even abortion. Thus, the pregnant woman should live a normal daily life with caution and arrange the daily schedule scientifically. She should rise early and go to bed early, and work, study and live regularly. Besides, she should modify her clothing to prevent cold and summer-heat in conformity to seasonal variations.

The strenuous exercise is not advisable for the pregnant woman. *Chan Yun Ji*, or *Collection of Labour and*

Pregnancy, puts forth "The pregnant woman should not climb high, walk fast, sit in a lateral position, bend over, limp along, lean against something, take an object from a high place, defecate and urinate in the out of-the-way places, stand, sit and lie long, expose herself to cold and heat." The pregnant woman should be cautious not to hit the abdomen, avoid being exposed to noxious substances like lead, mercury, benzol and arsenic as well as radioactive rays. It is not advisable for her to visit public places often to prevent infectious diseases causing the fetal injury or abortion.

The pregnant woman should maintain smooth defecation and urination. In the case of constipation without remission or dysuria, she should go to see a doctor in time.

5.2.4 Proper balance between work and rest

The pregnant woman should moderate her work and rest. "The pregnant woman should not have overrest, for overrest causes qi stagnation; the pregnant woman should not have overstrain, for overstrain results in qi deficiency." A proper amount of movement is beneficial to the fetal development and can prevent dystocia as well.

The pregnant woman can only do ordinary house work, but can not move and lift heavy objects due to the reaction of pregnancy at the early stage of pregnancy. Working at night and undertaking heavy physical labor are both not advisable. She should often go outdoors to take a walk, breathe in fresh air and receive sunlight.

At the stage of midpregnancy, the pregnant woman should not have overrest, but should undertake a certain amount of physical labor and a proper amount of exercise like Taijiquan and traveling. Nevertheless, she should avoid strenuous exercises such as riding a horse, cycling, swimming and running.

用力,毋疾行,毋侧坐,毋曲腰,毋跛倚、毋高处取物,毋向非常处大小便,毋久立久坐,毋久卧、毋犯寒热"。谨防碰撞腹部,避免接触铅、汞、苯、砷等有害物质和放射线辐射,不宜经常往来于公共场所,以防患传染病,导致伤胎或流产。

孕妇应保持二便通畅,若便秘不得缓解或排尿困难,应及时去医院治疗。

四、劳逸适度

孕妇应劳逸适度,"不可过逸,逸则气滞;不可过劳,劳则气衰"。适当运动有利于胎儿发育,还可避免难产。

孕早期,由于妊娠反应,只可做一般的家务劳动,切勿搬抬、举重。晚间操作、重体力劳动均不适宜。应常出户外散步,呼吸新鲜空气,接受阳光。

妊娠中期,不可过于安逸,应从事一定的体力劳动和适量的运动,如太极拳、旅游等,但应避免骑马、骑自行车、游泳、跑步等剧烈运动。

At the late stage of pregnancy, rest is mainly advisable. However, the pregnant woman should not oversleep with indulgence in it. She may take a walk regularly and have the proper exercise to await the right time for labor.

The pregnant woman should have sufficient sleeping time of 8 hours each night. This should be guaranteed. At the late stage of pregnancy, she should have bed rest of an hour at noon. The sleeping time should be further increased and the left lateral position assumed in sleeping several weeks before the parturient time.

5.2.5 Abstinence from sexual life

The pregnant woman should be free from avarice and wild fancy and recuperate quietly in a separate room away from her husband. Sexual life should be particularly forbidden at the early stage of pregnancy and three months at the prenatal period. Otherwise, it may give rise to fetal toxicosis, vaginal bleeding during pregnancy and abortion.

5.2.6 Using drugs with caution

Drugs should not be recklessly used so as to prevent the fetal injury if the pregnant woman is not ill; excessive administration of tonics may lead to dystocia due to oversized fetus. If the pregnant woman suffers from a disease, she should receive treatment as soon as possible. She should not only be fettered by the contraindications of administration in pregnancy, but also deal with them with caution. Some western medicines affect the fetus greatly such as diazepam, aspirin, tetracycline and antiepileptic. These drugs are not used in general. They should be administrated according to the doctor's advice.

5.3 Health care for children

Childhood refers to the stage from birth to the age of 12. The health preservation includes all the health measures from birth to school age, the characteristics of which attach equal importance to bringing up and education to preserve renal yang, the target of which is to educate the child to become a useful person.

Children are at the primary stage of growth and development. Physiologically, they are not only vigorous, but also insufficient in physique and qi. Due to weak body resistance against diseases, they are subject to diseases and the diseases develop fast. Because of the imperfect development in psychology, children are liable to be frightened, which gives rise to diseases. They are not emotionally stable. Besides, children have great plasticity and are easy to receive various influences and education.

5.3.1 Early education

The early education includes education of moral integrity, cultivation of healthy psychology, development of intelligence, health and aesthetics education.

Premature and abstruse education or instruction affects the child's health while delayed and plain education or instruction may postpone and affect, even hinder the child's development. The period from two to three years of age is the crucial stage for children to develop oral language and counting ability; the period from birth to four years of age is the critical stage to develop morphological perception; the period from four to five years of age is the key stage to study written language; the period from five to six years of age is the vital stage to master vocabulary with the quickest speed as well as the vital age to develop

第三节　少儿保健

从出生到12岁为少儿期。少儿养生，包括自出生至学龄期的一切保健措施。其特点是养教并重，以保养元真，教子成才为目标。

少儿处于生长发育的初期，在生理上，既有生机蓬勃的一面，又有形气未充的一面。其抗病力低下，易于发病，病情发展迅速。小儿的心理发育也未臻完善，易受惊吓致病，情志不稳，可塑性大，易于接受各方面的影响和教育。

一、早期教育

早期教育包括德行教育与健康心理的培养、智力开发、健康教育和美学教育。

教育过早过深有损孩子的健康，教育过晚过浅，会推迟、耽误甚至阻碍幼童的成长。2~3岁是儿童口头语言及计数能力发展的关键期；出生到4岁是形状知觉发展的关键期；4~5岁是开始学习书面语言的关键期；5~6岁是掌握词汇能力发展最快，又是数字概念发展的关键年龄。教育与训练的内容与要求，应与

digital concept. The content and requirement of education and training should be suited to the speed of the child's development. A large number of activities to learn characters and calculation are not generally advisable for children below five years old. The above-mentioned opportunities should be appropriately seized at the right time. Only in this way can the best effects be achieved.

5.3.2 Reasonable diet

Breast milk is the ideal natural food before the age of six months. Without breast milk, artificial feeding may be adopted with milk powder substitutes like milk, goat's milk, naigao (a baby food made of rice-flour, sugar, etc.) and soya-bean milk, of which fresh milk is the first choice.

Children are susceptible to calciprivia. The daily requirement of calcium for normal people is 800 mg. Nevertheless, the ordinary diet contains only 500 mg or so in general. If the children drink a bag of milk a day, the requirement can be met. After the Second World War, the Japanese government has supplied a bag of milk for every middle and primary school student every day free of charge. For many years, one generation of Japanese has surpassed another in height. The Japanese call this "One bag of milk vitalizes a nation". The British experts have been observing for 15 years on end and discovered that the children who drink one bag of milk a day are 2.8 cm taller than those children who do not drink. If children drink two bags of milk, they are 4.8 cm taller.

The secretion of growth hormone takes place at night. Thus, it is best for children to drink milk before bed time.

The food at the different stages of age should be sufficient in nutrition and suited to and promote the child's development. This is the principle.

Children are insufficient in the kidney qi, their teeth, skeleton and cerebral marrow are all under development. Thus, the supply of kidney-tonifying foods should not be ignored such as animal liver, kidney and cerebral marrow as well as Hetaoren (*Semen Juglandis*), Heizhima (*Semen Sesami*), Sangshenzi (*Fructus Mori*) and Heidou (*Semen Sojae Nigrum*). Warm-natured, tonifying, greasy and fine foods should be less eaten or contraindicated such as mutton, chicken, ham and sea cucumber. The following foods are more suitable for children.

5.3.2.1 Fishes

Various fishes promote cerebral development. Fish and shellfish contain more unsaturated fatty acid which is the raw material to produce nervous cells. These foods also contain high content of protein, vitamin and trace elements which can promote intelligent activities.

Fish scales contain a higher content of brain-tonifying substances, of which organic elements are even higher such as calcium and phosphorus. Fish scales have more lecithin which improves memory and controls cerebral cell decline. The method of eating fish scales: scrape the fish scales, wash them clean and pound them into small pieces. Then decoct the scales into colloid state with slow fire and cut the colloid substance into cubes. Add some condiments like vinegar, green Chinese onion and ginger to be stirred with the scales when eating.

5.3.2.2 Jinzhen mushroom

It is also called "Jingu" and "Pugu" in Chinese. The mushroom has a long and thin stipe with light yellow color. Accordingly, "Jinzhen" (golden needle) is used to describe it. Jinzhen mushroom is tender in quality, rich in nutrition, high in protein, low in fat and abundant in sugar. It also contains rich trace elements like calcium, iron and phosphorus and vitamin. The lysine and arginine containing in amino acid have the function of improving memory and developing intelligence. Therefore it is called "intelligence-improving mushroom". Jinzhen mushroom can be parched, stewed and used in cold dishes. The food is slippery, tender and delicious. As a result, Jinzhen mushroom is one of the required food for children' health care and development of intelligence.

5.3.2.3　Edible fungus

Fungus is divided into white fungus and black fungus. *Shennong Bencao Jing*, or *Shennong's Herbal Classic*, claims that it "benefits qi and makes people free from hunger, strengthens health and improves intelligence." The main nutritious constituents it contains include protein, lipid, sugar, calcium, phosphorus, iron, carotin, vitamin B1, vitamin B2, nicotinic acid, lecithin, cephalin, sphingomyelin, sterol and so on, of which unsaturated fatty acid like lecithin, vitamin, inorganic elements are the main constituents to strengthen health and benefit intelligence. It is better for children to eat white fungus.

5.3.2.4　Oyster

Its shell is used when oyster is used as a drug; its meat is used when oyster is used as a food. Every 100 g of the dry meat contains 63.5 g of glycogen, 1.3 g of various amino acids, as well as vitamin A, vitamin B_1, vitamin B_2, vitamin D, linolenic acid, linoleic acid, sterol, etc. In particular, oyster contains extremely rich trace elements (copper, zinc, manganese, barium, phosphorus, calcium, iodine, etc.), reaching up to 17.6 g/100 g. Besides, it also contains 1.3% of taurine and extremely rich glutathione.

The method of eating oyster: Wash it clean and put it into a pot with boiling water for a little while. Then scoop it up from the pot. The oyster may be parched with eggs, or cook soup, or be used in cold dishes after ginger is added.

5.3.2.5 Beef

As a food, beef makes people strong. It is most suitable for all children with weak physique and retarded development of intelligence.

Every 100 g of beef contains 20.1 g of protein, 10.2 g of fat, 7 mg of calcium, 170 mg of phosphorus, 0.9 g of iron, 0.07 mg of vitamin B_1, 0.15 mg of vitamin B_2 and 6 mg of nicotinic acid. Of these constituents, protein is the main tonic element. The types of protein constituting beef are various. The composition is reasonable, and it is the complete protein food.

Beef is the traditional food to benefiting intelligence. It was believed in ancient times that the heart of cattle had the best function.

5.3.2.6 Soybean

Soybean has intelligence-benefiting, anti-ageing and cosmetological actions. TCM classics carry that regular ingestion of soybean "makes people strong, complexion ruddy, permanently free from wan and sallow complexion". Generally speaking, people eat yellow soybean at ordinary times. They eat black less soybean. However, black bean is used more as a drug. In some aspects, black soybean surpasses yellow soybean in making people strong and benefiting intelligence.

The protein containing in soybean is abundant in quantity and good in quality. The composition of protein is similar to the requirement of the human body, and the composition proportion is similar to animal protein. The amino acid in soybean differs from that of cereal. For

出，然后可用来炒鸡蛋，或做汤，或加姜醋等凉拌。

5. 牛肉

牛肉是能使人强壮的食品，凡身体虚弱而智力发育较差的儿童，吃牛肉最为相宜。

每100 g牛肉中含有蛋白质20.1 g，脂肪10.2 g，钙7 mg，磷170 mg，铁0.9 mg，维生素B_1 0.07 mg，维生素B_2 0.15 mg，烟酸6 mg。其中的蛋白质是牛肉的主要滋补成分，组成牛肉蛋白质的氨基酸种类多，结构合理，为完全性蛋白质食品。

牛心是传统的益智食品，古代认为黄牛心作用最好。

6. 大豆

大豆具有益智、抗衰老、美容等功效。中医古籍记载，常食大豆可以"令人强壮，容貌红白，永不憔悴"。一般来说，平时食用以黄豆最普遍，黑豆较少食用，但黑豆入药较多，其强壮益智作用在某些方面超过黄豆。

大豆中所含的蛋白质，不仅量多，而且质好，其中氨基酸的组成与人体的需要比较接近，组成比例类似于动物蛋白。所含的氨基酸与谷物所

example, the lysine scanty in cereal is ample in soybean. Accordingly, children should be advocated to eat rice mixed with soybean or flour mixed with soybean in which the items complement each other.

Soybean fat has the richest linolenic acid. Besides, it also contains 1.64% lecithin. These are of significant importance for the development of children's brain and nervous system. Soybean has a high content of iron and is easy to be digested and absorbed. It is the suitable intelligence-benefiting food for children with anemia. It is more suitable for children to eat when soybean is made into bean curd because the addition of bittern or gypsum increases the content of inorganic elements such as calcium and magnesium.

There are many methods to eat soybeans. The bean products include delicate bean curd, tough bean curd, dried bean curd, sheets of bean curd, fermented bean curd, dried bean milk cream in tight rolls, fried bean curd, soya-bean milk, bean sprouts, jellied bean curd, etc. No matter what eating methods are used, bean products should be eaten after they are fully cooked. Otherwise, diarrhea would occur. This is because there exists an anti-trypsin factor in beans which inhibits the digestive function of trypsin to make it difficult for the protein in beans to be docomposed. As a result, digestion is affected. After the bean curd product is done, this factor will be destroyed and protein can be absorbed.

5.3.2.7 Honey

The chief constituents of honey are fructose, glucose, cane sugar, maltose, protein, amino acid as well as enzymes like invertase, reductase, oxidase, catalase and amylase, organic acids, acetylcholine, vitamins A, B_1,

B$_2$, B$_6$, C, D and K, nicotinic acid, pantothenic acid, folic acid and biotin, trace elements like copper, iron, magnesium and nickel. Honey is a good natural intelligence-benefiting product viewed from the five major nutrients of intelligence-benefiting diet.

The food honey may be drunk by watering it with boiled water or in the form of various beverages. It is the best for children and juveniles not to eat royal jelly, bee milk and their products. These things contain more hormones constituents, of which gonadotropic hormone may result in children's sexual prematurity. Therefore, they are not advisably eaten.

The children's spleen and stomach are not fully developed and they cannot regulate their diet by themselves. Slightly improper feeding may impair the spleen and stomach, affecting the growth and development. Therefore, the children's feeding should aim at protecting the spleen and stomach. Light diet should be selected. This is the principle. The stool should be instantly observed to find out the state of digestion and absorption. Modern children should prevent hypernutrition and regulate the diet accordingly. Namely, "The children should endure thirty percent starvation, be only seventy percent full and knead the belly frequently."

5.3.3　Rearing the children carefully

The clothing should be modified in conformity to seasonal changes of cold and heat, the criterion of which lies in the fact that the children's hands and feet are warm but do not sweat. The key points for keeping warm are that the head is advisably cool while the back, abdomen and feet are advisably warm. The children's clothing and quilt should particularly avoid being too thick and too warm while too much clothing should not be advisable at usual times.

Combing the hair often tonifies the brain. According to the theory of meridians and collaterals in TCM, the head is "the place where all yang meridians meet and all meridians communicate". The acupoint in the middle of the vertex is called Baihui (GV20). Combing the hair regularly makes people and the mind refreshed and overcomes fatigue. The process of combing the hair is actually massaging the every acupoint of the head, which regulates the excitement and inhibition of cerebral cortex via this stimulation of massage, improves blood circulation and the secretion of subcutaneous body of gland and improves nutritional metabolism. This is the so-called function of activating blood circulation and qi flow, dispelling wind and improving sight, nourishing and consolidating the hair, refreshing the mind and improving sleep.

It is advisable to comb the hair once in the morning and in the evening respectively. Comb the hair from the front to the back, and then from the back to the front, from the left to the right, and then from the right to the left. Repeat the cycles for from dozens of times to more than one hundred times until the feverish and contracting sensation appears on the scalp.

It is advisable to comb the hair more and wash it less. An ancient book says: "People should wash the hair once in five days except in summer." Take particular care not to expose the head to wind and cold. Otherwise, it would be susceptible to headache. In addition, it is not advisable for girls to have the hair permed. It is not even more advisable for girls to wear the hair-curling tube or hairpin to go to sleep in case the hair roots should be suppressed to affect blood circulation.

经常梳头,有健脑作用。按中医的经络学说,头部为"诸阳所会,百脉相通"之处,头顶正中的穴位就叫"百会"。经常梳理头发,会使人感到神志爽快,头脑清醒,消除疲劳。梳头的过程,实际上是在对头部各个穴位进行按摩,通过按摩的刺激,可以调节大脑皮质的兴奋和抑制过程,促进血液循环和皮下腺体的分泌,改进营养代谢。即中医所说的流通气血,散风明目,荣发固发,提神醒脑,改善睡眠。

梳头宜早上、晚上各1次,由前到后,再由后到前;由左向右,再由右向左。如此循环往复,梳数十遍至百余遍,以头皮出现发热和紧缩之感为止。

头发宜多梳,但不宜多洗。古书上说:"除夏以外,五日一沐"。尤其注意洗头后不要当风受凉,否则容易患头痛症。此外,女孩子不宜烫发,更不能戴着卷发筒或发夹睡觉,以免发根被压迫,影响血液循环。

5.3.4 Training physique

The natural sunlight and air should be fully utilized to train the physique. The outdoor activities should be ensured at least for two to three hours a day in children below 10. It is advisable to have such activities as gymnastics, swimming, playing games, short-distance running, Wushu, rope skipping and ball games. Children should play more intelligence-benefiting games to promote the development of intelligence. These games may be as follows.

5.3.4.1 Flexing fingers

Flex fingers of both hands simultaneously. Flex the thumb of the left hand and the little finger; or flex the index finger of the left hand and ring finger of the right hand. The movements proceed from slow ones to quick ones. After a period of exercise, alternate the left and right hands for more exercises.

5.3.4.2 Pointing to the nose and eyes

The parent holds an extending palm of the child with one hand and pats it with the other hand. The child uses the index finger of the other hand to point to the apex of nose. The other four fingers make a fist. Every time when the parents pat the palm of the child and shouts directions like "nose", "eye", "mouth" and "ear". When the parents shout the direction "nose", the child will keep his finger still. But the child should follow the parent's directions to point the index finger to the right place quickly the instance the other directions are given. The directions and the finger movements appear almost at the same times. Thus the child may point wrongly. This makes the people around laugh a lot. The game is very helpful to train the child's reactive, judging and emergency-meeting abilities.

四、体格锻炼

要充分利用大自然的日光、空气进行体格锻炼。10岁以内儿童,每天至少2～3小时的户外活动。以体操、游泳、游戏、短跑、武术、跳绳和球类运动为宜。儿童还应多做益智游戏,以促进智力的发育。如:

1. 屈指

左右双手同时做屈指运动,左手屈拇指,右手同时屈小指;或左手屈食指,右手屈无名指。动作由慢到快。做一段时间后,左右手交替再做。

2. 指鼻子指眼

家长握住孩子一只伸开的手掌,用另一只手拍打孩子手心,孩子的另一只手用食指按在鼻尖上,其余四指握拳。家长每打孩子手心一次,嘴里同时喊出"鼻子"、"眼"、"嘴巴"、"耳朵"等各种指令,除喊"鼻子"时手指不动外,其余所喊指令的瞬间,孩子要迅速地将食指指向所喊指令的部位。由于喊指令与手指移动几乎同时进行,所以孩子往往会乱指一气,逗得旁人哈哈大笑。这种游戏对训练孩子反应能力、判断能力、应变能力最有

5.3.4.3 Rubbing and striking the knees

Extend the left hand with the palm putting on the left knee-cap; make a fist with the right hand. After shouting "Begin!", rub the thigh forward and backward with the left hand, and strike the knee-cap upward and downward with the right fist at the same time. At the beginning of the game, the left hand subconsciously changes into the same movement of striking the knee-cap as the right hand, or the right hand shifts to the same movement of rubbing the knee as the left hand. After the people gradually get used to the game, his two hands will adapt to their respective movement step by step. At this time, another person may shout "Change!" to ask exerciser to exchange the movements of the left and right hands. At first, this exchange may cause the exerciser to be in a muddle and make other people around laugh merrily.

5.3.5 Developing good habits

5.3.5.1 Sleeping hygiene

The habit of going to bed and getting up in time should be developed from childhood. The habit of being carried in sleeping should not be cultivated. Teasing and joking with the child is not advisable before the child falls asleep while telling terrifying stories and playing exciting games are not allowable, either.

It is not suitable that the quilt is too heavy, excessively thick and extremely warm. Supination and lateral position are both acceptable while pronation is not advisable. The child should be often helped to change the sleeping posture and the direction of lateral position in case the cranial bone should develop into deformity. The pillow should not be too high.

5.3.5.2 Physical hygiene

Regular defecation and urination should be trained from about six months after the birth. The habit of washing hands before meals and after defecation and urination should be cultivated from about the age of one. The child should wash the face and feet while the vulva should be also washed in girls. The hair should be regularly washed, the body regularly bathed, the clothes frequently washed and replaced and the nails often trimmed. The child should rinse the month and brush the teeth after meals, but cannot go to sleep with the candy in mouth. At the age of four, the child should develop the ability to take care of himself and the correct postures. The common knowledge of health care should be instructed to prevent caries, myopia, trachoma, deformity of spinal column, tarsoptosis and infectious diseases. The preventive inoculation is regularly and quantitatively done, and the physical examination regularly conducted in order to prevent diseases and enhance immunity.

5.3.6 Benefiting intelligence with traditional Chinese drugs

There are many methods to promote the development of intelligence for children. Two effective prescriptions are listed here.

5.3.6.1 Sight-improving and Intelligence-developing Pill (cited from *Zheng Zhi Bao Jian*, or *Valuable Experiences of Diagnosis and Treatment*)

The prescription is composed of 9 tortoise hearts, 5 g of Longgu (*Os Draconis*), Yuanzhi (*Radix Polygalae*), Guiban (*Carapax et Plastrum Testudinis*), Zhusha (*Cinnabaris*), Shichangpu (*Rhizoma Acori Graminei*), Tianmendong (*Radix Asparagi*), Maimendong (*Radix Ophipogonis*), Baiziren (*Semen Biotae*),

2. 身体卫生

6个月左右，应该开始训练定时大小便的习惯。周岁左右，要养成饭前便后洗手的习惯，睡前洗脸、洗脚，女孩每晚洗外阴。定期洗头洗澡，衣服勤洗勤换，常剪指甲。饭后漱口刷牙，不可含着糖块入睡。到了4岁，要逐渐培养自理能力，注意培养正确的姿势，讲解卫生保健常识，预防龋齿、近视眼、沙眼、脊柱变形、扁平足和传染病的发生。为了防病增加免疫力，应定期定量做好预防接种，定期体检。

六、中药益智

中医有很多促进少儿智力发育的方法，现列举有效方剂两首：

1. 益明长智丸（《证治宝鉴》）

乌龟心9枚，龙骨、远志、龟版、朱砂、石菖蒲、天门冬、麦门冬、柏子仁、白茯苓、玄参、桔梗、人参、丹参、枣仁、胆南星、熟地黄、五味子、当归、茯神、甘草、熊胆（如无，以牛

Baifuling (*Poria*), Xuanshen (*Radix Scrophulariae*), Jiegeng (*Radix Platycodi*), Renshen (*Radix Ginseng*), Danshen (*Radix Salviae Miltiorrhizae*), Zaoren (*Semen Ziziphi Jujubae*), Dannanxing (*Arisaema cum Bile*), Shudihuang (*Radix Rehmanniae Praeparata*), Wuweizi (*Fructus Schisandrae*), Danggui (*Radix Angelicae Sinensis*), Fushen (*Poria cum Ligno Hospite*), Gancao (*Raix Glycyrrhizae*) and Xiongdan (*Fel Ursi*) [If it is not available, replace it with Niudan (*Fel Bovis*)] respectively.

Grind all the above ingredients into powder to make pills with honey with the size of a longan. Take one pill orally each time with the decoction of ten rush pithes and three dates. The prescription focuses on tonifying the heart and has better effects on congenital maldevelopment of intelligence. It is also effective for amnesia, frequent palpitation and insomnia.

5.3.6.2 Qisheng Pill (Pill of Seven Holy Ingredients) (cited from *Sheng Ji Zong Lu*, or *General Collection for Holy Relief*)

The prescription is composed of 60 g of Baifuling (*Poria*), 30 g of Rougui (*Cortex Cinnamomi*), Yuanzhi (*Radix Polygalae*), Renshen (*Radix Ginseng*), Tianmendong (*Radix Asparagi*), Shichangpu (*Rhizoma Acori Graminei*) and Digupi (*Cortex Lycii Radicis*) respectively.

Grind all the above ingredients into fine powder to make pills with honey with the size of a Chinese parasol seed. Take 10 to 20 pills each time. The prescription has the actions of invigorating the heart qi, clearing away heat from the heart and refreshing the mind. The book claims: "It benefits the heart and intelligence, makes people wise" and "treats amnesia".

胆代)各5 g。

上为末,炼蜜为丸,如桂圆大。每服1丸,用灯心10根,大枣3枚煎水送下。本方重在补心,对先天智力发育不良者较有效。若见有健忘而经常心慌、失眠的患者亦适宜。

2. 七圣丸(《圣济总录》)

白茯苓60 g,肉桂、远志、人参、天门冬、石菖蒲、地骨皮各30 g。

碾成细末,炼蜜为丸,如梧桐子大。每服10～20丸。本方有补心气、清心神的作用,原书称:"益心智,令人聪明",治疗"健忘"。

5.4 Health care for women

The physiological characteristics such as menstruation, pregnancy, labor and lactation, together with the psychological features like sentimentality and lack of emotional self control make women susceptible to the consumption of essence, blood, spirit and qi as well as diseases and premature ageing in women. Their health care should emphasize the hygiene and health care during the menstrual period, gestational period, stegmonth, lactation and climacterium in additional to the same points as men.

5.4.1 Health care during the menstrual period

Women should keep their pudenda clean and hygienic, avoid tension, fatigue, strenuous exercises and heavy physical labor. They cannot adopt the tub bath and swim. They should strictly abstain from sexual life, vaginal examination, etc. These are the basic content of health care in women. In addition, attention should be paid to the following aspects.

5.4.1.1 Keeping warm

Women should keep the body warm during the menstrual period and avoid attack by cold. They should not wade across a river, be drenched with rain, sit and lie on the damp ground and work in the paddy field. They should strictly abstain from swimming, cold bath and work with the scorching sun directly overhead and under intense heat. Otherwise, they are susceptible to menstrual disorders, dysmenorrhea, and amenorrhea, etc.

5.4.1.2 Abstaining from certain foods

Sthenia of the liver and asthenia of the spleen mostly exist during the menstrual period due to profuse discharge

第四节 妇女保健

妇女有月经、胎孕、产育、哺乳等生理特点,又有感情丰富,情不自制的心理特点,因此精血神气易于耗损,患病早衰。其养生保健,除了与男子相同者外,尚须注重经期、孕期、产褥期、哺乳期及更年期的卫生保健。

一、经期保健

保持阴部清洁卫生,避免紧张疲劳、剧烈运动及重体力劳动,不可盆浴、游泳,严禁房事、阴道检查等,是妇女保健的基本内容。此外,还需注意:

1. 寒温适宜

经期注意保暖,避免受寒,切勿涉水、淋雨、冒雪、坐卧湿地,下水田劳动。严禁游泳、冷水浴,忌在烈日高温下劳动。否则容易导致月经失调、痛经、闭经等证。

2. 饮食宜忌

月经期间,经血溢泄,多有乳房胀痛,少腹坠胀,纳少

of menstrual blood such as mammary distension and pain, distension of lower abdomen with bearing-down sensation, poor appetite and loose stool. Women should eat light and nutritious foods. They cannot eat more sour and pungent, pungent and hot-natured, aromatic and dry foods. Or this may give rise to hypermenorrhea; overeating of uncooked and cold foods may cause blood stagnation, giving rise to unsmooth menstruation, dysmenorrhea and amenorrhea; excessive drinking is not advisable either to keep the normal menstruation.

5.4.1.3 Regulating emotions

Women should remain at ease mentally and avoid excessive emotional activities. Otherwise, it may result in adverse and disorderly circulation of qi and blood. This may aggravate the discomfort during the menstrual period, lead to menstrual disorders in mild cases, and amenorrhea, tuberculosis, etc. in severe cases.

5.4.2 Health care during the puerperium

The puerperium refers to the period of six to eight weeks after the delivery. The organism needs longer careful recuperation because it is in a state of weakness and blood stasis due to the qi consumption and blood loss during the delivery.

5.4.2.1 Regular daily life

Adequate rest for recuperation is beneficial to the restoration of physiological functions. The living environment should be clean, quiet, warm, comfortable and well-ventilated. It is advisable for the parturients to keep warm in winter and not to shut the door and window tightly or wear very thick clothes in case sunstroke should occur. However, it is not advisable to lie in the draught in case pathogenic wind should take advantage of the physical weakness to attack the body.

便溏等肝强脾弱现象,应摄取清淡而富有营养之食品。不能多食酸辣、辛热、香燥之品,否则导致月经过多;过食生冷食物则血行凝涩,致使经行不畅、痛经、闭经。也不宜过量饮酒,以免影响经血的正常溢行。

3. 情志调和

保持心情舒畅,避免"七情"过度。否则,会引起气血运行逆乱,轻则加重经期不适感,导致月经失调,重则闭经、患痨瘵等症。

二、产褥期保健

产后6～8星期属产褥期。由于分娩时耗气失血,机体处于虚弱多瘀的状态,需要较长时间的精心调养。

1. 起居有节

充分休息静养,有利于生理功能的恢复。起居环境必须清洁安静,温暖舒适,空气流通。冬季宜注意保暖,夏季不宜紧闭门窗或衣着过厚,以免发生中暑,但不宜卧于当风之处,以免邪风乘虚侵袭。

It is not suitable to work hard and bear a heavy load too early so as to avoid puerperal metrorrhagia, hysteroptosis, etc. The parturients should not lie supine long to avoid retroversion of uterus. Generally, they may get up to move about 24 hours after the labor in case of normal labor, and gradually enlarge the space of activities to promote smooth lochial flow, uterine restoration, peristaltic restoration, smooth urination and defecation. This is beneficial to the recovery of the body.

5.4.2.2 Reasonable diet

Tonification should not affect the stomach and leave blood stasis during the supplementation of nutrients. The diet should not only be bland, delicious, light, and easy in absorption, but also contain rich nutrients, sufficient quantity of heat and water. The parturients should abstain from greasy diet, uncooked and cold fruits as well as the pungent and hot-natured foods consuming body fluids. The new parturients of one to three days after the delivery may eat millet gruel, soft rice, stewed egg, soup of lean meat, etc. Later on, they may ingest all egg, milk, meat, bone soup, bean products, coarse food grain and vegetables. Simultaneously, the parturients should be supplementarily treated with the dietary therapy. For instance, the patients with asthenia of the spleen and stomach may ingest Huaishanyao Biandou Jingmi Gruel (Gruel of Rhizoma Dioscorease, Semen Dolichoris and Semen Oryzae Sativae); the patients with lumbago due to renal asthenia may take Zhuyaozi Caimo Gruel (Gruel of Ren Suis and Minced Vegetable); the patients with lochiorrhagia may take Danggui Shengjiang Yangrou Soup (Soup of Radix Angelicae Sinensis, Rhizoma Zingiberis Recens and Mutton) or Yimucao Hongtang Liquid (Decoction of *Herba Leonuri* and Brown Sugar), etc.

不宜过早操劳负重，避免发生产后血崩、阴挺下脱等病。睡眠不宜长期仰卧，以免子宫后倾。一般顺产可在产后24小时起床活动，并且逐渐增加活动范围，以促进恶露畅流、子宫复元，恢复肠蠕动，令二便通畅，有利于身体康复。

2．合理饮食

加强营养，但必须注意补不碍胃，不留瘀血。饮食宜清淡可口，易于消化吸收，又富有营养及足够的热量和水分。忌食油腻和生冷瓜果，也不宜吃辛热伤津之食。产后1～3日的新产妇可食小米粥、软饭、炖蛋和瘦肉汤等。此后，凡蛋、奶、肉、骨头汤、豆制品、粗粮、蔬菜均可食用。并辅以食疗进补，如脾胃虚弱者可服怀山药扁豆粳米粥，肾虚腰疼者食用猪腰子菜末粥，恶露不畅者可服当归生姜羊肉汤或益母草红糖水等。

5.4.2.3 Keeping the vulva clean

Parturients should take sponge bath and shower regularly, and pay attention to keeping the vulva clean to prevent infection. They should wash and air the underclothes and sanitary belt regularly, abstain from sexual life within one hundred days. They cannot take tub bath during the four weeks after labor.

5.4.3 Health care during the breast feeding period

5.4.3.1 Health care of the breasts

Lactation may begin eight to twelve hours after the labor. The parturients should keep the nipples clean and dry and should not let the baby sleep with the nipple in the mouth. At the beginning of lactation, the parturients may often suffer from stagnation mastitis manifesting distension, hardness and pain of the breast. In this case, they may use local hot compress to dredge the mammary collaterals. They may take traditional Chinese drugs to promote lactation. In the case of cracked nipples or acute mastitis, the parturients may see a doctor in time.

5.4.3.2 Supplementing nutrients

The parturients should supplement the dietary nutrients, abstain from irritative foods and abuse of tonics. For example, in the case of scanty milk, the parturients may drink more fish soup, chicken soup, and soup of pig's trotters, etc. In the case of galactorrhea or hypogalactia, they should see a doctor.

5.4.3.3 Health care in daily life

The parturients should remain at ease in the mind, regular in daily life and a proper balance between work and rest. They should pay attention to contraception but should not take oral contraceptives to prevent the inhibition of milk secretion.

3. 清洁外阴

经常擦浴淋浴,特别注意外阴清洁,预防感染。内衣裤、月经带要常洗晒,百日之内严禁房事。产后4周不能盆浴。

三、哺乳期保健

1. 乳房保健

产后8~12小时即可开奶。保持乳头清洁和干燥,不要让婴儿含着乳头入睡。刚开始哺乳时,往往会出现蒸乳反应,表现为乳房胀硬疼痛,可做局部热敷,使乳络通畅。也可用中药促其通乳。若出现乳头皲裂或乳痈,应及时医治。

2. 加强营养

加强饮食营养,忌食刺激性食品,勿滥用补品。如乳汁不足,可多喝鱼汤、鸡汤、猪蹄汤等。若乳汁自出或过少,需求医诊治。

3. 起居保健

保持心情舒畅,起居有时,劳逸适度。要注意避孕,但勿服避孕药,以免抑制乳汁的分泌。

5.4.3.4 Being cautious of administration

Many drugs may enter milk by means of blood circulation in the feeding mothers. For instance, infantile diarrhea may result from the administration of large amount of Dahuang (*Radix et Rhizoma Rhei*). Besides, atropine, tetracycline, erythromycin, phenobarbital and sulfa drugs can be all discharged from the feeding mothers' mammary glands. Infantile poisoning may result from prolonged or large amount of administration of these drugs. Therefore, the administration should be handled with caution.

5.4.4 Health care during the climacterium

Women enter the climacterium at the age of 45 to 50. During climacterium, imbalance of yin and yang occurs due to the gradual deficiency of the kidney qi and deficiency of thoroughfare vessel and conception vessel, giving rise to light-headedness, headache, tinnitus, palpitation, insomnia, restlessness of the mind, irascibility or depression, menstrual disorder, fever, sweating, etc. These phenomena are called menopausal syndrome. The health measures at this stage are as follows.

5.4.4.1 Regulating emotions

Women should remain optimistic, open-minded and self-confident, actively adapt themselves to the various discomforts due to physiological changes.

5.4.4.2 Regulating the diet for recuperation

The women during climacterium suffer from profuse or scanty menstrual blood as well as short or prolonged menstrual cycle due to the gradual deficiency of the kidney qi. As a result, they are susceptible to anemia. In this case, they can selectively eat high-protein foods like egg, animal liver, lean meat and milk as well as vegetables and fruits such as spinach, rape, tomato, peach and orange to cure anemia. The patients with hypertension of hyperactive

4. 谨慎用药

许多药物可以经过乳母的血循环进入乳汁。例如,乳母服大黄可使婴儿泄泻。阿托品、四环素、红霉素、苯巴比妥及磺胺类,都可从乳腺排出,如长期或大量服用,可使婴儿发生中毒。故用药必须谨慎。

四、更年期保健

妇女在45～50岁进入更年期。更年期由于肾气渐衰,冲任二脉虚惫,可致阴阳失调,出现头晕目眩、头痛耳鸣、心悸失眠、烦躁易怒或忧郁、月经紊乱、烘热汗出等症,称为更年期综合征。保健措施如下:

1. 调节情志

要保持乐观情绪,胸怀开阔,树立信心,主动适应生理变异带来的各种不适应现象。

2. 饮食调养

更年期妇女肾气渐衰,月经量或多或少,经期或短或长,往往容易出现贫血,可选食鸡蛋、动物内脏、瘦肉、牛奶等高蛋白食物以及菠菜、油菜、西红柿、桃、橘等绿叶蔬菜和水果纠正贫血。患有阴虚阳亢型的高血压患者,可摄食

yang type due to yin deficiency may eat coarse food grain (including millet, ground maize, and oatmeal, etc), mushrooms, celery, apple, Chinese hawthorn, wild jujube, mulberry, and green tea, etc. They should eat less salt and abstain from drinking, coffee, strong tea, pepper and other irritative foods.

5.4.4.3 Regular physical examination

Women during climacterium are susceptible to genital tumor. If menstruation lasts more than ten days or profuse menstrual blood tends to cause anemia, the women should see a doctor. In the case of vaginal bleeding or profuse leukorrhea after menopause, the women should see a doctor in time to perform the relevant examination and timely treatment. Physical examination should be conducted in every half a year to every one year so as to discover the diseases as early as possible for early treatment. This includes cancer prevention.

5.5 Health care for old people

Old age means the age exceeds 60. Physiologically, old people are marked by the natural decline of viscera, qi, blood and spirit as well as the psychological changes due to physiological and social factors such as the commonly-seen loneliness, ageing, melancholy, suspiciousness, mania, restlessness of the mind and irascibility. When confronted with the bad environment and irritative factors, old people are susceptible to various diseases and it is more difficult for them to recover from these diseases.

5.5.1 Establishing the psychological state of being optimistic, open-minded, kind and enterprising

The aged should have deep love for life, maintain

self-confidence, make frequent use of the brain, do more good turns and treat others open-mindedly, magnanimously, modestly, kindly and gently. All these are beneficial to health.

The old people should avoid various unfavorable environments and mental stimulations. They should do their best to avoid the environments and scenes of the death, funeral, disaster, grief and depression. The revelrous, pretty and coquettish, frivolous and obscene occasions are not suitable for them. They should cultivate the happy and pleasing temperament according to the personal character and interest like tranquilizing the mind to sit quietly, chatting with friends, watching fish beside the pond and walking through the forest to listen to the bird's singing. This can make them content with their lot in life and is beneficial to health and longevity.

Senior citizens should acquire optimism and the confidence to defeat diseases, participate in some meaningful activities and training, actively cooperate with the doctor in treatment, have the physical examination regularly to discover the unfavorable signs as soon as possible for the timely prevention and treatment.

5.5.2 Taking the nutritious, bland, well-cooked, soft and various diet

5.5.2.1 Various diets

Old people should take in various diet with rich and complete nutrients to strengthen essence and qi and delay ageing. They should supplement the deficient nutrients of the organism appropriately. For instance, old people are subject to calciprivia. Accordingly, they should select the diet with rich calcium. Milk and dairy products, soybean and bean products are the ideal sources of calcium in diet. Also, celery, hawthorn fruit, coriander, etc. contain a

保持自信，勤于用脑，多做好事、善事，处世宜豁达宽宏、谦让和善，有益于身心健康。

老年人应回避各种不良环境、精神因素的刺激。尽量避免丧葬凶祸、悲哀忧愁的环境和场面，狂欢妖艳、轻薄淫秽的场所更不相宜。老年人应根据性格和情趣怡情悦志，如澄心静坐、益友清谈、临池观鱼、披林听鸟等，使生活自得其乐，有利康寿。

老年人应树立乐观主义精神和战胜疾病的信心，参加一些有意义的活动和锻炼，积极主动地配合治疗，定期进行体检，及早发现一些不良征兆，及时进行预防或治疗。

二、保持营养、清淡、熟软、多样的饮食

1. 食宜多样

摄食多样饮食，做到营养丰富全面，以补益精气延缓衰老。要适当补充机体缺乏的营养物质，如老年人容易缺钙，因此要在饮食中选用含钙高的食品。乳类及乳制品、大豆及豆制品是理想的食物钙来源，芹菜、山楂、香菜等含钙

large proportion of calcium. Besides, old people may regularly eat the foods strengthening the spleen and kidney, benefiting health and prolonging life such as lotus seed, Chinese yam, lotus root starch, water chestnut, walnut and black soyabean.

5.5.2.2 Bland diet

The old people's diet should be rich in protein, vitamin and fibrin but scanty in sugar, fat and salt. This is the quintessence of the so-called "bland diet". The spleen and stomach in old people are asthenic and declining, and weak in transportation and transformation. Consequently, old people should eat more fish, lean meat, bean products, fresh vegetables and fruits. But they should limit animal fat while vegetable oil is advisable such as sesame oil and maize oil.

5.5.2.3 Warm, well-cooked and soft diet

It is suitable for old people to eat warm diet, not uncooked and cold one in case the spleen and stomach should be impaired. However, it is not advisable to eat the very hot diet, either. The diet should be "warm but without scalding the lips, cold but without shaking the teeth." Old people with odontoseisis and odontoptosis have dysmasesia. Thus, it is suitable for them to eat the soft diet but abstain from sticky, hard and heavy foods. Gruel is the most suitable food for old people. It is not only light, but also strengthens the lung and promotes the production of body fluids. It is particularly suitable for old people's viscera.

5.5.2.4 Scanty food intake and slow feeding

The aged should not eat too much, but eat for more times, a small amount at each time. The feeding should not be too hurried and fast while careful mastication and slow swallowing are advisable. This can not only help digestion and absorption, but also prevent "gulping, cho-

量也较高。此外,可经常食用莲子、怀山药、藕粉、菱角、核桃、黑豆等补脾肾、益康寿之食品。

2. 食宜清淡

老人饮食的原则是"三多三少",即蛋白质多、维生素多、纤维素多;糖类少、脂肪少、盐少。该原则的精髓便是"清淡"。老年人脾胃虚衰,运化力弱,要多吃鱼、瘦肉、豆类食品和新鲜蔬菜水果,要限制动物脂肪,宜食植物油,如香油、玉米油。

3. 食宜温热熟软

老年人宜食用温热之品,勿食或少食生冷,以免损伤脾胃,但亦不宜温热过甚,以"热不炙唇,冷不振齿"为宜。老人牙齿松动脱落,咀嚼困难,故宜食用软食,忌食粘硬不易消化之品。粥是老人最宜之物,不仅容易消化,且益胃生津,对老年人的脏腑尤为适宜。

4. 食宜少缓

进食不宜过饱,应少量多餐。进食不可过急过快,宜细嚼慢咽,这不仅有助于饮食的消化吸收,还可避免"吞、呛、噎、咳"的发生。

king, dysphagia and cough".

5.5.3 Sports activities

Active physical training cannot only promote the circulation of qi and blood, delay ageing, but also produce a favorable mental stimulation to make people vigorous. This has the active actions of eliminating loneliness, ageing, melancholy, suspiciousness, mania, restlessness of the mind, irascibility, etc.

The physical training should be moderate in duration and amount, constant in efforts, and proceed in an orderly way and step by step in accordance with individual conditions. Before physical training, old people should have the overall physical examination to understand the health status and whether they have serious diseases or not. Under the guidance of the doctor, the aged may select the suitable sports events and properly control the intensity, speed and duration of the sports activity. It is suitable to have a small amount of exercise, slow and rhythmical movements. The suitable events include Taijiquan, five mimic-animal games, eight-section brocade, jogging, taking a walk, swimming, table tennis, badminton, gymnastic exercise for the aged, etc. Old people may have the above events once or twice a day. But they cannot have the physical training in bad climate, nor can they have it in starvation.

5.5.4 Reasonable administration

In health care administration, more tonic medicines but less purgative ones are advisable; neutral-and mild-natured drugs but small dosage are advisable; the stress is placed on the spleen and kidney with the five zang organs concurrently taken into account; the tonification is based on differentiation of physique with yin and yang regulated;

三、适宜运动

积极的体育锻炼可以促进气血运行,延缓衰老,并可产生一种良性心理刺激,使人精神焕发,对消除孤独垂暮、忧郁多疑、烦躁易怒等情绪有积极作用。

要遵循因人制宜、适时适量、循序渐进、持之以恒的原则。参加锻炼前,要进行全面体检,了解身体健康状况及有无重要疾病。在医生的指导下,选择恰当的运动项目,掌握好活动强度、速度和时间。运动量宜小不宜大,动作宜缓慢而有节律。适合的项目有太极拳、五禽戏、八段锦、慢跑、散步、游泳、乒乓球、羽毛球、老年体操等。每天1~2次,不能在恶劣气候环境中锻炼,更不能在饥饿时锻炼。

四、合理用药

保健用药宜多进补少用泻;药宜平和,药量宜小;注重脾肾,兼顾五脏;辨体质论补,调整阴阳;多以丸散膏丹,少用汤剂;药食并举,因势利导。如此才能适应老人生理特点,

more dosage forms of bolus, powder, plaster and pill are used but less decoction is applied; medication and dietary therapy are concurrently adopted according to the specific conditions. Only in this way can the old people's physiological characteristics be suited to, abuses rectified, diseases prevented and life prolonged.

收到补偏救弊,防病延年之效。

5.6 Health care for mental workers

Mental workers refer to the people who use the brain for a longer time for spiritual and thinking activities. These people often bend over their desks working and lack for movement of their limbs. Their working postures are simple and partial muscle remains in a tense state. This may easily cause qi stagnation and blood stasis. As a result, diseases often occur in limbs and joints. Particularly, overuse of the brain may lead to cerebral ischemia and anoxia, giving rise to dizziness, headache, palpitation and insomnia. Accordingly, mental workers should concentrate on exercising limbs, tonifying the heart and brain, with equal attention to psychosomatic health in their health preservation.

5.6.1 Scientific use of the brain

Overuse of the brain is not advisable. Otherwise, it would give rise to consumption of qi and blood. Therefore, mental workers should not surpass two hours each time when they bend over their desks working. It is advisable for them to take a rest once every hour for 10 to 15 minutes. The methods for rest may include exercising the body and limbs, taking a deep breathing or thinking long and hard with the eyes closed. When having prolonged mental work, take care to alternate the working

第六节 脑力劳动者的保健

脑力工作劳动者,是指较长时间使用大脑进行精神思维活动的人。这类人经常昼夜伏案,缺少肢体运动;姿势单一,部分肌肉处于持续紧张状态,气血容易瘀滞,产生四肢关节病。尤其是过度使用大脑,脑部缺血缺氧,会产生头晕、头痛、心悸、失眠等症状。因此,脑力劳动者养生的重点是运动肢节、养心健脑、心身兼顾。

一、科学用脑

大脑工作不宜过用,过用就会耗气损血。因此,每次伏案工作不应超过2小时,最好是每小时休息一次。每次10~15分钟。休息的方式,可以运动肢体,也可以连续进行深呼吸,或者闭目冥想。长时间进行脑力劳动时,应注意交替变换工作内容,如阅读、朗

contents. For example, alternate the activities of reading, reading aloud, listening to music and watching pictures. Mental workers may also select the light, soft and slow music as the background to balance the activities of the work of the left brain and the right brain. As a result, the pressure of the thinking center can be relieved.

5.6.2　Protecting eyesight

When using the brain, mental workers use the eyes at the same time as well. TCM believes prolonged use of the eyes may consume the liver blood. Stop using the eyes when the tiredness is felt in the eyes. Then sit in repose with the eyes closed. Or "wiping the eyes with the fingers" (Please refer to Section 4 of Chapter 7 of the book). Look at the remote sights after wiping the eyes with the fingers.

5.6.3　Living in a suitable environment

The brain consumes a great deal of oxygen. Therefore, the living environment should be well-ventilated to ensure plentiful supply of oxygen. Besides, it is the best for the working environment to be in a natural light with moderate brightness. Intense or weak light may impair eyesight. The working environment should be kept quiet and free from noises. The brain may be injured when the noise surpasses 60 dB. Apart from the above, the room temperature of 16℃ is the most beneficial to maintaining the brain in a refreshing state.

5.6.4　Tonifying the brain with drugs

Fat, glucoprotein, calcium, phosphorus, etc. are the essential substances for the activities of the brain. The simplest method to supplement these substances is to obtain them from foods.

读、听录音、看图象等活动交替进行,还可以选用轻柔舒缓的音乐作背景,以平衡左右脑的活动,减轻思维中枢的压力。

二、保护目力

脑力劳动者在用脑的同时,也会大量使用目力。中医认为,长时间用眼会耗损肝血。应在眼睛感到疲乏时宜停下来闭目养神,或"运睛"(参见本书第七章第四节),运睛结束后眺望远景。

三、居处适宜

大脑的耗氧量十分巨大,因此居处环境需要空气流通,保证充足的氧气供应。其次,工作环境最好具备明暗适中的自然光线,光线过强或过弱会对视力产生损害。工作场所要保持安静,杜绝噪音。当噪音超过60dB时,大脑就会受到伤害。此外,16℃左右的室温最利于大脑保持清醒状态。

四、食物补脑

脂肪、糖蛋白、钙、磷等物质　是大脑活动时必不可少的,补充这些物质的最简单的途径,是从食物中摄取。

Walnut is the traditional brain-tonifying food. TCM holds walnut is warm-natured, sweet and free from toxin. It tonifies blood, preserves vitality and prolongs life for longevity. The phospholipid in walnuts has better health care effect on the cerebral nerves. Walnut oil contains unsaturated fatty acid. It is the important constituent of the cerebral tissue and prevents cerebral arterosclerosis. Walnut kernel contains the essential trace elements of cerebral activities like zinc, magnesium and chromium.

Fish and shellfish contain more unsaturated fatty acid. Unsaturated fatty acid is the important raw material to produce and protect cerebral cells. It should be eaten more.

Carrot   It contains rich vitamin B_1. Those who lack vitamin B_1 may suffer from thinking retardation and melancholia.

Spinach   It contains rich Vitamin A and vitamin C. It is particularly important because it contains vitamin B_6 and vitamin B_{12} that are beneficial to the cerebral function of memory. Lack of vitamin B_6 and vitamin B_{12} may result in neuritis, obstruction of nerve conduction, with the symptoms of amnesia and restlessness. Besides, spinach contains chlorophyll, and mineral substances like calcium, iron and phosphorus. These substances have brain-tonifying effect as well.

Kelp   It contains the rich mineral nutritious substances essential to the human body such as phosphorus, magnesium, sodium, kalium, calcium, iodine, iron, silicon, manganese, zinc, cobalt and molybdenum. Some of these substances are the ones some terrestrial vegetables lack. In addition, kelp also contains rich taurine. Taurine has significant actions of protecting sight and cerebral functions.

核桃　是传统的健脑食品。中医认为核桃性温，味甘，无毒，有补血养神、延年益寿功效。核桃中的磷脂，对脑神经有良好保健作用。核桃油含有不饱和脂肪酸，是脑组织的重要组成成分，且能防止脑动脉硬化。核桃仁中含有锌、锰、铬等大脑活动不可缺少的微量元素。

鱼和贝类　含有较多的不饱和脂肪酸，而不饱和脂肪酸是制造和维护脑细胞的重要原料，应该多食。

红萝卜　含有丰富的维生素 B_1，而缺乏维生素 B_1 的人，会发生思维迟缓和忧郁症状。

菠菜　含维生素 A、C，尤为重要的是它含有对大脑记忆功能有益的维生素 B_6 和 B_{12}。缺乏维生素 B_6 和 B_{12} 会导致神经炎、神经传导受阻，出现健忘和不安症状。此外菠菜中还含有叶绿素和钙、铁、磷等矿物质，也具有健脑益智作用。

海带　含有丰富的人体必需的矿物质营养，如磷、镁、钠、钾、钙、碘、铁、硅、锰、锌、钴、钼等，有些是陆生蔬菜所没有的物质，而且它还含有丰富的牛磺酸，对保护视力和维护大脑功能有重要的作用。

Crowndaisy chrysanthemum It has rich nutritious constituents. Both its stems and leaves are edible. It contains rich carotin. Every 100 g contains 2.54 mg of carotin. This is 15 to 30 times of that of the same amount of cucumber and eggplant.

Besides, nut kernel, milk, eggs, fresh fish, internal organs of animals and marine products contain calcium, phosphorus, and magnesium essential to nervous activities. Lack of these elements may cause nervousness, insomnia, declining memory, anxiety and spasm. Fresh milk, fresh mushroom, fresh liver and monosodium glutamate as well as other fresh foods contain glutamic acid essential to cerebral thinking activities. In addition, leafy vegetable, coarse food grain, malt, beans, yoghurt and beer contain vitamins B_1, B_6 and B_{12} that have catalytic effects on energy metabolism of cerebral substances and can improve memory.

5.6.5 Eyesight-protecting drugs and foods

Brain workers overuse their eyes. This is susceptible to tiredness of eyes with manifestations of dryness and foreign-body sensation in the eyes and blurred vision after slightly long use of eyes. For some people, they cannot even write or read, suffer from dizziness and headache. They may have nausea and vomiting in severe cases.

5.6.5.1 Eyesight-improving decoction

15 g of black bean powder, 15 g of walnut kernel, 250 ml of milk and 19 ml of honey. Grind black beans into powder after the beans are parched until they are done. Parch the walnut kernel until it is slightly burnt. Then remove the covering and pound the kernel to paste. Take out 15 g of the above two foods and put them into the boiled milk and add the honey to the milk. Take the pre-

茼蒿 营养成分丰富。茎与叶均可食。含丰富的胡萝卜素。每100 g含2.54 mg,是黄瓜、茄子含量的15～30倍。

此外,坚果仁、牛奶、蛋类、鲜鱼、动物内脏及海产品中,含有神经活动不可缺少的钙、磷、镁,缺少时将发生神经过敏、失眠、记忆力减退、焦躁和痉挛症。鲜奶、鲜蘑菇、鲜肝、味精及其他鲜味食品中含有大脑思维活动所必需的谷氨酸(智慧酸)。而叶菜、粗粮、麦胚、豆类、酸奶、啤酒中富含对大脑物质能量代谢有催化作用的维生素B_1、B_6、B_{12},可增加脑力。

五、护眼药食

脑力劳动者过度使用视力,易产生眼睛疲劳,表现为眼睛干涩,视物稍久则模糊,有的甚至无法写作或阅读,头昏头痛,严重时可出现恶心、呕吐。

1. 增视汤

黑豆粉15 g,核桃仁15 g,牛奶250 ml,蜂蜜19 ml。黑豆炒熟后磨成粉,核桃仁炒微焦,去衣,待冷后捣如泥。取以上两种食品各15 g,冲入煮沸过的牛奶,加入蜂蜜。早晨服。

5.6.5.2　Eye-nourishing decoction

10 g of Gouqizi (*Fructus Lycii*), 10 g of Sangshenzi (*Fructus Mori*), 10 g of Shanyao (*Rhizoma Dioscoreae*) and 10 Chinese dates. Decoct the ingredients in two different times. Mix the two decoctions and take the mixed decoction in two different times.

Besides, it is advisable to eat the following foods regularly to protect the eyes.

Foods with rich vitamin A　For instance, yolk, milk, goat's milk, animal liver, green leafy vegetable, and maize. These foods prevent corneal dryness and degeneration.

Foods with rich carotin　For example, carrot, pumpkin, red potato, green leafy vegetable, green soya bean and tomato.

Foods with rich vitamin B_2　For instance, flour, peanut, egg, lean meat, milk and green leafy vegetable.

5.6.6　Brain-tonifying and intelligence-benefiting drugs

It is advisable for mental workers to take brain-tonifying drugs regularly. This is especially true for those who often have dizziness, amnesia and insomnia. The following drugs may remedy hypotension, hypoglycemia, malnutrition of cardiac muscle and angina pectoris due to overuse of the brain. As for old people, these drugs may prevent and treat retardation of reaction as well as hypomnesia of senile dementia.

5.6.6.1　Yangshen Decoction, or Spirit-nourishing Decoction (cited from *Ren Shu Bian Lan*, or *Benevolent Skills for Handy Reading*)

The prescription is composed of 3 g of Tianmendong

2. 养目汤

枸杞子10 g,桑椹子10 g,怀山药10 g,红枣10枚。水煎2次,药汁混合后分2次服。

此外,保护眼睛宜常食以下食物

富含维生素A的食物。如蛋黄、牛奶、羊奶、动物肝脏、绿叶蔬菜、玉米等。这类食物可防止角膜干燥退化。

含胡萝卜素较多的食物。如胡萝卜、玉米、南瓜、红薯、绿叶蔬菜、青豆、西红柿等。

含维生素B_2较丰富的食物。如面粉、花生、鸡蛋、瘦肉、牛奶、绿叶蔬菜等。

六、健脑益智药物

脑力劳动者宜常服健脑药物。经常头晕、健忘、失眠者尤其必要。以下方药可纠正用脑过度而产生的低血压、低血糖、心肌营养不良、心绞痛等病症,对于老年人可防治反应迟钝、记忆力减退的老年痴呆症。

1. 养神汤(《仁术便览》)

天门冬、麦门冬、当归身

(*Radix Asparagi*), Maimendong (*Radix Ophiopogonis*) and Danggui (*Radix Angelicae Sinensis*) respectively, 1.5 g of Danshen (*Radix Salviae Miltiorrhizae*), 3 g of Beimu (*Bulbus Fritillariae Thunbergii*), 1.5 g of Huanglian (*Rhizoma Coptidis*), 3 g of Baizhu (*Rhizoma Atractylodis Macrocephalae*), Zhimu (*Rhizoma Anemarrhenae*) (parched with spirit) and Chenpi (*Pericarpium Citri Reticulatae*) respectively, 1.5 g of Shichangpu (*Rhizoma Acori Graminei*), Wuweizi (*Fructus Schisandarae*) (9 in number), 3 slices of Shengjiang (*Rhizoma Zingiberis Recens*). Decoct the ingredients for oral administration. Take it on a semi-empty stomach.

The prescription nourishes the heart yin and concurrently clears away asthenic fire. As for its actions, the book says "The prescription makes those diligent brain workers refreshed." It can be used as the health care drug for mental workers for prolonged administration. It is generally free from side effects. However, prolonged administration is not advisable for those with loose stool due to qi deficiency of the spleen and stomach.

5.6.6.2　Da Yizhi Powder, or Powder for Greatly Benefiting Intelligence (cited from *Qian Jin Yao Fang*, or *Valuable Prescriptions*)

The prescription is composed of 60 g of Shudihuang (*Radix Rehmanniae Praeparata*), Renshen (*Radix Ginseng*), Baifuling (*Poria*) and Roucongrong (*Herba Cistanchis*) respectively, 25 g of Tusizi (*Semen Cuscutae*) and Yuanzhi (*Radix Polygalae*) respectively and 7.5 g of Shechuangzi (*Fructus Cnidii*). Grind all the above ingredients into fine powder. Take the powder 3 g each time with rice soup after the meal, twice a day. The dosage may also be reduced proportionally and decocted for oral administration.

The prescription invigorates the kidney qi and

benefits the kidney yin. It is especially applicable to dizziness, tinnitus, retardation of reaction, amnesia and mental retardation. The prescription also has better effects on those with concurrent symptoms of seminal emission, dizziness, fatigue, general tiredness and trance. The book records that hare meat and pork are contraindicated during the administration. This is only for the readers' reference.

5.6.6.3 Kai Congming Prescription, or Intelligence-promoting Prescription (cited from *Chuan Ya Wai Bian*, *Treatise* on *External Folk Medicine*)

The prescription is composed of a proper amount of Hehuageng (*Petiolus Nelumbinis*) and Heshouwu (*Radix Polygoni Multiflori*). Dry Hehuageng (*Petiolus Nelumbinis*) in the sun and grind it into powder, Then soak the powder and Heshouwu (*Radix Polygoni Multiflori*) together in boiling water. Take the drug frequently as tea.

Hehuageng (*Petiolus Nelumbinis*), the chief ingredient in the prescription, raises the pure qi. When pure qi is raised, phlegm retention will disappear by itself, inducing resuscitation consequently. Therefore, the book says "Prolonged administration makes ordinary people intelligent, and even the weak-minded become wise."

Of the patent Chinese drugs sold in the markets, Tianwang Buxin Bill (Cardiotonic Pill), Kongsheng Zhenzhong Pill (Pill in Confucius' Pillow), Guipi Pill (Pill for Invigorating the Spleen and Nourishing the Heart), Liuwei Dihuang Bolus (Bolus of Six Drugs Including Rehmannia), etc. all have the action of tonifying the brain and may be selected for use according to the specific symptoms.

效。对头晕耳鸣，反应迟钝，健忘愚钝等症状尤为适宜。对兼有遗精，头晕乏力，浑身疲软，精神恍惚者也有较好疗效。据原书记载，服本方期间应忌食兔肉和猪肉，供参考。

3. 开聪明方(《串雅外编》)

荷花梗、何首乌各适量。将荷花梗晒干为末，与何首乌一起用沸水冲泡，当茶频饮。

此方以荷梗为主，有升清气之效。清气一升，痰饮自化，心窍随开。故"久服则令人聪明，虽至愚者亦心灵生慧也"。

市售成药中，天王补心丹、孔圣枕中丹、归脾丸、六味地黄丸等，均有脑力保健作用，可对证选用。

5.6.7 Health care with sports and massage

5.6.7.1 Sports activities

Running is the most commonly selected training event. It helps the improvement of blood circulation and functions of internal organs to accordingly ensure the plentiful supply of cerebral oxygen. Ball games like table tennis and tennis raise the speed of cerebral information conduction and feedback to improve cerebral dexterity accordingly. These events may be selected according to the individual's interest and specialty

5.6.7.2 Standing upside down walking backwards

Standing upside down effectively increases cerebral blood flow volume, eliminates tinnitus, dizziness and cerebral ischemia; backward walking moves the muscular ligament of the back, regulates the function of spinal nerves and may prevent and cure the commonly seen diseases of brain workers like cervical spondylosis, joint diseases of the waist and legs and periarthritis of shoulder.

5.6.7.3 Massaging the scalp

Massaging the vertex: Rub the scalp with both hands from the front hairline to the back hairline like the movement of combing the hair. Massaging the cephalic region: Press the temples with the thumbs. Then massage the two sides of the head upwards and downwards in a line with the other four fingers of both hands. Again, press and knead the temples clockwise and anticlockwise for several times respectively. At this time, wipe the face with the hands and massage the eyes. After rubbing the two hands together until the hands get warm, massage the face from the upper part to the lower part, from the inside part to the outside part for several times. Afterwards, do the health care exercise for the eyes. This method is ap-

七、运动按摩保健

1. 体育运动

跑步是最常选用的锻炼项目,有助于改善血液循环状态和内脏功能,从而保证大脑充足的氧气供应。乒乓球、网球等球类运动可以提高大脑信息传导、反馈的速度,从而增强大脑反应的敏捷性。可根据兴趣和特长选择。

2. 倒立与倒行

倒立可以有效地增加脑血流量,消除耳鸣、眼花及脑缺氧状态;倒行则活动背部的肌肉韧带,调节脊神经功能,可以防治脑力劳动者的常见病,如颈椎病、腰腿关节病、肩周炎。

3. 脑部按摩

头顶按摩:以两手搓头皮,从前发际到后发际作梳头动作。头侧按摩:用两手拇指按住太阳穴,其余四指从头两侧由上至下做直线按摩,再按揉太阳穴,顺时针与逆时针方向各数次,浴面摩眼。两手搓热后,从上至下,从内至外摩面数次,然后做眼部保健操,此法可消除工作后大脑疲劳。

plicable to ease cerebral fatigue after work.

5.7 Health care for physical workers

Physical workers concentrate on the movements of the tendon, bone and muscle, the characteristics of which are more consumption of energy and vigorous metabolism of internal substances. Physical workers with different types of work often assume a certain fixed posture or repeat one simple action. This makes the local tendon, bone and muscle tense for a long time and may cause internal injury due to physical overstrain. *Huangdi Neijing*, or *Canon of Medicine*, says "Prolonged looking impairs blood, prolonged lying qi, prolonged sitting muscle, prolonged standing the bone, prolonged walking the tendon." Besides, some physical workers may suffer from occupational diseases as a result of long exposure to hazardous factors like noises, radioactive substances, high temperature as well as lead, mercury, benzol, methyl alcohol, ethyl alcohol, organic phosphorus and dust.

5.7.1 Moving the limbs

Assuming the standing position for a long time makes the muscle of the waist and leg tense and tired. As a result, physical workers often feel exhausted, aching pain of the waist and leg. They are also susceptible to hump back and injury of lumbar muscle due to physical overstrain. In addition, due to gravity, blood circulation is not smooth. Consequently, phlebeurysma of lower limbs occur easily. Accordingly, participate in more activities at usual times such as taking a walk, jogging, practicing Taijiquan, swaying legs and performing gymnastics.

When working in the sitting position for a long time,

第七节 体力劳动者的保健

体力劳动者以筋骨肌肉活动为主,其特征是消耗能量多,体内物质代谢旺盛。不同工种的劳动者往往采取某个固定姿势或重复单一的动作,局部筋骨肌肉长时间处于紧张状态,可能引起劳损。《黄帝内经》有"久视伤血,久卧伤气,久坐伤肉,久立伤骨,久行伤筋"之说。此外,某些体力劳动者长期接触噪声、放射性物质、高温以及铅、汞、苯、甲醇、乙醇、有机磷、粉尘等危害因素,导致职业病的发生。

一、活动肢体

长时间处于站立姿势,腰腿肌肉紧张疲劳,常感筋疲力尽,腰腿酸痛,还容易发生驼背、腰肌劳损。又因重力作用,血液循环回流不畅,容易发生下肢静脉曲张。因此,平时可多做些散步、慢跑、打拳、摆腿、体操等活动。

长时间坐姿工作,可选择

select the events of exercising the whole body like ball games. These games improve the flexibility and sensitivity of the fingers and wrist. Besides, the games also tonify the brain, benefit intelligence and improve microcirculation.

Those who engage in high-temperature operation consume a lot of physical strength. They may take part in more activities such as walking, jogging, fencing and keep-fit gymnastics to increase the adaptive capacity and tolerance of high temperature of the organism.

Those workers who engage in highly technical jobs not only consume their physical strength, but also use the brain, for instance, long-distance drivers and technical workers in an assemble line. These people's brains are highly tense, and they are susceptible to insomnia, headache and nervous hypertension. It is advisable for them to choose the traditional Chinese keep-fit sports events with small amount of exercise and mild movements like Taijiquan and eight-section brocade. These events regulate breathing, tranquilize the mind, exercise the body, which not only relax mental tension, but also promote qi flow, relax the muscle and tendon and activate blood circulation. These people may also participate in some ball games and gymnastic games on or with apparatus to improve the ability of quick and flexible reactions of the body.

5.7.2 Balancing the diet

Adequate supply of quantity of heat should be firstly guaranteed in the diet of physical workers. Secondly, select the food which can counteract or eliminate the hazardous factors in the food according to the different types of work. Supply salt-containing drink, vitamins B and C to supplement the loss of organic salt and water due to perspiration for those who engage in high-temperature operation; increase the proportion of fat in diet for those who

全身性活动,如球类运动,可增强手指、手腕的灵巧、敏感度,并可健脑益智,改善微循环。

从事高温作业者,体力消耗大。可多散步、慢跑、击剑,多做保健体操等,以提高机体对高温的适应与耐受力。

从事技术性强,既耗体力又费脑力的工作者,如长途汽车驾驶员及连续流水作业的技术工人,此类人员大脑高度紧张,易患失眠、头痛、神经性高血压等病,宜选择运动量小、动作柔和的运动,如太极拳、八段锦等中国传统健身运动。能起到静息、安神、动形,既可放松精神,又可行气、舒筋活血的作用。也可参加一些球类及器械体操运动,以提高身体快速灵巧的反应能力。

二、平衡膳食

体力劳动者的膳食,首先要保证足够热量的供给。其次要根据不同工种,选择能抵消或解除有害因素的食物。从事高温作业者,要补给含盐饮料、维生素 B、C 等,以补充因出汗损失的无机盐和水分。在冷冻环境下工作的劳动者,

engage in freezing environment; take care to supplement vitamin A and vitamin D for those who engage in the environment lacking sunlight like mines, tunnels and places under water; increase the intake of protein, carbohydrate and vitamin C in the diet for those who are long exposed to benzol to limit the intake of fat.

5.7.2.1 Bone-strengthening medicinal diets

5.7.2.1.1 Guishen Shanyao Soup with Pig Kidneys

The diet includes 10 g of Danggui (*Radix Angelicae Sinensis*), 10 g of Dangshen (*Radix Codonopsis Pilosulae*), 10 g of Huaishanyao (*Rhizoma Dioscoreae*), 2 pig kidneys (remove the fasciae and impure substance) and a proper amount of seasoning (soy sauce, ginger, green Chinese onion, garlic, vinegar and sesame oil). Put Danggui (*Radix Angelicae Sinensis*), Dangshen (*Radix Codonopsis Pilosulae*) and Huaishanyao (*Rhizoma Dioscoreae*) into a gauze bag. Then add a proper amount of water to decoct bag for 30 minutes. Next, scoop out the bag. At this time, place a small amount of vinegar, green Chinese onion together with pig kidneys into a pot and decoct these items with slow fire. Cut the kidneys into slices when they are cold. Afterwards, put the slices into the Guishen Shanyao Soup to be decocted for a while. Eating methods: Scoop out the kidney slices first and put them into a plate. Mix the slices with seasoning. Eat the slices and drink Guishen Shanyao Soup. Or leave the pig kidney slices in the soup. Then, add some seasoning. Eat the slices with the soup.

5.7.2.1.2 Eucommia fried with Kidneys

The diet includes 12 g of Duzhong (*Cortex Eucommiae*), two pig kidneys (remove the fasciae and cut them into slices) and a proper amount of seasoning (cooking wine, ginger and green Chinese onion). First, add some clear water to Duzhong (*Cortex Eucommiae*) to be decocted for 30 minutes until the decoction is 50 ml. Then, add the cooking wine, 15 g of the seed powder of Gorgoneuryale and a proper amount of refined salt to the decoction. After stirring the decoction, mix the kidneys with the decoction. Next, put the decoction with all the ingredients into the pot to be stir-parched. When the meat is to be done, add the seasoning. The whole process is finished at this time.

5.7.2.1.3 Soup of Bone Marrow and Achyranthes

The diet includes 500 to 1,000 g of pig bone (the leg bone with marrow referred), 20 g of Huainiuxi (*Radix Achyranthis Bidentatae*) and 1,000 ml of clear water. Put the bone and Huainiuxi (*Radix Achyranthis Bidentatae*) into the water simultaneously. Decoct until the water boils. Then, add 50 ml of millet wine to the decoction. After that, decoct the ingredients again with slow fire for 30 minutes. Finally, put a small amount of ginger, green Chinese onion and refined salt to the decoction. The prescription may be used as drink. It not only relieves thirst, but also strengthens the tendon and bone.

5.7.2.2 Muscle-strengthening medicinal diets

5.7.2.2.1 Gruel of Wheat and Round-grained Nonglutinous Rice

The diet includes 150 g of wheat, 60 g of round-grained nonglutinous rice, 15 g of Guiyuanrou (*Arillus Longan*), 10 Chinese dates, 60 g of refined sugar and 1 000 ml of clear water. Cook thin gruel with all the above ingredients. Eat it when it is warm.

5.7.2.2.2 Shenyao Chinese dates Gruel

The diet includes 20 g of Dangshen (*Radix Codonopsis*

30 分钟,约至 50 ml,然后加料酒适量、荛粉 15 g、盐适量,调和后再拌入腰花,放锅内拌炒,将熟时,入调料即成。

3. 骨髓牛膝汤

猪骨(腿骨中带骨髓者最好)500～1 000 g,怀牛膝 20 g,清水 1 000 ml。将骨头与牛膝同时入水,煮沸后加黄酒 50 ml,再用小火煮 30 分钟,入姜、葱、精盐少许。本方可代饮料,既可解渴,又能强壮筋骨。

(二) 壮肌药膳

1. 小麦米粥

小麦 150 g,元米 60 g,桂圆肉 15 g,大枣 10 枚,白糖 60 g,清水 1 000 ml,共煮成稀粥,温服。

2. 参药红枣粥

党参 20 g,怀山药 30 g(研

Pilosulae), 30 g of Huaishanyao (*Rhizoma Dioscoreae*) (ground into powder), 30 g of Chinese dates, 50 g of round-grained nonglutinous rice and 1,000 ml of water. First, put Dangshen (*Radix Codonopsis Pilosulae*) into water to be decocted for 30 minutes. Then, scoop out it. Afterwards, place Chinese date and round-grained nonglutinous rice in the decoction and cook them together until the decoction boils. At this time, decoct the ingredients again with slow fire for 15 minutes. After that, put the powder of Huaishanyao (*Rhizoma Dioscoreae*) into the decoction and decoct the decoction once more for a while. The whole process is finished. Add a proper amount of refined sugar when eating the gruel.

5.7.2.3 Tendon-strengthening medicinal diet

5.7.2.3.1 Tendon Paste

Soak 500 g of pork tendon or ox tendon in warm water for a day and night. Then, cook it until it gets pulpy. At this time, add a proper amount of salt to it. Finally, wait until the tendon is cold and turns into colloid substance. Take 2 to 3 spoonfuls of it each time with boiled water.

5.7.2.3.2 Eucommia Wine

Cut 50 g of Duzhong (*Cortex Eucommiae*) into slices and soak the slices in the bottle of 500 g of red wine. Keep the bottle airtight. Shake it once a day for 7 to 15 days. Take 20 to 30 ml of the wine each time, once or twice a day.

5.7.3 Reasonable use of the brain

Physical workers should also use the brain frequently so as to achieve the balance between physical and mental activities. Develop their interest in study, and take some courses selectively according to the features of their

粉),红枣 30 g,元米 50 g,水 1 000 ml。先将党参入水煮 30 分钟,捞出,再入红枣、元米同煮,沸后小火再煮 15 分钟左右,调入山药粉,再煮片刻即可。食时加适量白糖。

(三) 强筋药膳

1. 蹄筋膏

猪筋或牛筋 500 g,温水泡 1 昼夜,小火煮至糜烂,加适量盐,待冷如胶状。每次服 2~3 匙,开水冲服。

2. 杜仲酒

杜仲 50 g,切片,浸泡于 500 g 红葡萄酒内。密封,每日振摇 1 次,7~15 日即可服用。每服 20~30 ml,每日 1~2 次。

三、合理用脑

体力劳动者也要勤用脑,做到体、脑运动的平衡。要培养自己的学习兴趣,结合职业特点选修不同的课程。如学

occupation like gardening, cooking, sewing and painting. Also, train memory consciously. Read more books and newspapers when going off work. They may participate in some head-using games like playing chess and guessing riddles.

5.8 Life cultivation for handicapped people

Handicapped people refer to the people who have lost partial or all abilities of individual life or social life as a result of the loss or abnormality in psychology, physiology and certain tissues of the human body.

5.8.1 Health care for visual disabilities

5.8.1.1 Regulating the emotions

Those with visual disabilities are susceptible to negative emotions like tension, impetuosity, depression and pessimism. It is advisable to adopt the methods of straightening them out, checking one emotion with another and suggestion therapy so as to remove bad emotional reactions. They may also use the recreational methods like music, singing and drama to make themselves cheerful. This can stabilize their emotions and improve their life quality.

5.8.1.2 Training the body

Daoyin Close the eyes and aim at the eyes with the palms in turn. Namely, the right palm aims at the right eye first. Then, imagine that a bright light is penetrating into the eyeball from the palm center. The left hand repeats the same movements. Do the daoyin with the alternating hands for 7 to 8 minutes, but no more than 10 minutes in general. Afterwards, "wipe the eyes with the

第八节 残疾人群的养生

残疾人是指因为心理、生理或人体结构上某种组织功能丧失或不正常,从而部分或全部失去个人生活能力或社会生活能力的人。

一、视力残障

(一)情志保健

视觉障碍者容易出现紧张、急躁、抑郁、悲观等消极情绪,可采用说理开导、情志相胜、暗示等方法,消除不良情志反应。也可采用音乐、歌咏、戏剧等娱乐方式,怡心悦志,以安定情绪,改善生活质量。

(二)锻炼形体

导引:闭眼,双手手掌依次轮流对准眼睛,即先右掌张开,掌心对准右眼,默想光明由掌心透入眼球。再用左手做同样动作。交替导引,作7~8分钟,一般不超过10分钟。然后"运睛"(见本书第七

fingers" (Please refer to the relevant content in Chapter 7). If there exist mild sensations like soreness, numbness and itching in the eyes, these are normal reactions.

Practice eight-section brocade or Taijiquan everyday. Generally, the simplified Taijiquan is advisable. People with better physical strength may select the forty-eight-section Taijiquan or Yang's Taijiquan.

5.8.1.3 Rehabilitation with the diets

Generally people with visual disabilities mostly select sight-improving foods like Baihe (*Bulbus Lilii*), Juhua (*Flos Chrysanthemi*) and animal livers.

5.8.1.3.1 Wolfberry Vegetable

Wolfberry vegetable, also called "Gouqitou", "Gouqimiao" and "Gouqiye" in Chinese, is the tender leaf of wolfberry. The leaf can be used to stir-fry dishes, make tea, cook gruel and thick soup. Wolfberry is bitter and sweet, cool-natured and acts upon the liver meridian and kidney meridian. It has the actions of clearing away heat, curing deficiency, nourishing the liver and improving sight. The drug is applicable to declining sight, night blindness, etc. It is advisable to decoct 60 g of wolfberry leaves, 30 g of Juemingzi (*Semen Cassiae*), 9 g of Yemingsha (*Faeces Vespertilionis*), 120 g of pork liver together. Eat the liver.

5.8.1.3.2 Abalone

Abalone, also called "Jiukongbao" and "Fuyu", is salty and warm-natured, acting upon the liver meridian. It nourishes blood, liver and yin, clears away heat, benefits essence and improves sight. The fish contains protein and over 20 nutritious constituents like amino acid as well as Baolingsu Ⅰ and Baolingsu Ⅱ. These substances can inhibit cancer cells, streptomycin, staphylococci, flu viruses, simple herpes viruses, keratitis viruses, type 12 adenovirus, etc. The meat can be made into dried abalone for food. The food is a rare delicacy and the good food for patients with eye diseases or hypertension.

5.8.1.3.3 Carrot

Carrot is sweet and neutral-natured. It benefits qi and produces blood, strengthens the stomach to remove food retention, improves sight and nourishes the liver. It is advisable to eat for those who have poor sight.

5.8.1.3.4 Gouqizi Wine (Wine of Fructus Lycii)

When brewing rice wine at home, put a proper amount of Gouqizi (*Fructus Lycii*) (1/10 of the rice) into the round-grained nonglutinous rice. After the wine is brewed, drink 20 ml of the wine when having supper or at bed time every day. The wine is applicable to declining sight and blurred vision due to blood deficiency of the liver.

5.8.1.3.5 Wolfberry Leaves Stewed with Pig Kidney

Add a proper amount of water to 100 to 150 g of wolfberry leaves and a pair of pig kidneys (remove the fasciae, wash them clean and cut them into small cubes) to cook soup. Then add some seasoning to eat the meat. The dish has the actions of strengthening the kidney and benefiting essence, improving hearing and sight. It is applicable to visual disabilities due to renal essence deficiency in old people.

5.8.1.3.6 Wolfberry Stewed with Beef

The diet includes 250 g of meat of cattle leg, 10 g of Huaishanyao (*Rhizoma Dioscoreae*), 20 g of Gouqizi (*Fructus Lycii*), 6 g of Guiyuanrou (*Arillus Longan*), a proper amount of cooking wine, refined salt, gourmet powder, segments of green Chinese onion, slices of ginger and edible oil respectively. First, wash the Shanyao

干供食用，为名贵珍肴，亦为眼科及高血压病患者的适宜食品。

3. 胡萝卜

性味甘平。功能益气生血，健胃消食，明目养肝。视力不佳者可常食。

4. 枸杞子酒

家中自酿米酒时，在元米中兑入适量干枸杞子（约为米的 1/10）。酒酿成后，每天晚餐或睡觉前饮用 20 ml 左右。适用于肝血不足所致的视力减退，视物模糊。

5. 枸杞叶煲猪腰

取枸杞叶 100～150 g、猪腰 1 对（去筋膜，洗净，切成小块），加水适量煲汤，调味食之。有补肾益精，聪耳明目之效。适用于老年肾精亏虚之视力残障。

6. 枸杞炖牛肉

牛腿肉 250 g，怀山药 10 g，枸杞子 20 g，桂圆肉 6 g，料酒、精盐、味精、葱段、姜片、生油各适量。将山药、枸杞子、桂圆肉洗净，放入盅内。将牛肉放入沸水锅中氽约 3

(*Rhizoma Dioscoreae*), Gouqizi (*Fructus Lycii*) and Guiyuanrou (*Arillus Longan*) clean and put them into a handleless cup. Secondly, put the beef into a boiling pot to be cooked for 3 minutes and scoop it out. After washing the meat clean, cut it into the chips with a diameter of 4 cm. Thirdly, heat the iron pot until it is hot. Fourthly, pour the peanut oil into the pot. Fifthly, pour the beef chips into the pot and fry them quickly with strong fire. Sixthly, boil the cooking wine and put it into the cup with the ginger and green Chinese onion on it. Seventhly, pour boiling water and salt into the cup. Then, put the cup on the water and heat it until the beef is very tender. At this time, take out the meat and remove the ginger and green Chinese onion. Finally, add the gourmet powder to the meat. The whole cooking process is finished. The meat has the actions of strengthening the kidney to benefit essence, invigorating qi and blood, nourishing the liver to improve sight. It is applicable to blurred vision due to deficiency of qi and blood resulting from insufficiency of the liver and kidney. It can also delay ageing, strengthen tendons and improve sight for healthy people.

5.8.1.3.7 Shouwu (*Radix Polygoni Multiflori*) Stewed with Liver Chips

The ingredients are 250 g of pig liver, 10 g of Heshouwu (*Radix Polygoni Multiflori*), 75 g of edible fungus (fermented in water), 50 g of green vegetable, 25 g of soya sauce, 10 g of cooking wine, 1 g of gourmet powder, 15 g of water starch, 5 g of green Chinese onion, 5 g of ginger and a proper amount of water. First, cut Heshouwu (*Radix Polygoni Multiflori*) into chips. And cook the drug in water to extract 100 ml of the concentrated liquid of Heshouwu (*Radix Polygoni Multiflori*). Secondly, cut the pig liver into chips with the shape of a willow leaf, the green Chinese onion into slivers and the

分钟捞起,洗净后切成直径约4 cm 的肉片,铁锅烧热,下花生油,倒入牛肉片爆炒,烹料酒,炒匀后放进盅内,姜、葱放在上面。白开水、盐、料酒共倒入盅内,隔水蒸2小时,至牛肉软烂取出,去掉姜、葱,加入味精即成。有补肾益精,益气益血,补肝明目之效。适用于肝肾不足,气血虚弱所致的视物模糊。健康人食用能抗衰、强筋、明目。

7. 首乌肝片

猪肝 250 g,何首乌 10 g,水发木耳 75 g,青菜 50 g,酱油 25 g,料酒 10 g,味精 1 g,水淀粉 15 g,葱 5 g,姜 5 g,清汤适量。将何首乌切片,按水煮提取法,提取何首乌浓缩液 100 ml。将猪肝切成柳叶片,葱切丝,姜切片,水发木耳摘干净,青菜洗净切成片,用开水焯一下。用木耳、青菜、葱丝、姜片、酱油、料酒、味精、盐、

ginger into slices. Thirdly, Cut the edible fungus and green vegetable into slices after washing them clean and scald the two ingredients in boiling water for a little while. Fourthly, extract the juice of the edible fungus, green vegetable, slivers of green Chinese onion, ginger slices, soya sauce, cooking wine, gourmet powder, salt, vinegar, and water starch. Use the juice and a proper amount of soup to make starch juice. Fifthly, put vegetable oil into a pot and heat the pot until the oil is 70%—80% done. Sixthly, scald the pig liver in boiling water and then remove the water in the liver. Seventhly, dip the liver in the oil in the pot until it is completely done. Eighthly, Place the cooked liver in a strainer, leave the oil in the pot. Next, put the pig liver into the pot again and fry it with strong fire. At this time pour the starch juice, cook the ingredients and stir them evenly. Finally, strain some cooked oil, and the whole cooking process is finished. This prescription nourishes the liver and improves sight. It is applicable to premature ageing, night blindness, blurred vision, etc. due to asthenia of the liver and kidney.

5.8.1.4 Health care with drugs

5.8.1.4.1 Mingmu Dihuang Pill, or Rehmannia Pill for Improving Sight(cited from *Yi Lue Liu Shu*, or *Six Books for Brief Introduction to Medicine*)

The prescription is composed of 150 g of Shudihuang (*Radix Rehmanniae Praeparata*), 60 g of Shanyurou (*Fructus Corni*), 30 g Zexie (*Rhizoma Alismatis*), 45 g of Mudanpi (*Cortex Mouttan Radics*), 60 g of Fuling (*Poria*) (wood removed), 90 g of Shanyao (*Rhizoma Dioscoreae*), 60 g of Danggui (*Radix Angelicae Sinensis*), 30 g of Chuanxiong (*Rhizoma Ligustici Chuanxiong*), 90 g of Maimendong (*Radix Ophiopogonis*) (core removed) and 90 g of Shihu (*Herba Dendrobii*). Grind all

醋、水淀粉、何首乌提取汁和适量的汤，兑成芡汁。锅内放植物油，旺火上烧至七、八成熟，先把猪肝在热水中焯一下，控净水分，下油锅内一过，熟透后倒漏勺里，锅底留油，用旺火，把猪肝倒回炒锅，随即把芡汁烹入，搅拌均匀，淋入少许明油即成。本方养肝明目。适用于肝肾亏虚所致的早衰，夜盲症，视物昏花等。

（四）药物保健

1. 明目地黄丸（《医略六书》）

熟地黄150 g，山萸肉60 g，泽泻30 g，牡丹皮45 g，茯苓60 g（去皮），山药90 g，当归60 g，川芎30 g，麦门冬90 g（去心）、石斛90 g。上为末，炼蜜为丸。每次9 g，用滚水送服。本方滋阴补血，养肝明目。可用于肝肾阴亏所致的羞明畏光，迎风流泪，视物昏花等症。球

the above ingredients into powder and make the powder into pill with honey. Take the pill with boiling water, 9 g each time. The prescription nourishes yin and enriches blood, nourishes liver and improves sight. It is applicable to photophobia, wind-induced lacrimation and blurred vision due to yin deficiency of the liver and kidney. Prolonged administration of the drug is also advisable for patients with visual disabilities due to eyeground diseases like orbital optic neuritis, optic atrophy, central retinitis and chronic glaucoma.

5.8.1.4.2 Huma Yanshou Pill, or Pill of Sesame and Qiushi (*Halitum Praeparatum*) for Prolonging Life (cited from *Fu Shou Jing Fang*, or *Excellent Prescriptions for Promoting Longevity*)

The prescription is composed of 120 g of sesame, 120 g of Qiushi (*Halitum Praeparatum*), 120 g of Heshouwu (*Radix Polygoni Multiflori*), 120 g of Baifuling (*Poria*) and 30 g of Gancao (*Radix Glycyrrhizae*). Grind all the above ingredients into fine powder and make it into pills with the size of a Chinese parasol seed with 500 g of honey. Take the pills with rice wine, 5 g each time, three times a day. The prescription has the actions of blackening the hair and beard, improving hearing and sight, preserving health and prolonging life. It may be used as the health care drug for those with visual disabilities in summer.

5.8.2 Health care for hearing disabilities

5.8.2.1 Regulating emotions

Deafness affects normal life and work, makes the patients susceptible to psychic disturbances, with the manifestations of impetuosity, irascibility, passivity and pessimism. This may aggravate the state of illness. For some patients the onset of disease is just related to emotional factors. Therefore, importance should be attached to regulating emotions.

Straightening out the patients: Get ready for explaining the situation to the patient and the family members so that they have better understanding of the onset and prognosis of deafness. As for impetuous and irascible patients, it is advisable to tell them the protracted nature of the course of disease and rehabilitation treatment. Ask them to cultivate the mind, overcome impetuosity and irascibility and be patient and perseverant in treatment. For those patients who are passive and pessimistic, encourage them positively, build up their confidence, bestir themselves, overcome their mental burden. Ask the patients to appreciate music, practice calligraphy and painting, watch fish and raise flowers. These activities may make people have ease of mind and overcome bad emotions.

5.8.2.2 Sports daoyin

5.8.2.2.1 Daoyin for Deafness (cited from *Zhu Bing Yuan Hou Lun*, or *General Treatise on the Causes and Symptoms of Diseases*)

Sit on the ground with the feet crossed. Then, extend the hands into the place where the feet bend. Afterwards, lower the head and put crossed hands on the back of the neck. Do the exercise twice a day, 5 to 10 minutes each time.

5.8.2.2.2 Taijiquan and Eight-section Brocade

The two events may be done respectively every day in the morning and evening. Increase the amount of exercise gradually. The games are to strengthen physique and cultivate the mind.

5.8.2.2.3 Self-control Therapy

After getting up in the morning and going to bed in the evening, stand in a place with fresh air with the eyes closed and attention concentrated. Then, place the tongue

因此,养生应重视调节情志。

语言开导:对病人及其家属做好解释工作,使他们了解耳聋的发病和预后。对急躁易怒患者,当告之本病病程及康复医疗的长期性,嘱其涵养精神,戒躁戒怒,耐心坚持医疗。对消极悲观患者,应给予积极鼓励,唤起信心,振作精神,消除不必要的思想负担。欣赏音乐、书法绘画、观鱼养花等娱乐活动,能舒畅病人心情,消除不良情绪。

(二)运动导引

1. 耳聋导引法(《诸病源候论》)

坐在地上,交叉两脚,用两手从脚腕子中伸入,低头把手交叉放在项部,每日2次,每次5~10分钟。

2. 太极拳和八段锦

可分别安排在每天早、晚进行,运动量逐渐增加,旨在增强体质,怡养精神。

3. 自控疗法

早起后、晚睡前,站立于空气新鲜之地,闭目凝神,舌尖抵上腭,意念集中耳内。腹

tip against the upper palate, and concentrate the mind on the inner part of the ear. Assume abdominal respiration and keep silent for 2 minutes. After that, rub the two hands against each other until they get warm. Next, press the external auricular tract with the palms and rotate clockwise for 100 times. Afterwards, press the auricles and cover the auricular tracts with the middle fingers of the both hands. Snap the middle finger with the index finger downwards and strike the mastoidea of the ear root for 100 times. At this moment, the sound of "ge! ge!" (cluck! cluck!) can be heard to reach the auricular drum membrane directly. Finally, swallow the saliva in the mouth slowly and move the mind to Dantian.

5.8.2.3　Self-massage

Adopt the methods of Ming Tian Gu, or massaging the auricles (Please refer to the relevant content in Section 5 of Chapter 7 of this book). Besides, knead and press Tinggong. Namely, knead and press Tinggong (SI 19) acupoints with the two index fingers, with the middle fingers overlapping on the index fingers until there appears the feeling of the sound "rumble" inside the ears. Knead and press the part upwards while inhaling; knead and press the part downwards while exhaling. This is a cycle. Repeat the cycle for 8 times continuously.

The method is advisable for those who have otopiesis of covering the ears and drawing the air from the ears with the palms. Namely, press the two ear roots with the two palms respectively, with the palm root facing the front and the fingers pressing close to the back hairline. First, Apply force into the ears with the two palms. Then pull away the palms quickly from the ears to draw air inside the ears. Do the exercise for 5 to 10 times. Afterwards, adopt the method of bulging the mouth with air. Namely, the patient holds the nose be-

式呼吸，静默2分钟，然后搓两手使热，用手掌按住外耳道顺时针方向旋转100次。又用两手中指各按耳郭贴盖耳道，用食指从中指上弹滑下来敲打耳根乳突部100次，只听见"咯、咯"的声音直射耳鼓膜。最后将口中唾液徐徐咽下，用意念引至丹田。

（三）自我推拿

采用鸣天鼓、按摩耳郭等（见本书第七章第五节）。另可揉按听宫，即两手食指在听宫处揉按，并以中指叠加其上，以感到耳内有隆隆声为宜。吸气时向后向上揉按，呼气时向下揉按，连做8次。

对鼓膜内陷者，可施窝耳拔气法。即两手掌心分按两耳，掌根向前，手指贴后发际，两手掌先向耳内慢压用力，随即迅速向外拔起，计5～10次。然后，可加用自身鼓气法。即让病人捏鼻闭口，用力鼓气，每日1次，以促使内陷鼓膜向正常位变化（患感冒及鼻炎者忌用）。

tween the fingers and close the mouth. Then bulge the mouth forcefully with air. Do the exercise once a day to promote the normal changes of the ear with otopiesis (This method is contraindicated in the case of common cold and rhinitis).

5.8.2.4 Health care with the diet

It is advisable for deafness patients to eat more kidney-strengthening foods like black-bone chickens, animal kidneys and black beans.

5.8.2.4.1 A proved recipe

The recipe includes a pair of pig kidneys (with the fasicae removed and the meat cut into slices), 200 g of Jingmi (*Fructus Oryzae Sativae*), 2 segments of Congbai (*Bulbus Allii Fistulosi*), 7 segments of Xiebai (*Bulbus Allii Macrostemi*), 5 g of Renshen (*Radix Ginseng*) and 3 g of Fangfeng (*Radix Ledebouriellae*). Grind all the ingredients into powder. Cook gruel with the powder. It is especially applicable to asthenic deafness.

5.8.2.4.2 Deer Kidney Gruel (cited from *Taiping Shenhui Prescriptions*, or *Peaceful Holy Benevolent Prescriptions*)

The Gruel includes a deer kidney, 30 g of Roucongrong (*Herba Cistanchis*), 100 g of Jingmi (*Fructus Oryzae Sativae*), a proper amount of Congbai (*Bulbus Allii Fistulosi*), pepper powder and table salt respectively. First, remove the fasciae and wash the deer kidney clean. Then cut the kidney into pieces. Next, soak Roucongrong (*Herba Cistanchis*) in yellow rice wine for a night. After that, remove the creased bark and from Roucongrong (*Herba Cistanchis*) and cut it into pieces. Afterwards, wash the nonglutinous rice clean and put it in a pot. Cook the rice until it is half-done. At this time, add the deer kidney, Roucongrong (*Herba Cistanchis*), Congbai (*Bulbus Allii Fistulosi*), pepper powder and salt to

（四）饮食保健

耳聋患者，宜多食乌骨鸡、动物肾脏、黑豆等补肾食物。

1. 验方

猪肾1对（去膜，切），以粳米200 g、葱白2根、薤白7根、人参5 g、防风3 g为末，同煮粥食。尤适合虚证耳聋。

2. 鹿肾粥（《太平圣惠方》）

鹿肾1具，肉苁蓉30 g，粳米100 g，葱白、胡椒粉、食盐各适量。将鹿肾去除筋膜，冲洗干净切碎。肉苁蓉用黄酒浸泡一宿，刮去皱皮，切碎。粳米淘洗干净，放入锅中，煮至半熟，加鹿肾、肉苁蓉、葱白、胡椒粉、食盐，再煮至粥成。本品有补肾壮阳、益精填髓功效。适用于虚弱劳损，耳聋耳鸣。

cook gruel. The gruel has the actions of strengthening the kidney yang, benefiting essence and supplementing marrow. It is applicable to weakness, internal injury due to physical overstrain, deafness and tinnitus.

Deafness patients should moderate the diet and avoid craputence. It is advisable for them to have bland diet, more melons, fruits and vegetables, to drink less wine and quit smoking.

5.8.2.5 Health care with drugs

Prolonged administration of the following proved recipes has better protective effects on hearing.

5.8.2.5.1 The recipe includes 30 g of Huangqi (*Radix Astragali seu Hedysari*), 15 g of Baijili (*Fructus Tribuli*), 15 g of Qianghuo (*Rhizoma seu Radix Notopterygii*) and a pair of sheep kidneys. Dry all the ingredients over a fire and grind them into powder. Make the powder into pills with honey with the size of a Chinese parasol seed. Take the pills before the meal with the soup of stewed green Chinese onion and salt, 3 g each time. It is applicable to deafness due to asthenia of the kidney.

5.8.2.5.2 Grind 45 g of Qiuyin (*Pheretima seu Allolobophora*) and Chuanxiong (*Rhizoma Ligustici Chuanxiong*) into powder. Take the powder with Maimendong Decoction (Decoction of Radix Ophiopogonis), 6 g each time and one dose a night. After the administration, bendover the desk to sleep with the head lowered. It is applicable to deafness with concurrent the symptoms of blood stasis.

5.8.2.6 Nursing in daily life

Keep the living environment comfortable, regular schedule of work and rest and plentiful sleep. Attach importance to physical training to enhance physique. As for senile deafness, it is in particular advisable to avoid fatigue; as for noise-induced deafness, it is advisable to reduce or control noises so as to avoid aggravating the disease. It is forbidden to pick the ears so as to keep the ear tract clean. In the case of deafness due to drug poisoning, greatest effects should be exerted to avoid further use of these drugs.

5.8.3 Health care for linguistic disabilities

Linguistic disabilities include two major groups: aphasia (like the loss of linguistic function after apoplectic seizure) as well as deafness and dumbness. Deafness and dumbness mostly are due to the severe deafness of two ears as a result of congenital factors or various causes during infancy. This results in the inability to learn speech, giving rise to deafness and dumbness. Of deafness and dumbness, deafness is the main cause which leads to dumbness. Deafness and dumbness are divided into congenital one and acquired one. The former includes the three major factors of hereditary, gestational and perinatal factors; the latter includes loss of hearing function due to infectious diseases, drug poisoning or certain accidental factors which may further develop into deafness and dumbness.

5.8.3.1 Regulating emotions

Due to the loss of communicative function with language, aphasia patients are susceptible to bad emotional reactions like impetuosity, irascibility or dispiritedness and pessimism. They are liable to sense of inferiority. Accordingly, people should adopt gesture language or other means of images to straighten them out. During their daily life and study, use encouraging methods such as awarding and praising to overcome their bad emotions like depression and pessimism. Organize the patients to participate in games, dances, fishing, flying the kite as well as

量减少或限制噪音,以免加重病情。禁止挖耳,保持耳道清洁。对药物中毒性耳聋,应尽可能避免再次使用耳毒性药物。

三、语言残障

语言功能障碍,包括失语(如中风后的语言功能丧失)和聋哑两大类。聋哑多系先天因素或婴幼儿时期多种原因使双耳发生重度耳聋,致无法学习言语,造成既聋又哑状态。两者关系是以聋为主,因聋而哑。又可分为先天性聋哑和后天性聋哑。先天者,有遗传、孕期和产期三类因素。后天者,则是由于传染病、药物中毒,或某些意外而失去听觉功能,变成聋哑。

(一)调节情志

失语患者由于语言交流功能的丧失,容易产生急躁易怒或消极悲观的不良情志反应。聋哑患者容易出现自卑心理。因此,应采用手势和其他形象化手段来实施开导。平时的生活学习要多用奖励、表扬等鼓励方法,以消除抑郁悲观等不良情绪。组织患者经常参加游戏、舞蹈、钓鱼、放

appreciating calligraphy and painting. These activities may make them be in a cheerful frame of mind and increase joys of life.

5.8.3.2 Sports Daoyin

5.8.3.2.1 The method of "swallowing saliva" recorded in Chinese ancient books has better healthcare effect on aphasia patients. Do the exercise once in the morning and in the evening respectively. The methods are as follows. ① Assume the erectly standing posture, with the feet being as wide as the shoulder. Bend the knees slightly with the neck straight and shoulder dropped. Draw in the chest and lift the back. Put the overlapped hands on the place one cun below the navel [Qihai (CV6)], with the left hand inside and the right hand outside. Close the mouth, with the lingual tip touching the upper palate. Close the eyes slightly, with natural breathing. Enter a quiet state, with all distracting thoughts removed, and mindwill concentrated on Dantian. ② Stir the tongue in the mouth endlessly. This is the so-called "The Red Dragon Stirring the Sea". This makes the saliva in the mouth increase steadily. Wait until there is a mouthful of saliva and swallow it slowly in three divided doses. Meanwhile, send the saliva down to Yongquan (KI1) with the mindwill. Do the exercise for 6 times. ③ Put the crossed hands in the front, with the thumbs fixing the chin. Open the mouth slightly and loosen the lower jaw. Move mindwill from Dantian to Yongquan (KI1). Afterwards, shake the hands towards the anterosuperior direction endlessly so that the loosened lower jaw loosens and shuts as the hands shake. This causes the lower teeth to tap the upper teeth, producing the sound of "snapping". Generally, the advisable tapping speed is 120 times a minute. Wait until there is a mouthful of saliva and swallow it slowly in three divided doses. Send the saliva to Dantin

风筝活动及观赏书画等，使其心情愉快，增强生活乐趣。

（二）运动导引

1. 中国古籍中的"咽唾法"对失语者有较好的保健效果，每天早晚各练一次。其方法是：① 身体直立，两脚与肩同宽，膝稍曲，项直，沉肩，含胸拔背。左手里，右手外，相叠置于脐下1寸半（气海穴）处，闭口，舌抵上腭，微闭眼，自然呼吸，入静，排除一切杂念，意守丹田。② 将舌在口中不停搅动，此谓"赤龙搅海"，使口中唾液不断增生。待唾液满口，分三口随气徐徐咽下，用意送到丹田。连做6次。③ 双手合十置于面前，以两手大拇指扣住下巴，微张嘴，放松下颌，意念从丹田移守涌泉穴，然后双手向前上方不停颤动，使放松的下颌随手的颤动一松一合，带动下齿叩击上齿，发出"叩叩"声响，一般以每分钟120次左右为宜。待唾液满口，则分三口随气徐徐咽下，用意送到丹田。连做3次。④ 用双手搓面、摩头各36下后结束。

with mindwill. Do the exercise for three times. ④ Rub the face and massage the head with the hands respectively for 36 times. The whole process is finished by now.

5.8.3.2.2　Taijiquan and eight-section brocade
The two events may be done respectively in the morning and in the evening, and the amount of exercise is gradually increased. The events make the patients be at ease of the mind and enhance physique.

Please refer to the relevant content in "7.8.2 Hearing disabilities" as for healthcare with sports for people with deafness and dumbness.

5.8.3.3　Life cultivation with the diet

Aphasia patients should eat bland diet, avoid greasy, fine, sweet, dampness-promoting and fire-generating foods. It is advisable to eat more fruits like haws, apples, and bananas as well as more vegetables like celeries, radishes, wax gourds and potatoes. Quit smoking and drinking.

5.8.3.3.1　As for asthenia of the liver and kidney, it is advisable to select Er Mu Yuan Yu, or Soft-shelled Turtle Stewed with Zhimu (*Rhizoma Anemarrhenae*) and Beimu (*Bulbus Fritillariae*) (cited from *Fu Ren Liang Fang*, or *Effective Prescriptions for Women*) The ingredients include one soft-shelled turtle (roughly 500 g), 5 g of Beimu (*Bulbus Fritillariae*), Zhimu (*Rhizoma Anemarrhenae*), Qianhu (*Radix Peucedani*), Chaihu (*Radix Bupleuri*) and Xingren (*Semen Armeniacae Amarum*) respectively and a proper amount of table salt. Add water to cover the meat. Steam the ingredients in a steamer for an hour. Eat the meat while it is warm after it is done.

5.8.3.3.2　As for blood stasis due to qi deficiency, it is advisable to select Peach Kernel Gruel (cited from *Duo Neng Bi Shi*). The ingredients are 15 g of Huangqi

2. 太极拳和八段锦　可分别安排在每天早、晚进行，运动量逐步增加，一则调畅情志，二则以增强体质。

聋哑患者的运动保健，参见本节"二"。

（三）饮食养生

失语患者的饮食以清淡为宜，应避免油腻厚味、肥甘助湿生火之品。宜多食山楂、苹果、香蕉等水果，多食芹菜、萝卜、冬瓜、西红柿等蔬菜。并戒烟酒。

1. 肝肾亏虚证，可选二母元鱼（《妇人良方》）：元鱼（鳖）1只（约重500 g），贝母、知母、前胡、柴胡、杏仁各5 g，黄酒适量，食盐少许。宰杀元鱼，去头、内脏，洗净切块，加入贝母、知母、前胡、柴胡、杏仁及适量黄酒、少许食盐，加水没过肉块，置蒸锅中蒸1小时，于蒸熟后趁热食用。

2. 气虚血瘀证，可选桃仁粥（《多能鄙事》）：黄芪15 g，桃仁10～15 g，粳米100 g，先

(*Radix Astragli seu Hedysari*), 10 to 15 g of peach kernel and 100 g of Jingmi (*Fructus Oryzae Sativae*). First, pound the peach kernel to paste. Then, add water to grind the juice and remove the dregs. Finally, cook thin gruel with the juice and the rice.

It is suitable for the patients with deafness and dumbness to eat more liver-and kidney-tonifying foods like animal kidneys, sea cucumbers and eels. As for the diet prescriptions, please refer to the relevant content of "7.8.2 Hearing disabilities".

5.8.3.4 Health care with drugs

It is advisable to regularly take Chinese patent medicines for tonifying the liver and kidney, promoting blood circulation and inducing resuscitation like Liuwei Dihuang Bolus (Bolus of Six Drugs Including Rehmannia) and Jie Yu Pill (Aphsia-curing Pill) at usual times.

5.8.3.5 Nursing in daily life

Participate in suitable sports activities to enhance physique. At the same time, take care to combine work and rest to avoid overfatigue. It is advisable to select light and nutritious foods. People should pay attention to the patients' psychological trends to ensure their safety during daily life.

5.8.4 Health care for disabilities of limbs and the body

Disabilities refer to the functional disturbances or loss due to trauma and diseases of limbs and the body like hemiplegia, paraplegia, fracture and amputation. In addition, severe multiple neuritis, myelitis, progressive myoatrophy, myodystrophy and hysterical paralysis. The disease is called "wei zheng"(flaccidity syndrome) in TCM. Here all these diseases are discussed together.

Disabilities of limbs and the body may occur in many

把桃仁捣烂如泥,加水研汁去渣,同粳米煮为稀粥。

聋哑患者宜多食补养肝肾之品,如动物肾脏、海参、鳝鱼之类。食疗方参见本节"二"。

（四）药物保健

日常保养宜常服六味地黄丸、解语丹之类补养肝肾、活血开窍成药。

（五）起居护理

参加合适的体育活动,增强体质,并注意劳逸结合,避免过分疲劳。饮食宜选易消化,富有营养之品。生活中注意其心理动向,以保障安全。

四、肢体残障

肢体因伤、因病导致功能障碍或丧失,如偏瘫、截瘫、骨折、截肢等,均属此列。此外,多发性神经炎重症、脊髓炎、进行性肌萎缩、肌营养不良症、癔病性瘫痪等,中医称为"痿证"者,在此一并论述。

肢体残障可发生于身体

parts of the body such as limbs, vertebrae and trunk. Flexible treatment and proper methods are advisable according to the specific pathological sites in the health preservation of the disabilities.

5.8.4.1 Regulating emotions

The patients are susceptible to bad emotions like pessimism, melancholia and impetuosity because of the functional loss resulting from disabilities of limbs and the body. It is advisable for them to select proper psychological health preservation methods in accordance with the patients' mental states. Various toys are suitable for children and juveniles with disabilities of limbs and the body as a means of recreation, and also beneficial to the rehabilitation of the functions of their hands and feet. Besides, reasonable arrangement of the colors, objects, flavors, light and sounds may have the imperceptible psychological actions of health preservation as well. For further information, please refer to the relevant content of Chapter 2.

5.8.4.2 Health care with sports

Select the proper patting methods in health preservation in accordance with the different sites of disabilities. For example, the patient or the doctor may pat the patient's left upper limb from the upper part to the lower part, from the front to the back, from the left to the right with the right palm or fist for 25 times respectively (in 5 different times, 5 times of patting each time). Afterwards, pat the right upper limb with the left palm or fist in the same way as the above method. The patient or the doctor may also pat the patient's lower limbs. Pat the left thigh and leg from the upper part to the lower part with the left palm or fist for 5 times each time. Pat the upper, lower, medial and lateral sides 5 to 10 times respectively, 100 to 200 times in all; then pat the right thigh and leg

诸多部位,如四肢、脊椎、躯干等,应根据病理部位的不同,灵活处理,采用合适的养生方法。

(一) 调节情志

由于肢体残障而功能缺失,患者易产生悲观、忧郁、急躁等不良情绪。应根据病人精神状态,选择适当的心理养生法。如书法、绘画、弹琴等有利于平静心情,同时可促进上肢功能的恢复。各种玩具是少年儿童肢体残障者适应的娱乐方式,也有利于手足功能的康复。此外,室内色彩、景物、气味、光线、声音的合理搭配,也能起到潜移默化的心理养生作用,可参阅本书第二章的有关内容。

(二) 运动保健

根据残障部位的不同,适当采用拍打健身的方法。如:拍打上肢,可由患者或医者,用右掌或握拳拍打左上肢,从上而下,前后左右,每面拍打25下(分5次,1次5下)。然后用左手掌或握拳拍打右上肢,方法同前。拍打下肢,亦可由患者或医者进行。用左手掌或握拳拍打左侧大腿和小腿,从上往下拍打,一次5下,拍打上、下、内、外四面,每面拍打5至10次,100~200下;然后右手拍打右侧大腿小

with the right hand in the same way as the above method.

For those with the activity disturbances of upper limbs except paraplegia, they may practice to write characters, throw objects, catch a ball, use an abacus, play a musical instrument and knit a sweat; for those with activity disturbances of lower limbs, they may practice to ride a tricycle, do some sewing, etc.

In addition, other health preservation methods with traditional sports events are advisable according to the patients' specific conditions like state of diseases, interest and individual conditions. Take care to follow in order and advance step by step when having physical training on the basis of their abilities.

5.8.4.3 Life cultivation with loutrotherapy

Bathing in spring water is more suitable. It is advisable to drink spring water and bathe in spring water simultaneously. It is suitable to drink sweet spring water and to bathe in low temperature spring water in combination with massage for the promotion of qi flow and blood circulation as well as functions of limbs and the body. Generally speaking, bathe in the water of salt springs or carbonic acid springs with the suitable temperature of 39 to 42℃ for 20 to 30 minutes; bathe in the water of hydrogen sulfide springs or radon springs with the suitable temperature of 38 to 40℃ for 15 to 20 minutes, 3 or 4 times a day. Bathing massage is mostly done by a doctor while the patient is bathing. The patient may use the buoyancy of water to exercise his or her affected limbs. Hot water may be used as the substitute in the place where there are no springs.

Besides, the patient may use hot sand therapy, sunlight therapy and air therapy as he thinks the method is practicable.

Medicated bath is also the commonly-used health

腿与前同。

除截肢者外,若上肢活动障碍者,采用写字、投掷、接球、拨算盘、弹琴、编织等;下肢活动受限,采用踏三轮车、缝纫等方法运动。

此外,还可结合病人具体情况,如病情、兴趣及个人条件等,采取其他传统体育养生法。锻炼时要注意循序渐进,量力而行。

(三) 沐浴养生

泉水浴较适宜,可采取泉饮与泉浴双管齐下的方法。泉饮以甘泉水为宜,泉浴则以低温度水浸浴为宜,并结合浴中按摩,以流通气血,促进肢体功能。一般而言,食盐泉或碳酸泉,水温宜39~42℃,浸浴20~30分钟;硫化氢泉或氡泉,水温宜38~40℃,浸浴15~20分钟,每日可烫浴3~4次。浴摩法多由医者在浴中施行按摩。患者可利用水的浮力活动病肢。无泉水的地方,可用热水代替。

此外,尚可酌情选用热沙疗法、日光疗法、空气疗法等。

药浴也是肢体残障者常

preservation method for those with disabilities of the limbs and body. Decoct Cangzhu (*Rhizoma Atractylodis*), Huangbai (*Cortex Phellodendri*), Niuxi (*Radix Achyranthis Bidentatae*), Heshouwu (*Radix Polygoni Multiflori*), black bean, Taoren (*Semen Persicae*), Honghua (*Flos Carthami*) and Danggui (*Radix Angelicae Sinensis*). Use the decoction to fumigate and steam, or bathe the affected part, or wash and bathe the whole body for 15 to 20 minutes each time, once or twice a day.

5.8.4.4 Dietary therapy with the medicinal diet

Dry 300 g of cattle bone marrow over a fire and grind it into powder. Parch 300 g of black sesame until it smells fragrant and grind it into powder. Then add a proper amount of sugar to the powder and mix and stir the types of powder evenly. Take the powder twice a day, 9 g each time. Or cook 200 g of fresh pig bone marrow, 30 g of soybeans and 100 g of Jingmi (*Fructus Oryzae Sativae*) together. Eat the food. Besides, it is also advisable to dry pig spinal cord or cattle spinal cord over a fire. Then, grind it into powder. Mix it with rice powder. Take the powder after mixing it with sugar water. Also, The powder of human placenta may be taken, twice a day, 3 g each time.

In addition, patients with deficiency of qi and blood may eat Hen Stewed with Danggui (*Radix Angelicae Sinesis*) and Gruel of Huangqi (*Radix Astragali seu Hedysari*) and Dazao (*Fructus Ziziphi Jujubae*); patients with blood stasis may eat Peach Kernel Gruel or Haw Gruel.

5.8.4.5 Health care with drugs

The ingredients include 300 g of slices of Lujiao (*Cornu Cervi*) (soaked in wine for 12 hours first), 120 g of Shudihuang (*Radix Rehmanniae Praeparata*) and 45 g of slices of Fuzi (*Radix Aconiti Praeparata*). First, steam the ingredients until they are done. Then, dry the ingredients over a fire and grind them into powder. Make the powder into pills with barley gruel. Take the pills with rice soup, 3 times a day, 7 g each time. The pill is applicable to asthenia of the liver and kidney.

5.8.4.6 Nursing in daily life

Patients lying in bed may adopt the clinostatic passive physical training, the postures of which are changed at any time to prevent deformities. Then, they may adopt active physical training like the sitting, standing and walking exercise.

Patients lying in bed should take care to keep them warm to avoid invasion by exogenous pathogenic cold and wind. Turn over body frequently and change the postures to prevent pneumonia and bed sore.

5.8.5 Health care for intellectual disabilities

Intellectual disabilities refer to the decline, even loss of the patient's intelligence (including the abilities to observe, memorize, concentrate attention, comprehend, judge, orientate, calculate and imagine), which makes the patient incompetent to work, and difficult to manage household duties and daily life. At the same time, the patient is accompanied by personality changes with the manifestations of depression, mechanical and queer life, or impetuosity, confrontation with others due to trifle affairs, or susceptibility to suspicion and anxiety, increase of speech which is long-winded and repeated. The typical symptom is weak-mindedness and dementia.

Intellectual disabilities are mostly due to cerebral trauma, sudden cerebral stroke, anoxic cerebral injury, toxic cerebropathy and senile degenerative cerebral diseases

熟,焙干为末,大麦粥和为丸,每日3次,每次7g,米汤送服。适用于肝肾亏损证。

(六) 起居护理

卧床患者可采用卧位被动形体训练,随时变换姿势,防止畸形发生。继则采用主动训练,如坐、立和步行练功。

卧床者要注意保暖,避免冷风外邪的侵袭。经常翻身,改变体位,以防并发肺炎及褥疮。

五、智力残障

智力残障,是指患者的智力(包括观察力、记忆力、注意力、理解力、判断力、定向力、计算力、想像力等)衰退,甚至完全丧失,难以胜任工作、家务,生活自理困难。同时伴有人格改变,表现为抑郁寡欢,生活刻板怪异,或情绪急躁,易因小事与人冲突,或善疑多虑,语言增多,啰唆而重复。而最典型的症状为弱智、痴呆。

智力残障,除少部分是先天导致,大部分是因为脑外伤、脑卒中、缺氧性脑损害、中

except a small number of congenital factors.

5.8.5.1 Regulating emotions and art cultivation

Family members and physicians should be considerate of and care for patients, comfort and encourage them to induce their active will for rehabilitation. On this basis, perform intellectual rehabilitation for them. Doctors should try their best to discover the still existing intellectual factors. Then adopt the behavior therapy and repeatedly intensify this to delay or remedy the continuous decline of intelligence. The artistic forms like music are the very good methods to improve the patients' emotions. Certain people with intellectual disabilities often have exceptionally good artistic abilities. Therefore, doctors should take care to discover and cultivate these talents.

5.8.5.1.1 Life cultivation with music

Music has better effects on promoting intelligence and should be often applied in daily life. For the patients mainly with depression, select the music for expressing emotions and arousing feeling; for the patients with susceptibility to impetuosity and irascibility, select the light and melodious music for tranquilizing the mind. As for old people, it is suitable to select the songs the patients were familiar with or liked when they were children or youths to slow down the decline of their memory and delay their ageing. This is helpful for the rehabilitation of patients with senile dementia. As to children, select simple, easy, happy and lively children's musical compositions suitable for children's psychological features.

5.8.5.1.2 Watching or performing plays

In plays, there exist the music, dances, plots and

毒性脑病、老年变性脑病等所致。

（一）调节情志和艺术养生

家人和医师对待智力残障患者应采取体贴、关心的态度，生活中多采用安慰、鼓励的方式，诱导患者产生康复的积极愿望，在此基础上进行智力的康复。应尽量发现患者尚存智力的因素，采用行为疗法，反复予以强化，以延缓或纠正智力的继续衰退。音乐等艺术形式是改善患者情志的很好方式，某些智力残障者往往具有艺术方面的超常才能，应注意发现并加以培养。

1. 音乐养生

音乐对促进智力有较好的效果，可在日常生活中经常使用。对以抑郁为主的患者，可选用抒解心情、激昂情绪的乐曲；对急躁易怒的患者，则选用镇静安神、轻松悠扬的乐曲。对老年人，应采用患者幼时与年轻时熟悉和喜欢的歌曲，可以减缓记忆力的衰退，推迟智力老化，有助于老年性痴呆病人的康复。对儿童，则应选择符合儿童心理特点，浅显易懂、轻松活泼的儿歌类乐曲。

2. 观赏或表演戏剧

戏剧有音乐舞蹈，还有情

roles which greatly move people and provoke people's thinking. Accordingly, watching or performing plays may regulate the patients' emotions and delay the decline of cerebral functions. Middle-aged and old people should often watch plays, and the patients may also be organized to rehearse and perform plays if the conditions permit.

5.8.5.1.3 Practicing calligraphy, painting, playing a musical instrument and chess

People should be absorbed in practicing calligraphy and painting, playing a musical instrument and chess to bring the thinking and creative abilities of their brains into full play in pursuit of the aesthetic artistic conception. Therefore, these activities may promote intellectual development and train the fine movements of hands as better means of intellectual health preservation. A part of children with intellectual disabilities have exceptionally good artistic talents. This may also be discovered by the daily training.

5.8.5.2 Meditation and enhancement of health

5.8.5.2.1 Meditation

Meditation surely promotes intellectual activities. Its mechanism lies in the fact that the purpose of improving physiological functions is achieved by means of the psychological self suggestion. Its method is as follows: Get rid of all distracting thoughts and suggest to yourself that there exists a red sun, shining over your head. Your vertex feels hot gradually. The warm current enters your brain, every part of your brain. Then the warm current penetrates into your limbs, even throughout the whole body.

The detection of the cerebral blood flow chart shows that for those with intellectual disabilities, the supply of blood volume of cerebral cortex increases greatly if they often practice meditation. This indicates that the cerebral

节、角色,能感人肺腑,引人思考,因而能调节患者情绪,减缓大脑功能的衰退,中老年人应经常观赏戏剧,有条件者还应当组织患者排练、表演戏剧。

3. 书画弹琴弈棋

从事书画弹琴弈棋等活动,务必全神贯注,集中发挥大脑的思维创造能力,追求美的意境,因此能促进智力发展,还能锻炼手的精细动作,是较好的智力养生手段。部分智力残障儿童在艺术方面有超常的才能,也可以通过日常训练而发现。

(二) 冥想和健身

1. 冥想

对促进智力活动有肯定的效果。其原理,是通过心理学上的自我暗示,以达到改善生理功能的目的。做法为:排除头脑中的一切杂念,暗示自己的头顶有一轮红日照耀,头顶渐渐发热,热流进入大脑,进入大脑的每一个部位,然后进入四肢,乃至全身。

脑血流图的检测表明,经常练习冥想的智力残障者,大脑皮质的供血量有较大幅度的增加,表明大脑的血液循环

blood circulation has been improved.

5.8.5.2.2 Health-enhancing ball

Health-enhancing ball is applicable to the intellectual disabilities due to maim and disease-induced handicap. As for training methods, the patients may use the simple movements like rotating one ball clockwise and anticlockwise on one palm at first. Then, gradually shift to complicated movements like rotating two balls on two palms, rotating two balls in an inside-outsidely leaping way, rotating many balls in a mutually circling way and rotating balls once after every three times of dribbling balls. The patients may shift to new methods continuously to achieve the state of high proficiency and frequent variations. This may effectively delay decline of the brain. Balance the left and right hands, and alternate the two hands when practicing the balls with two hands. Do not ignore to use the left hand in particular. This measure may ensure equal development of the functions of the two cerebral hemispheres.

In addition, the patients may practice the simplified Taijiquan, eight-section brocade and five-mimic games. Playing games is also the suitable training item for patients with intellectual disabilities. Please refer to the methods introduced in Section Two of this chapter.

5.8.5.3 Life cultivation with diets

Brain-tonifying Tea: The ingredients include Hegeng (*Petiolus Nelumbinis*), Heshouwu (*Radix Polygoni Multiflori*), Dandouchi (*Semen Sojae Praeparatum*), Huajiao (*Pericarpium Zanthoxyli*), Gouqizi (*Fructus Lycii*), Dazao (*Fructus Ziziphi Jujubae*) and crystal sugar. Drink it as beverage at usual times. The tea has unique taste and can be used regularly as a daily drink.

Brain-tonifying Gruel: Grind Hetaoren (*Semen*

2. 健身球

适用于伤残、病残导致的智力残障。锻炼的方法,可由单球正反旋转等运动逐步向双球双手旋转、里外跳跃旋转、多球互绕旋转、三带一旋转等高难动作发展,使玩球的花样不断翻新,以达到得心应手、变化无常的境界,这样便会有效地延缓大脑的衰退。左右手锻炼健身球要注意平衡,交替使用,尤其不要忽视左手玩球,以保证大脑两个半球的功能水平得到均衡发展。

此外,还可选练简化太极拳、八段锦及五禽戏等。游戏也是智力残障者的适宜锻炼项目,可参考本章第二节介绍的方法。

(三) 食疗养生

健脑茶 荷梗、何首乌、淡豆豉、花椒、枸杞子、大枣、冰糖,平时作为饮料服用。该茶有独特的口味,可作为日常饮品常用。

补脑粥 用核桃仁、莲

Juglandis), Lianzi (*Semen Nelumbinis*), Gouqizi (*Fructus Lycii*), Xingren (*Semen Armeniacae Amarum*), Taoren (*Semen Persicae*), Baiziren (*Semen Biotae*), Zaoren (*Semen Ziziphi Jujubae*) and Shichangpu (*Rhizoma Acori Graminei*) into pieces. Cook gruel with the ingredients and oatmeal. Eat the gruel as the main food in the morning and in the evening.

Heart-marrow Soup: Cook soup with pig heart and spondylous bone. A proper amount of Shengdihuang (*Radix Rehmanniae*), or a small amount of Xiyangshen (*Radix Panacis Quinquefolii*) may be added. Use the soup as an assistant food.

According to TCM theory, "The kidney controls bones, generates marrow and communicates with the brain." and "The teeth are the outward manifestation of the bones." Therefore, strengthening the dental masticating movement and improving the oral masticating ability are the supplementary measure to promote cerebral functions. It is advisable to encourage the patients to eat more coarse and hard foods at usual times.

5.8.5.4 Health care with drugs

5.8.5.4.1 Lingzhi Tablet (Lucid Ganoderma Tablet) or Lingzhi Syrup (Lucid Ganoderma Syrup) Take 4 tablets or 5 ml each time, three times a day.

5.8.5.4.2 Shenrong Extract (Extract of Radix Ginseng and Cornu Cervi Pantotrichum) Take it three times a day, 3 to 5 drops each time.

5.8.5.4.3 Grind equal amount of Sangshenzi (*Fructus Mori*), Heizhima (*Semen Sesami*), Hutaoren (paste of *Semen Juglandis*) and Wuzao (*Fructus Ziziphi Jujubae*) with the pit removed respectively. Take 3 g of the powder each time, three times a day.

5.8.5.4.4 Yishen Ningxin Prescription (Kidney-benefiting and Mind-tranquilizing Prescription) The ingredients include Dangshen (*Radix Codonopsis Pilosulae*), Huangqi (*Radix Astragali seu Hedysari*), Shengdihuang (*Radix Rehmanniae*), Shudihuang (*Radix Rehmanniae Praeparata*), Shanyurou (*Fructus Corni*), Fuling (*Poria*), Huaishanyao (*Rhizoma Dioscoreae*), Yuanzhi (*Radix Polygalae*), Zaoren (*Semen Ziziphi Jujubae*), Longgu (*Os Draconis*), Guiban (*Carapax et Plastrum Testudinis*), Zexie (*Rhizoma Alismatis*), Wuweizi (*Fructus Schisandrae*) and Shichangpu (*Rhizoma Acori Graminei*). Take the drug for 2 to 3 months. It is applicable to patients with deficiency of healthy qi intermingled with phlegm.

5.8.5.5 Nursing for life cultivation

At usual times, the nursing staff should communicate more with patients, and encourage them to speak more, listen more and move more. Ask the patients to tell stories, recite short articles, read books and newspapers and retell what they have read. These methods may gradually improve their abilities to distinguish, memorize and judge things.

The rich perfume of flowers refreshes the brain. Accordingly, flowers like roses, jasmines and narcissuses can be placed in the living environment.

5.8.6 Health care for mental disabilities

Mental disabilities mainly refer to mental diseases such as schizophrenia, manic-depressive psychosis and involutional psychosis. The disease, called "dian kuang" (a general term for manic-depressive psychosis), is a category of mental disorder and mental abnormality. "Dian" manifests as depressive state, and "kuang" as state of excitement.

4. 益肾宁心方：党参、黄芪、生地黄、熟地黄、山萸肉、茯苓、怀山药、远志、枣仁、龙骨、龟版、泽泻、五味子、石菖蒲，服用2～3个月。适用于正虚挟痰者。

（五）养生护理

平时护理人员应多与患者交流，鼓励患者多说、多听、多动。讲故事，背诵短文，读书看报，并复述所读内容，以及逐步增加其识别、记忆、判断的能力。

浓郁的花香有醒脑作用，因此，居住环境中可陈设玫瑰、茉莉、水仙等花草。

六、精神残障

精神残障主要是指精神分裂症、躁狂抑郁性精神病、更年期精神病等精神病患者，中医称为"癫狂"。是一类精神错乱、神志失常的疾病。"癫"表现为抑郁状态，"狂"表现为兴奋状态。

5.8.6.1 Regulating emotions and art cultivation

Excite the depressive patients and tranquilize the excited ones according to the differences of the patients' emotional states. The principle is to make the patients relaxed, sanguine, happy and calm for the purpose of emotional stabilization. However, avoid great anger, great joy and great fright. It is advisable to adopt various methods. For example, light blue, green and pink are the suitable colors of the living environment. The flowers and plants indoors should be the quietly elegant, strong orchids, chrysanthemums and plum blossoms. Change the living environment occasionally and go to mountains and forests to tranquilize the mind in the peaceful and secluded environments if the conditions permit. Proper arrangement of study, work and physical labor is also advisable to divert emotions and get joys from these activities in accordance with the patients' conditions. Straightening the patients out is also the commonly-used measure aiming at the pathogenic psychic factors. Try to overcome their hang-up and make them happy and cheerful. The patients' family members and people around should not discriminate, be indifferent to, ridicule and cold-shoulder the patients.

Health preservation with art mainly attaches importance to the recreational functions like listening to music, learning to sing, seeing movies, watching TV, dancing, playing games, playing chess, reading books, newspapers and magazines. The patients may also visit parks and places of historical interests if the security is ensured. These activities may increase the patients' love and interest of the real life, enhance the confidence and courage of their life.

（一）调节情志与艺术养生

应根据患者情绪状态的不同,抑郁者予以兴奋,亢奋者予以镇静。原则是使其精神轻快、开朗、恬愉、平静,以保持其情绪稳定,切忌大怒、大喜、大惊。可采用多种方法,如家居环境的色彩以淡蓝、青色、粉红色为宜。室内外花草或香味,宜淡雅悠远的兰草、菊花、梅花等为宜。有条件的可经常更换环境,前往山区、森林,取其幽静宁神。也可以根据病人的情况,适当安排学习、工作和劳动,以转移情志,从中获得乐趣。针对致病的精神因素,心理疏导也是经常性的养生措施,尽量解除心头死结,使其心情舒畅,精神愉快。其家属及周围人员对病人切不可歧视、冷漠、嘲笑、嫌弃。

艺术养生主要注重其娱乐功能,如听音乐、学歌咏、看电影、看电视、跳舞、做游戏、下棋、阅读书报杂志。在保证安全的情况下,还可以游览公园和名胜古迹。以提高患者对现实生活的爱好和兴趣,增强其对生活的信心和勇气。

5.8.6.2 Strengthening health with sports

It is suitable for patients with depressive psychosis to practice eight-section brocade and five-mimic games, the purpose of which is to promote qi flow and blood circulation. It is suitable for patients with manic psychosis to practice the events with light and slow movements. At first, practice the simplified Taijiquan. Later on, practice half of a set of or the whole Taijiquan.

Various ball games and track and field events may be arranged if they are suitable for the patients.

5.8.6.3 Life cultivation with the diet

TCM believes that the pathological site of mental disabilities lies in the heart. Therefore, the patients should eat more foods acting on the heart meridian such as lotus roots, green beans, red beans, edible gourds, wheat, arrowheads, lotus leaves, lilies, peach kernels, watermelons, muskmelons, dried fruit of longan, jujube kernels, lotus seeds, pig skins and sea cucumbers.

Cook donkey meat and fermented soya beans together and add seasoning to the food. Eat the food at usual times. The food tranquilizes the mind, benefits qi and relieves fright. The patients may eat it regularly.

Of the prescriptions of medicated diets, Ganmai Dazao Decoction (Decoction of *Radix Glycyrrhiae*, Wheat and *Fructus Ziziphi Jujubae*), Renshen Gruel (Gruel of *Radix Ginseng*), Yimi Gruel (Gruel of *Semen Coicis*), Baihe Gruel (Gruel of *Bulbus Lilii*), Taoren Gruel (Gruel of *Semen Persicae*) and Shanzha Gruel (Gruel of *Fructus Crataegi*) are also the proper foods for life cultivation for the patients with mental disabilities.

The diets for patients with mental disabilities should be soft and delicious, free from irritating substances. When distributing foods, take care to prevent the patients from eating secretly, overeating, hiding food for them-

（二）体育健身

癫证患者以八段锦、五禽戏为宜，旨在流畅气血，增进胆识。狂证则以轻慢活动为宜，先练单式太极拳，以后再练半套或全套太极拳。

各种球类运动、田径运动等活动也可酌情安排。

（三）食疗养生

中医认为精神残障的病位在心，故平时宜多食入心经的食物，如莲藕、绿豆、赤小豆、瓠瓜、小麦、慈姑、荷叶、百合、桃仁、西瓜、甜瓜、龙眼肉、酸枣仁、莲子、猪皮、海参等。

驴肉与豆豉合煮，加入调味品常食，有宁静安神、益气定惊的作用，可常食之。

在药膳方中，甘麦大枣汤、人参粥、薏苡仁粥、百合粥、桃仁粥、山楂粥等粥类，也是精神残障者适合的养生食品。

精神病人的饮食，要求松软可口，无刺激性。在分配食物的时候，要防止偷食、饱食、藏食、漏食。宜多食新鲜蔬

selves and missing meals. It is suitable to eat more fresh vegetables and fruits, forbid pungent, fat, sweet and roasted foods which may transform into phlegm and fire.

5.8.6.4 Nursing for life cultivation

If one person lives in a single room, the light inside the room should be slightly dark, the arrangement of things should be simple and practicable. Take great care to prevent the falling object stored in the room from hitting people. Also, keep the inside and outside environments of the patient' room quiet and clean. Simultaneously, avoid various psychic irritations to aggravate the disease.

菜、水果,禁食辛辣、肥甘、炙煿食品,以免生痰化火。

(四) 养生护理

单人单间住宿,室内光线宜偏暗,陈设宜简单、实用,尽量避免存放一切可以打伤人的物品,并要注意保持病室内外环境的安静和清洁。同时要避免各种精神刺激,以免加重病情。

6 Examples of TCM Life Cultivation in Accordance with Seasonal Conditions

This means regulating the mind, living conditions, and diet, etc. to achieve the purposes of strengthening health, preventing diseases and prolonging life according to the principles and features of the climatic variations and the waxing and waning of yin and yang during a year.

The ancient Chinese solar calendar regards the four solar terms as the beginning of the four seasons respectively, namely, Lichun (the Beginning of Spring), Lixia (the Beginning of Summer), Liqiu (the Beginning of Autumn) and Lidong (the Beginning of Winter). TCM holds that human, as a part of nature, is between the heaven and the earth and closely related to nature. On the other hand, the climatic variations in nature may influence the human body directly or indirectly, causing the corresponding physiological or pathological changes. Man lives in the natural environment and all the vital activities should conform to the objective principles of the seasonal waxing and waning and transformation of yin and yang. Only in this way can man be healthy and enjoy a long life. Otherwise, unconformity to the seasonal changes and violation of the natural principles will incur nature's punishment and harm the health, giving rise to diseases and failure to enjoy a long life. The life cultivation experts through the ages have required that people should arrange their daily life, regulate their mental activities and diet in

第六章 因时制宜的养生实例举隅

因时制宜，就是根据一年四季时令气候阴阳消长变化的规律和特点，从精神、起居、饮食等方面进行调摄，从而达到强身健体、预防疾病、延年益寿的目的。

中国古代历法把立春、立夏、立秋、立冬作为四季的开始。中医学认为，人处于天地之间，与自然界息息相通，自然界的气候变化可直接或间接地影响人体，使机体产生相应的生理或病理变化。人们生活在自然环境中，一切生命活动，必须顺应四时阴阳消长、转化的客观规律，这样才能健康长寿。否则如果不顺应四时的变化，违背自然规律，就会受到自然的惩罚，给身体带来危害，而变生疾病，不能尽享天年。历代养生家都要求人们根据四时的变化安排起居作息，调节精神活动和饮食。不仅养生者宜顺应自然，即使康复医疗也不能忽视这一环节。只有保持内外

the light of the seasonal variations. Not only should the life cultivation people conform to nature, but also rehabilitation cannot ignore this point. Only when the balance and harmony between the internal and external environments are maintained can the normal physiological functions be guaranteed. If the abnormal changes occur in the climate, and the human being can not adapt his functions to these changes in time, then, this will destroy the unity between the internal and external environments of the human body and consequently give rise to diseases. In this case, it is even more impossible for the sick to recover from the disease.

6.1 Life cultivation in spring

The Beginning of Spring, the first one of the 24 solar terms, is regarded as the beginning of spring by the Chinese folks. Spring refers to the period from the Beginning of Spring to the previous day of Beginning of Summer which includes the other solar terms of Rain Water, the Waking of Insects, Pure Brightness and Grain Rain chronologically. It is the time to germinate and grow during the three months of spring. It shifts from cold to warmth; ice and snow melt; yang qi ascends; various living things come to life and develop, with a new face. Everything under the heaven and on the earth overflows with vigor and everywhere seems a picture of prosperity. At this time, the yang qi of the human body also conforms to nature to disperse upwards and outwards. Therefore, health preservation and rehabilitation should conform to the characteristics of "germination and growth" in spring.

6.1.1 Regulating the daily life

The theory of TCM life cultivation and rehabilitation

环境的平衡协调，才能保证生理功能的正常，如果自然界气候发生异常变化，而人体的功能又不能调节适应，其内外环境的统一性遭到破坏，便会导致疾病；有病之人，更因此而不能康复。

第一节 春季养生

立春，是二十四节气中的第一个节气，在我国民间被作为春季开始的日子。从立春始，历经雨水、惊蛰、清明、谷雨至立夏前一天为春季。春三月是生发的季节，天气由寒转暖，冰雪消融，阳气升发，自然界各种生物萌生发育，弃故从新，天地生机盎然，一派欣欣向荣的景象。此时人体的阳气也顺应自然，向上向外疏发，所以春季养生保健和医疗康复都应适应春季这种"生发"特性。

一、起居调养

中医养生康复理论历来

has been believing that people should go to bed late at night and rise early in the morning to be fully bathed in the spring sunlight, let the hair hang down, loosen the clothes and belt, limber up the body and take a hike in the courtyard to make the mind natural and at ease just like the germination and growth in spring. Yang qi ascends in spring. But at this time, wind prevails and the climate changes greatly. Especially during the early spring, yang qi appears before long while cold still does not disappear completely. Thus, the climate changes even more dramatically. Cold wave often attacks people and the climate changes abruptly from warmth to cold. In addition, the yang qi of the human body begins to reach the exterior and the skin striae become loose. Accordingly, the body resistance against pathogenic cold weakens relatively. At this time, the temperature changes dramatically and abnormally, people should avoid the attack of pathogenic wind in time. Especially old people, children and people with weak physique should modify their clothes instantly to keep the body warm. These people should not wear less clothes and use less quilts too early or cut down on clothes abruptly. The ancients' so-called "muffling the body in spring and freezing the body in autumn" is indeed the wise remark of experienced people. Wearing a proper amount of clothing keeps the body warm to resist wind and cold, makes the human body conform to the climatic changes gradually in spring. This can promote the ascending of yang qi of the human body and nourishment of yang.

6.1.2　Regulating emotions

In spring, everything on the earth comes to life and is full of vitality. When spring is approaching, the human metabolism becomes more and more vigorous as well. The spring corresponds to the liver. As a result, the functional

认为，春天应当晚睡早起，充分沐浴春日阳光，并披散头发，松缓衣带，形体舒展，漫步于庭院中，以使意志像春天生发之气一样条达舒畅。春季阳气生发，但此时风气当令，气候变化较大，尤其是早春，阳气初生，阴寒未尽，气候变化更大，常有寒潮来袭，多出现乍暖乍寒的气候，再加上人体的阳气开始趋向于表，皮肤腠理较为疏松，对寒邪的抵御能力相对减弱，当此之时，气温骤变无常，应及时做到"虚邪贼风，避之有时"。特别是老年人、小儿和身体虚弱的人，要随时注意增减衣被，注意保暖，切忌过早地脱衣减被，衣服更不可顿减。前人所说的"春捂秋冻"的确是经验之谈。着衣保暖以防风寒，使人体逐渐适应春天的气候变化，才有助于人体阳气的升发而养阳。

二、情志调节

春季，万物萌生，生机勃勃，人的新陈代谢也随着春季的到来而日趋旺盛，春气通于肝，所以春季是肝气活动旺盛

activities of the liver are most vigorous in spring. The liver controls the regulation of qi and blood and prefers free movement. But it is averse to depression and related to anger. If the liver qi is free to regulate qi and blood, then people can adapt themselves to the climatic changes in winter. Consequently, they are healthy and free from diseases. On the contrary, if the liver qi fails to be free, the liver will fail to regulate qi and blood. In this case, people cannot adapt themselves to the climatic variations, giving rise to the corresponding pathological changes such as dizziness, headache, excitement, fatigue, lassitude, thoracic and hypochondriac distending pain and anorexia. Some patients with the mental disease and hepatic disease are subject to the onset in spring. Therefore, particular attention should be paid to the conformity to the hepatic regulation of qi and blood during the mental regulation in spring. People should be mentally easeful, broad-minded and optimistic so that the yang qi inside the body can be dispersed and the harmony between the body and the outside environmental changes maintained. It is not advisable for people to sleep and sit alone, remain depressed and withdrawn. Furthermore, they should avoid becoming impetuous and angry because fury easily impairs the liver and may induce hypertension, hepatic diseases, apoplexy, etc. as well. If people, together with their families can go for a walk in the country, appreciate flowers and scenery, go on trips to different scenic spots, sing and dance cheerfully to express their emotions and become harmonized with nature during the days of the sunlit and enchanting scene with gentle breeze, this will be even more beneficial to the hepatic regulation of qi and blood and the ascending of the spring yangqi.

的季节。肝主疏泄，性喜条达，而恶抑郁，其志在怒。如果肝气疏泄条达，就可以适应春季的气候变化而健康无病。反之，肝气失于条畅，不能适应春季的气候变化，就会出现相应的病变，如头晕、头痛、情绪激动、疲劳倦怠、胸胁胀痛、不思饮食等等。一些精神病及肝病患者，也容易在春季发病。所以春季精神调养，尤应注意顺应肝气的疏泄条达。做到心情舒畅，心胸开阔，情绪乐观，使体内阳气得以疏发，保持与外界环境变化的协调和谐。不宜孤眠独坐，忧思沉闷，更忌急躁恼怒，暴怒容易伤害肝脏，也可诱发高血压病、肝病及中风等。在春光明媚、风和日丽的日子里，若能与家人或亲友一道，去踏青问柳，观花赏景，游山戏水，行歌舞风，抒发情怀，与大自然融为一体，则更有益于肝气条达，春阳的升发。

6.1.3 Regulating the diet

Yangqi ascends in spring. The liver prefers smooth regulation of qi and blood but is averse to depression. Therefore, it is suitable for people to eat pungent, sweet and yang-ascending food to conform to the hepatic regulation of qi and blood such as green Chinese onion, coriander, jujube and peanut. On the other hand, sour flavor acts on the liver and is astringent in nature, which is not beneficial to the generation and ascending of yangqi as well as the hepatic regulation of qi and blood. Accordingly, people should eat less sour-flavored foods. Besides, the liver functions vigorously in spring. In this case, the hyperactive liver easily subjugates and restricts the spleen, or reversely restricts the lung. Thus, splenogastric and pulmonary diseases are liable to occur or worsen in spring. Therefore, health preservation or rehabilitation with the diet and drugs should take these climatic factors into consideration. Dietetically , "less sour-flavored foods and more sweet-flavored foods" are followed to nourish the spleen qi. People may select some sweet-flavored and neutral-natured foods to strengthen the spleen and prevent the hyperactive liver from restricting the spleen and stomach such as jujube, honey, lotus seed, Chinese yam and coix seed; the people with poor digestive function of the stomach and intestine may eat more radishes to regulate qi, resolve phlegm and regulate the stomach; the decoction of Jupi (*Pericarpium Citri Reticulatae*) can resolve phlegm, quench thirst, regulate qi and the stomach; drinking the tea infused with Maogen (*Radix Rubi Parvifolii*) and Lugen (*Rhizoma Phragmitis*) or the decoction of peeled Yali pear and water chestnut can clear away heat from the lung, prevent disease of respiratory and enterogastric tracts like common cold.

三、饮食调养

春季阳气升发,肝气喜疏泄而恶抑郁,宜食辛甘发散为阳之品,以顺应肝之疏泄,如葱荽、大枣、花生等;酸味入肝,其性收敛,不利于阳气的生发和肝气的疏泄,故应少吃。又春季肝气旺盛,肝旺则易乘克脾土,或反侮肺金,在这一季节里,脾胃和肺系病症易于发作或加重。因此,运用饮食、药物进行养生或康复,也要考虑到这些节气因素。在饮食上应"减酸增甘"以养脾气。可选用一些甘平之物,如红枣、蜂蜜、莲子、怀山药、薏苡仁等食物,以培补脾土,防止春季肝气过旺以戕克脾胃;胃肠消化功能差者,可多吃萝卜,以理气化痰和胃;煮橘皮水喝可以化痰止渴,理气和胃;茅根、芦根沏茶,或鸭梨、荸荠去皮煮水喝,可清热润肺,预防感冒等呼吸道和肠胃道疾患的发生。

6.1.4 Physical training

Winter goes and spring comes. Ice and snow melt. Everything comes to life and is full of vigor in nature. "Man adapts to nature relevantly." With the arrival of spring, the yang qi of the human body begins to ascend and qi and blood tend to reach outwards. At this time, people should often exercise the body to accelerate the circulation of qi and blood. This can promote the realization of this tendency to inspire the enthusiasm. In severe winter, the air is dirty and the amount of exercise is also greatly reduced because people often stay indoors and seldom open the door and windows. Accordingly, people should leave indoors for the places with fresh air like the garden, square, forestry, riverside and mountain slope. They may play ball games, run, shadowbox, and do exercises. People should not stick to the forms as long as they can exercise as much as possible according to personal likes. However, the point is that the amount of exercise should be moderate. This may be determined by the fact that people feel happy, relaxed and comfortable after the training. This can make the spring qi ascend and yang qi increase in an orderly way which meets the requirement of "nourishing yang in spring and summer". As far as old people are concerned, they may select some simple, easy and effective exercises like Taijiquan and eight-section brocade to promote the functional activities of qi of the human body.

6.2 Life cultivation in summer

Summer refers to the period from the Beginning of Summer to the previous day of the Beginning of Autumn which includes the solar terms of Grain Full, Grain in

Ear, the Summer Solstice, Slight Heat and Great Heat in time order. In summer, the scorching sun shines everywhere and the ground is burning. As yang qi grows, it gradually supersedes yinqi. This climatic environment is very beneficial to the growth and development of all living things. All living things grow luxuriantly and many plants blossom and bear fruit. This is a season of luxuriance and beauty in nature during a year. The feature of this season is "growing". The functions of the human body also change correspondingly due to the influence of the scorching climate in summer during the integration of yangqi with yinqi. The yangqi inside the human body tends to release outwards. Therefore, people should pay attention to the protection of yangqi and conform to the feature of "growing" during the summer life cultivation.

6.2.1 Regulating the daily life

In summer, everything grows and everywhere is a picture of prosperity. This is the easiest time for the yang qi of the human body to release outwards. The science of TCM health preservation holds that people should sleep late and rise early and should not be averse to the long daytime and high temperature in summer. They should have the physical training outdoors facing the rising sun in the early morning every day. This can promote the timely excretion of waste inside the body, inspiration of fresh air and metabolism. People had best go to the high mountains, forestry and seashore for convalescence. They may take sunbath and receive a proper amount of fresh air so as to conform to the principle of growing in summer. Bathing with warm water once a day is a keep-fit measure which is worth advocating under the intense heat in midsummer. Taking a bath can not only wash away the sweat and dirt to make the skin cooling and

夏季艳阳当空，地热蒸腾，天地之气交合，这种气候环境对生物的生长发育非常有利；万物生长茂盛，许多植物开花结果，这是一年自然界万物繁荣、争芳斗艳的季节。这个季节的特点是"夏长"，即生长之意；人在气交之中，受夏季炎热气候的影响，机体内在机能也发生相应变化，人体阳气易于向外发泄，所以夏季养生保健，要注意顾护阳气，顺应"夏长"的特性。

一、起居调养

夏季，万物生长，一派欣欣向荣的景象，此时人体的阳气也最易向外发泄。中医养生学认为，夏季人们应晚睡早起，不要厌恶夏天昼长天热。每天早晨迎着初升的太阳到户外进行锻炼，使体内的废物得到及时排泄，吸入新鲜的空气，促进体内的新陈代谢。最好能到高山森林、海滨地区去疗养，适当进行日光浴、空气浴，以顺应夏天养生之道。酷暑盛夏，每天洗1次温水澡，是一项值得提倡的健身措施。洗澡不仅能洗掉汗水、污垢，使皮肤清爽，清暑防病，而且能够锻炼身体。因为温水在

refreshing and prevent sunstroke and diseases, but also exercise the body. Because the pressure of the warm water during the bathing as well as the mechanical massage can lower the excitability of the sympathetic nerve, dilate the superficial blood vessels, accelerate blood circulation, improve the nutrition of the skin and tissues, reduce muscular tension, eliminate fatigue, improve sleeping and enhance body resistance.

Daytime is longer than nighttime in summer, and the sleeping time is shorter at night. Besides, the scorching weather affects the sleeping quality. Accordingly, people should take a nap after lunch appropriately to get rid of fatigue and maintain vigorous energy.

In terms of clothing, people should select light, soft, light-colored, well-ventilated and hygroscopic material. The wide and loose clothes should be tailored to meet the requirement of the scorching weather and profuse sweat in summer. The ideal material for summer clothing includes silk and linen fabrics which are light, thin and well-ventilated and also are suitable for tailoring underwear. Pure cotton cloth absorbs water well, but it is poor in heat dissipation. In addition, it easily sticks to the skin after perspiration. Thus, it is not suitable for tailoring summer clothes and underwears.

6.2.2 Regulating emotions

Summer controls fire and the heart is the organ of fire which governs emotions. Thus, the summer-heat easily acts upon the heart to cause uprising of the heart fire, giving rise to restlessness of the mind, irascibility, anxiety, uneasiness, even insomnia, etc. Particularly, old people have the poor ability to endure the climatic variations. They are often in an anxious state of mind. This affects their health, even induces diseases. Accordingly, in

冲洗时的水压及机械按摩作用,能使交感神经兴奋性降低,体表血管扩张,加快血液循环,改善肌肤和组织的营养,降低肌肉的张力,消除疲劳,改善睡眠,增强抵抗力。

夏季昼长夜短,晚上睡眠时间较短,又因天气炎热而影响睡眠质量,因此要适当午睡,以利消除疲劳,保持旺盛的精力。

在衣着方面,选料要质轻而软,色彩浅淡,透气性好,吸湿性强,裁制衣服要宽松,以适应夏天炎热多汗的需要。最理想的夏季衣料是真丝和麻织品,轻薄、透气好,也适用于做内衣。纯棉布的吸湿性好,但散热性差,出汗后易粘附在皮肤上,不宜做夏衣和内衣。

二、情志调节

夏日主火,而心为火脏,主神志,故暑气容易内应于心,致使心火上炎而出现烦躁易怒、焦急、不安,甚至失眠等症状。特别是年老之人,对气候变化的承受能力较差,常因情绪波动而影响健康,甚至诱发疾病。所以夏季情志调节

summer emotional regulation, people should tranquilize the mind, treat people and deal with things calmly, avoid anger and vexation so as to cultivate temperament in a quiet state. Some classics repeatedly mention that in summer people should "cultivate the temperament peacefully and avoid being restless in the mind" and "Cultivation of temperament is more important than health preservation", etc. Only in this way can people conform to the principle of summer health preservation.

6.2.3 Regulating the diet

Summer-heat acts upon the heart. The heart is the organ of fire and the cardiac fire easily rises. Therefore, in summer it is advisable to eat foods of clearing away heat from the heart, purging fire, clearing away heat and removing summer-heat such as bitter gourd, chrysanthemum leaf, towel gourd, water melon, musk melon and mung bean which are the first choice. Besides, people may prepare some health beverages, medicated gruel and medicated food like Baihe Lüdou Soup (Soup of Bulbus Lilii and Semen Phaseoli Radiati), Bohe Lüdou Soup (Soup of *Herba Menthae* and *Semen Phaseoli Radiati*), Bitter Gourd Tea, Juemingzi Soup (Soup of *Semen Cassiae*), Jinyinhua Distilled Medicinal Water (Distilled Medicinal Water of *Flos Lonicerae*), Suanmei Decoction (Decoction of *Fructus Mume*), Heye Gruel (Lotus Leaf Gruel), Huaishanyao Biandou Gruel (Gruel of *Rhizoma Dioscoreae* and *Semen Dolichoris*) and Juhua Gruel (Gruel of *Flos Chrysanthemi*). However, they should never overingest cold drink, iced water, unripe and cold melon and fruit due to addiction to cool so as to prevent the splenogastric injury because of the excessive cold. In late summer, dampness is more excessive and dampness often intermingles with heat. This may often affect the digestive

要安定自己的思想，待人处事应心平气和，避免生气和烦恼，在清静之中怡养神志。一些古籍反复提到夏季须"静养勿躁"以及"养生莫若养性"等，这样才能适应夏天养生之道。

三、饮食保健

暑气通于心，心为火脏，易于上炎，故夏季宜食用清心泻火，清热解暑之品，如苦瓜、菊花叶、丝瓜、西瓜、甜瓜、绿豆等为首选佳品，并可根据各人的口味，自制一些有保健作用的饮料、药粥、药膳等。如百合绿豆汤、薄荷绿豆汤、苦瓜茶、决明子汤、金银花露、酸梅汤、荷叶粥、怀山药扁豆粥、菊花粥等。切忌因贪凉而暴吃冷饮、冰水、生冷瓜果等，以免寒凉达过伤及脾胃。夏季中的长夏时节，湿气较重，湿热交蒸，常会影响脾胃的消化功能，在食物选择上应以清淡易消化为原则，可酌情多食冬瓜、薏苡仁、黄瓜、红豆等，忌食肥腻、辛辣、燥热等品，以免助阳化火，酿生湿热。在饮食调配方面，要力求品种多样化，并注意菜肴的色、香、味、形，以醒脾开胃，增进食欲。

function of the spleen and stomach. When selecting foods, people should follow the principle of being bland and light. They may eat more wax gourd, Yiyiren (*Semen Coicis*), cucumber, love pea, etc. But they should abstain from fat, greasy, pungent and hot-natured foods accordingly in order to prevent yang from transforming into fire as well as the generation of dampness and heat. When preparing foods, people should try their best to seek for varieties. Meanwhile, they should emphasize the color, smell, taste and appearance so as to activate the spleen, promote the gastric function and improve appetite.

6.2.4 Physical training

Physical training is beneficial to health. Nevertheless, people should stress the methods and have physical training flexibly in accordance with the features of the external scorching environment and the more physical consumption in summer, etc. For instance, it is better to have physical training in the morning and evening with more indoor activities. Besides, large amount of exercise is not suitable. Especially in midsummer, people should not select the events which consume more physical strength. This can avoid profuse sweat due to the strenuous exercise. Excessive perspiration not only impairs yin, but also makes yang qi release outwards. In this case, people violate the principle of "nourishing yang in spring and summer". Therefore, people had best select some physical training events which are moderate in amount of exercise or prevent sunstroke and lower temperature in summer such as swimming, taking a walk, jogging, setting-up exercises, Taijiquan, billiard ball and bowling. Besides, they may select the events on the basis of personal tastes and hobbies.

四、运动锻炼

运动锻炼对健康有益,但夏季应根据外界的炎热环境和机体消耗较大等特点,讲究方法,灵活变通。比如锻炼时间以早晚为好,可多从事室内活动;运动量不宜过大,尤其是盛夏时节,不可选择体力消耗较大的项目,以免剧烈运动导致大汗淋漓,汗出过多,不仅伤阴,也可使阳气随之外泄,违背了"春夏养阳"的原则。因此,夏季体育锻炼的形式,最好选择一些运动量适中或有防暑降温的项目,如游泳、散步、慢跑、体操、太极拳、台球、保龄球等,并可以根据自己的兴趣爱好进行选择。

6.3　Life cultivation in autumn

　　Autumn refers to the period from the Beginning of Autumn to the previous day of the Winter Solstice which includes the solar terms of Limit of Heat, White Dew, the Autumnal Equinox, Cold Dew and Frosts Descent chronologically. The three months of autumn are a season of maturity and harvest. At this time, the yang qi gradually decreases while yin and cold increase step by step. The autumnal wind is crisp. The climate turns cooler and cooler. The temperature varies greatly between day and night. The four seasons change from yang into yin. Everything declines gradually as yinqi increases. Qi and blood of the human body constrict inwards accordingly in order to adapt to the changes of yin and yang from "summer growth" to "autumnal harvest". Consequently, life cultivation in autumn should conform to the changes: gradual decrease of yang qi and decline of all things. This can make the lung qi clean and descend, qi and blood harmonious. Simultaneously, people should protect the internally-lodged yinqi to follow the principle of "harvesting and storing the vital essence."

6.3.1　Regulating the daily life

　　Autumn is a transitional season from summer to winter in which it turns from cool to cold. The yang qi in nature shifts from outward dispersion to inward constriction. This creates the conditions to store the vital essence in winter. Sleeping rhythm should be also adjusted in conformity to the seasonal changes. The ancient Chinese health preservation experts believed people should get up early and go to bed early in autumn. Getting up early promotes free circulation of the lung qi; going to bed early prolongs the sleeping time slightly in conformity to the storage of yin and essence and the gathering of qi by means of nourishment. The early risers may have physical training according to their interests. In the early morning, the autumn wind blows gently and the air is fresh. People may come to the lakeside and garden to jog, practice Taijiquan, etc. This can remove the inhibitory state of the brain after sleeping, activate every organ of the body, make people more energetic and more resourceful, consequently creating the good physical conditions for physical labor, work and study.

"Muffling the body in spring and freezing the body in autumn" is a Chinese folk saying and the summarization of Chinese people's experience in health preservation as well. The saying means that people should not add clothing and quilts too early. At the beginning of autumn, summer heat does not vanish completely. When cool wind blows, people should add garments and quilts gradually, and never add too many at a time to muffle the body. In late autumn, though the wind soughs and signs, people should control clothing as well and consciously to let the body be slightly frozen deliberately. This can avoid perspiration due to wearing too many garments which cause sweat to consume yin and body fluids, make yangqi release outwards, and conform to the internal accumulation of yin and essence as well as the internal gathering of yangqi in autumn and prepare the conditions to store essence in winter as well.

Generally speaking, the climatic variations are relatively stable in autumn. But in late fall, particularly in September in the north, the cold wind and excessive rain, together with the increasingly intensified cold air make the temperature lower and lower. In this case, people are susceptible to common cold. Especially, the slow metabolism and poor circulation in old people make them fear

"收"气。早起者可根据自己的爱好进行早练。清晨,秋风习习,空气新鲜,人们来到湖边、公园慢跑、打太极拳等,可以消除睡眠后大脑的抑制状态,使身体各器官活动灵活起来,使精力更充沛,头脑更机敏,为一天的劳动、工作、学习准备良好的身体条件。

"春捂秋冻"是一句中国的民间俗语,也是中国人民长期养生经验的总结。说的是秋天不要急忙添衣加被。初秋,暑热未尽,凉风时至,衣被要逐渐添加,切不可一下加得过多,捂得过严。晚秋,虽然秋风萧瑟,但穿衣也要有所控制,有意识地让人体逐渐适应向寒冷季节转换的环境变化。这样,可以避免因多穿衣服产生的身热汗出,阴津耗伤,阳气外泄,顺应了秋天阴精内蓄,阳气内收的养生需要,也为冬季藏精做好了准备。

一般来说,秋天的气候变化相对稳定,但深秋时分,特别是北方的九月凄风苦雨,冷空气势力日渐增强,气温日降,容易使人感冒,特别是老年人代谢低,循环差,既怕冷又怕热,对天气变化很敏感,

both cold and heat. They are very sensitive to weather changes. More autumnal garments should be prepared to keep the body temperature constant by modifying the number of clothes instantly. Old people should pay more attention to keeping the hands and feet warm because of their poor peripheral circulation.

6.3.2 Regulating emotions

Autumn acts upon the lung. The lung takes charge of qi, governs respiration, and emotionally relates to grief and grief easily impairs the lung. The autumnal climate turns cooler and cooler. The grass withers; the leaves fall; the flowers and trees are withered, fallen and scattered about. At this time, the sight easily strikes a chord in people's hearts. Some of them have the feeling of being desolate, dreary, unfrequented, old and feeble. As a result, the emotional changes occur such as depression and restlessness of the mind. Accordingly, in autumnal health preservation, people should first develop optimism, think of the joy of the fruitful harvest to be psychologically relieved. They should tranquilize the mind and stabilize the emotions so as to withhold the essence and vitality and avoid the influences of the autumnal weather and sight on the human body. This can conform to the autumnal bleakness and create the good conditions to hide yangqi in winter. Failing to keep the motions stable and excessive melancholy and anxiety may impair the lungqi. This can not only cause the pathological changes of the lung, but also make the adaptive capacity of the human body for hiding in winter lower and people liable to diarrhea with undigested food.

6.3.3 Regulating the diet

The autumnal climate is always marked by dryness,

要保持体温恒常,就应多准备几件秋装,及时增减更换。老年人的末梢循环差,更应注意手部、足部的保暖。

二、情志调节

秋季内应于肺,肺主气,司呼吸,在志为忧,悲忧易伤肺。秋天气候逐渐转凉,草枯叶落,花木凋零,此时人们容易触景生情,产生萧条、凄凉、冷落、垂暮之感,从而导致忧郁、烦躁等情绪变化。因此,秋季精神调养首先要培养乐观情绪,静想收获累累硕果的喜悦,维持心理平衡,做到内心恬静,神志安宁,以收敛神气,免受肃杀之气凋零景象对人体的影响,以适应秋季容平之气,并为冬季阳气潜藏作好准备。如果不能保持神志安宁,忧思多虑,就会损伤肺气,不仅秋季罹患肺脏病变,而且还会使人体适应冬季潜藏的能力降低,容易发生完谷不化的泄泻。

三、饮食调养

秋季总的气候特点是干

hence the term "autumnal dryness". The lung governs respiration, associates with the skin and hair and exterior-interiorly relates to the large intestine. Therefore, when the humidity in the air drops, the lung, large intestine, skin and hair are the first target to be affected. Pathogenic dryness injures people, consumes the human yin and body fluids easily, giving rise to the phenomenon of dryness in everything. This is the so-called "excessive dryness causing xerosis". For example, the skin and mucosa become tight, even desquamation, rhagadia, withered and lustreless hair, increase of dandruff, dry or cracked lips, excessively dry throat, constipation, etc. may occur. Autumnal xerosis is divided into heat xerosis and cool xeroisis according to the differences of clinical manifestations. The main symptoms of the pulmonary injury due to heat xerosis include cough with scanty sputum, dry throat and nose, thirst, headache, anhidrotic fever, etc; the clinical manifestations of cool xerosis includes cough with thin sputum, dry throat and lips, nasal obstruction, anhidrosis, aversion to cold, headache, slight fever, etc. The recuperation with the diet and drugs involves the following aspects. Firstly, drink more liquid things such as boiled water, weak tea, fruit juice beverage, soya bean milk and milk to nourish yin, moisten dryness and remedy the consumed yin and body fluids. Secondly, eat more fresh vegetables and fruits, especially the ones moistening the lung and promoting the production of body fluids. For instance, pears can be eaten uncooked or cooked. Eating the ones uncooked clears away heat and promotes the production of body fluids while eating the steamed ones nourishes yin. If the conditions permit, eat some yin-nourishing and lung-moistening products like autumnal pear paste, paste of nourishing yin and clearing away heat form the lung and pear paste candy. These things are all

燥,故常称之为"秋燥"。由于肺司呼吸,外合皮毛,与大肠相表里,当空气中湿度下降时,肺、大肠与皮毛首当其冲。燥邪伤人,容易耗人阴津,使人出现一派燥象。所谓"燥胜则干",如皮肤黏膜变得紧绷绷的,甚至起皮脱屑、皲裂,毛发枯而无泽,头皮屑增多,口唇干燥或裂口,鼻咽冒火,大便干结等。根据临床表现不同,秋燥又有温燥、凉燥之别。温燥伤肺的主要症状是咳嗽少痰,咽干鼻燥,口渴头痛,无汗发热等;凉燥的表现是咳嗽痰稀,咽干唇燥,鼻塞不通,无汗、恶寒,头痛以及轻微发热等。在药食方面,可从以下几个方面进行调养:一是多喝开水、淡茶、果汁饮料、豆浆、牛奶等流质以养阴润燥,弥补阴津的损伤。二是多吃新鲜蔬菜和水果,尤其是具有润肺生津作用的蔬菜和水果,如梨,生熟皆宜,生品清热生津,蒸熟能滋阴,有条件的可吃些秋梨膏、养阴清肺膏、梨膏糖等滋阴润肺之品,对于防秋燥均有益处。三是经常食粥,米粥能补胃健脾,润养肺燥,若在粥中加入梨、胡萝卜、芝麻、百合等润肺之药食,则益肺润燥效果更佳。四是药膳调养,如含有麦门冬、天门冬、沙参等

beneficial to the prevention of autumnal xerosis. Thirdly, eat gruel regularly. Rice gruel can strengthen the stomach and spleen, nourish the lung and moisten the pulmonary dryness. The rice gruel is more effective for strengthening the lung and moistening dryness if mixed with the lung-moistening drugs and food like pear, carrot, sesame and lily. Fourthly, recuperate with the medicinal diet. For instance, the medicinal diet with the traditional Chinese drugs such as Maimendong (*Radix Ophiopogonis*), Tianmendong (*Radix Asparagi*) and Shashen (*Radix Glehniae*) has the actions of nourishing yin, moistening dryness, promoting the production of body fluids to supplement body fluids and prevent dry cough. Besides, Yinei Lianzi Soup (Soup of Tremella and Semen Nelumbinis), Yiner Bingtan Soup (Soup of Tremella and Saccharum), etc. are the commonly-used health foods to moisten the lung and promote the production of body fluids.

6.3.4 Physical training

In autumn, the wind blows gently and the weather is delightful. It is the best period to have physical training during a year. At this time, people should have the cold tolerance training or cold acclimatization training as early as possible to enhance the body resistance against cold and improve the comprehensive quality of the body. This can help them defeat cold and protect themselves. The cold tolerance training includes various ways like morning exercises, running in the early morning, Taijiquan, mountaineering, swimming and cold water bath. People may choose the training forms suitable for themselves according to personal conditions. Of the above events, mountaineering has been very popular since the ancient times in China. Old people are organized to climb the mountain on lunar September 9 every year. This event can not only

中药的药膳，有滋阴润燥、生津补液、防止干咳等作用。此外如银耳莲子羹、银耳冰糖羹等也是常用的润肺生津保健食品。

四、运动锻炼

秋天，金风送爽，气候宜人，是一年中锻炼的最好时期。此时应尽早地进行耐寒或冷适应锻炼，增强人体抵御寒冷的能力，提高身体的综合素质。耐寒锻炼的方式很多，如早操、晨跑、太极拳、散步、爬山、游泳、冷水浴等，可因人而异，选择适合自己的运动方式。其中登山旅游这种运动，在我国古代就十分盛行，每年农历九月九日，组织老年人进行登山活动，既可锻炼身体，也能愉悦情绪，这项活动一直延续至今，现在已成为群众性

exercise the body, but also make people cheerful. Therefore, the event has lasted so far and has already become the popular folk custom and mass sports activity.

6.4 Life cultivation in winter

Winter refers to the period from the Beginning of Winter to the previous day of the Beginning of Spring which includes the solar terms of Slight Snow, Great Snow, the Winter Solstice, Slight Cold and Great Cold chronologically according to the Chinese lunar calendar. Winter, the coldest season in a year, is a season of excessive yinqi and the hiding of everything. At this time, yinqi is in excess while yangqi conceals. It is a world of ice and snow everywhere. All things hide the vitality. The grass and trees are withered, fallen and scattered about. The insects hibernate. The yangqi of human body also stays inside accordingly. The human metabolic function is in a slow state relatively. Health preservation in winter should conform to the features of concealment of yangqi and hibernation to avoid cold and approach heat, preserve yang and yin. This is in agreement with "the principle of nourishment and hiding".

6.4.1 Regulating the daily life

In winter, going to bed early is advisable to nourish the human yangqi while getting up late is suitable for protecting yin and essence. This is because that retiring to bed early and rising late can help yangqi descend and conceal, yin and essence accumulate so as to maintain the balance of yin and yang of the human body. Do not work until the sun rises; avoid cold and approach heat to prevent external cold from impairing yang. In addition, adopt the heating devices to maintain a proper room temperature.

Very low room temperature may impair human yangqi and make people subject to common cold; very high room temperature makes the skin striae open, yangqi unable to conceal, but pathogenic cold easily invade the body, giving rise to affection by exopathogen and other diseases.

In terms of clothing, wear more or less clothes constantly as the climate changes. The cotton fabrics are the best for tailoring the underwear because they are soft, comfortable and good in heat preservation; the outer clothing should be slightly larger. Excessively thin clothing may easily impair yang, make people susceptible to common cold or numbness and pain of the waist and legs; excessively thick clothing may stir yangqi to affect its concealment. The shoes and socks should be a little larger so as to keep qi flow free and harmonious, limbs comfortable and warm. The hands and feet are liable to chilblain, so particularly in need of heat preservation.

6.4.2 Regulating emotions

Winter corresponds to the kidney internally. The kidney controls the storage of essence and is the congenital base of life and emotionally associated with fear and fright. Excessive or sudden fear and fright may impair the kidney and cause the pathological changes of the kidney. Accordingly, in winter, the time of hiding, people should stabilize emotions and cultivate the mind. They should be emotionally implicit, quiet and happy to avoid excessive emotional activities; fear, fright and dysphoria should be avoided most so as to guarantee that the normal physiological feature of the hiding of yangqi is not interfered with. Only when the mind is tranquilized, can yangqi inside the body be hidden, yin and essence accumulated. This can create the conditions to generate and develop spring yang for the coming year.

过高则腠理开泄,阳气不得潜藏,寒邪则易侵入而引起外感或其他疾病。

在衣着方面,要随气候变化及时增减衣服。内衣以棉织品为佳,其柔软舒适且保暖性好;外衣要稍宽大。着衣过薄则易伤阳、感冒或患腰腿痹痛;过多过厚则会扰动阳气影响其敛藏。鞋袜宜稍大一点,以便气血流通,四肢舒畅温煦,冬季手脚易发生冻疮,尤宜保暖。

二、精神调养

冬季内应于肾,肾主藏精,为先天之本,其在志为恐与惊,过度或突然的惊恐会伤害肾脏,引起肾脏的病变。所以在冬季闭藏之时,应潜藏心志,保养精神。做到心平气和,情绪要安静、愉快,避免情志过激,最忌恐惧、惊吓和烦躁,以保证冬令阳气潜藏的正常生理功能不受干扰。只有做到内心清静平和,体内阳气才能闭藏,阴精才能积蓄,为来年春阳生发作好准备。

6.4.3 Regulating the diet

Ingestion of tonics in winter has been the traditional life cultivation method in China for several thousands of years. Modern researches believe winter is the season in which nutrients are most easily accumulated in a year. Therefore, nutrients can be transformed into energy to the greatest extent and stored inside the body by means of recuperation with the proper diet to nourish viscera, limbs and bones. Ingestion of tonics in winter includes the two types of tonification with the diet and tonification with drugs. Tonic foods include mutton, chicken, beef, dog meat, and so on; tonic drugs include Ejiao (*Colla Corii Asini*), Renshen (*Radix Ginseng*), Lurong (*Cornu Cervi Pantotrichum*), etc. However, it should be stressed that the ingestion of tonics should be based on the requirement of one's own body no matter what methods are adopted, and that the tonification should be in combination with the constitution and the state of illness. Otherwise, the tonification is harmful, not beneficial and just opposite to the intended result. In terms of tonification with the diet, the people with yang deficiency or relative yang deficiency should eat sweet, warm-natured and yang-promoting foods like shrimps, dog meat and Lurong (*Cornu Cervi Pantotrichum*); the people with yin deficiency or yin deficiency syndromes should eat sweet and cool-natured or sweat and moist-natured foods such as rabbit meat, tortoise meat, soft-shelled turtle meat, Baihe (*Bulbus Lilii*) and Yin'er (*Tremella*); the people with deficiency of qi and yin should eat duck meat and goose meat. In terms of tonification with drugs, more attention should be paid to the fact that the tonification should be under the guidance of the doctor, free from arbitrary and excessive tonification to avoid the adverse effects on the

三、饮食保健

冬令进补是中国数千年来用以防病强身的传统养生方法。现代研究认为，冬季是一年四季中营养物质最易蓄积的时期。所以通过合理的饮食调补，能使营养物质转化的能量最大限度地贮存在体内，以滋养五脏六腑、四肢百骸。冬天进补的方式主要有食补和药补二种，食补诸如羊肉、鸡肉、牛肉、狗肉等，药补如阿胶、人参、鹿茸等。但应注意，无论哪种补法，均应根据自己身体需要而进补，并结合体质、病情的情况，进行调补。否则有害无益，适得其反。就食补而言，如素体阳虚者宜或偏于阳虚证的患者，宜进食甘温助阳的食物，如虾肉、狗肉、鹿茸等，素体阴虚者或阴虚证的患者宜进食甘凉或甘润之品，如兔肉、龟肉、鳖肉、百合、银耳等，气阴不足宜进食鸭肉、鹅肉等。在药补方面，更应引起注意，切不可乱补蛮补，应该在医生指导下进行，以免对身体产生不良作用。如体质虚弱、气虚之人可服人参，阴血不足者可服阿胶，肾阴虚者宜常服六味地黄丸，肾阳虚者宜用金匮肾气丸、鹿茸膏等，气血双亏者可

body. For example, the people with weak constitution and qi deficiency may take Renshen (*Radix Ginseng*); the people with deficiency of qi and blood may take Ejiao (*Colla Corii Asini*); the people with asthenic kidney should take Liuwei Dihuang Bolus (Bolus of Six Drugs with Rehmannia) regularly; the people with yang deficiency of the kidney should take Jinkui Shenqi Pill, Lurong Paste (Paste of *Cornu Cervi Pantotrichum*) and so on; the people with deficiency of both qi and blood should take Renshen Guipi Pill (Spleen-Invigorating and Heart-Nourishing Pill Including Ginseng) or Shiquan Dabu Bolus (Bolus of Ten Powerful Tonics), etc.

6.4.4 Physical training

Though it is cold in winter, people should still persevere in their physical training. This is the basic method to strengthen health. The sports events should be flexibly selected in accordance with the individual's and local conditions in the physical training in winter. The events suitable for indoor physical training in winter include health-strengthening massage, keep-fit qigong, Taijiquan, setting-up dance, and so on; the outdoor training events include long-distance running, heel-toe walking race, gymnastics, ball games, iceskating, and skiing, etc. The climate in winter is severely cold. All the living things in the universe are in the state of hiding. People should pay attention to prevention of cold and heat preservation to make yin and essence hide inside, yangqi not release excessively. This is in agreement with the natural climate in winter. Only in this way can "yin be even and well and yang firm", diseases eliminated and life prolonged. It is best to select the movements with large amount of exercise and to make the body sweat slightly when the sun rises. It is not advisable to rise early so as to avoid stirring

服人参归脾丸或十全大补丸等。

四、运动锻炼

冬日虽寒,但仍需持之以恒地进行自身锻炼,这是强身健体的根本方法。冬季活动锻炼,当因人因地制宜,灵活选择运动项目。适宜于冬季室内锻炼的项目有强身按摩、保健功、太极拳、健身舞等;室外锻炼项目有长跑、竞走、武术、体操、球类、滑冰、滑雪等。冬季气候严寒,宇宙万物都处于收藏状态,冬季健身应注意防寒保暖,使阴精潜藏于内,阳气不致妄泄,而与冬天的自然气候相适应。这样才能"阴平阳秘",祛病延年。最好是等待日光出来以后,且宜选择活动量较大的动作,使身体出些微汗为宜,不宜起得过早,以免扰动人体的阳气。同时要避免在大风、大寒、大雪、雾

up yangqi of the body. Meanwhile, avoid the training in strong wind, bitter cold, heavy snow, fog and dew. This can not only reach the purpose of avoiding cold and warming the body, but also maintain a cheerful frame of mind to gather essence, qi and vitality inside. This is in agreement with the principle of "preserving health by hiding" in winter. Violating this principle may incur the impairment of the kidney qi and flaccidity with cold limbs when spring comes to result in the weakening of the body's adaptation to the spring sprouting.

It should be emphasized that temperature inversion often exists in the morning due to the influence of cold high pressure. Namely, the temperature of the upper atmospheric layer is high while the temperature of the terrestrial surface atmospheric layer is low, with weakened convective activities. Consequently, the chemical atmospheric pollutants from factories, domestic kitchen ranges, etc. cannot easily diffuse into the upper atmospheric layer. As a result, these pollutants accumulate and stay in the breathing belt of the lower atmospheric layer. At this time, the people having the outdoor physical training exactly become the victims. Accordingly, it is not suitable to have the outdoor physical training in the early morning, especially for some old people, viewed from the angle of atmospheric pollution.

露中锻炼。这样既可达到避寒取暖的目的，也可保持心情愉快，使精、气、神得以内收。这就是适应冬季"养藏"的道理。如果违逆了这个规律，就会损伤肾气，到了来年的春天，就要发生痿厥一类的疾病，使人体适应春天升发之气的能力降低。

必须强调指出，在冬天冷高压影响下的早晨，往往会有气温逆增的现象，即上层气温高，而地表气温低，大气对流活动减弱，因而工厂、家庭炉灶等排出的化学性大气污染物不易向大气上层扩散。因此，从大气污染的角度来看，早晨室外锻炼是不适宜的，尤其是对一些老年人更不适宜。

7 Examples of TCM Health Care for Specific Regions

Every region of the human body is a component part of the human body such as the head, face, five sense organs, nine orifices, skin, trunk, limbs and viscera. Any local part in an unhealthy or dysfunctional state inevitably affects the functions of the whole body. As far as modern people are concerned, it is wise to select certain key regions purposely for protection and health care under the guidance of "starting with the local health care from the view point of wholism." This can achieve the purpose of getting twice the result with half the effort.

7.1 Oral health care

The oral cavity is the organ to control ingestion, digestion and speech as well as the important component part of the facial beauty. Good oral health care can prevent not only oral and dental diseases, but also many general diseases effectively like acute and subacute bacterial endocarditis, nephritis, rheumatic fever, arthritis and respiratory tract disease (These diseases are secondary to oral diseases).

7.1.1 Consolidating the teeth

7.1.1.1 Rinsing the mouth regularly

Rinsing the mouth can remove the turbid qi and food

第七章 特定部位的养生实例举隅

人体的各个部位,如头部、颜面、五官九窍、皮肤、躯干、四肢、五脏六腑等,都是人体的组成部分。任何局部的不健康或功能障碍,势必影响其整体功能。对于现代人而言,采用"从整体出发,从局部入手"的策略,有针对性地选择重点部位进行防护保健,有事半功倍之效。

第一节 口腔保健

口腔是完成进食、消化、语言的器官,也是颜面美观的重要组成部分。做好口腔保健,不仅可以预防口腔、牙齿疾病,而且可以有效地预防多种全身性疾病,如急性和亚急性细菌性心内膜炎、肾炎、风湿热、关节炎、呼吸道疾病等(这些疾病可以由口腔疾病所继发)。

一、固齿

1. 口宜勤漱

漱口能除口中的浊气和

residues and clean the mouth and teeth. The mouth should be rinsed every time after the ingestion. There are many ways to rinse the mouth such as rinsing the mouth with water, rinsing the mouth with tea, rinsing the mouth with salty water, rinsing the mouth with vinegar and rinsing the mouth with the water soaked with traditional Chinese drugs. People may select the method according to their specific conditions.

7.1.1.2 Tapping the teeth regularly

Tapping the teeth is an important method to promote health and longevity, particularly it is of more significance in the morning. The method is as follows. Get rid of all stray thoughts to relax mentally. Then, close the mouth and lips gently. Next, tap the back teeth for 50 times. Afterwards, tap the incisor teeth for 50 times. Finally, tap the molar teeth with the upper and lower teeth staggered for 50 times. Do the exercise once in the morning and evening respectively, or the number of tapping the teeth may be increased as well.

7.1.1.3 Massaging the lips

Close the mouth and lips tightly. Then, use the four closed-up fingers of the right hand to gently knead and rub the outside margins of lips clockwise and anticlockwise until the local part becomes slightly hot and congested. This method promotes the oral and gingival blood circulation, makes the teeth healthy and firm, prevents dental diseases and has the actions of facial beautification and healthcare as well.

7.1.1.4 Health care with the diet

Oral and dental diseases are related to the imbalance of nutrients to a certain degree. People should often eat fresh vegetables and fruits rich in vitamin C as well as foods rich in vitamin A, vitamin D and vitamin C like animal livers, kidneys, yolk and milk. Women during the

食物残渣，清洁口齿。进食之后皆需漱口。漱口的方式很多，如水漱、茶漱、津漱、盐水漱、食醋漱、中药泡水漱等，可根据实际情况选用。

2. 齿宜常叩

叩齿是健康长寿的重要方法，尤其清晨叩齿意义更大。方法是：排除杂念，思想放松，口唇轻闭，先叩臼齿50下，次叩门牙50下，再错牙叩大齿部位50下。每日早晚各作一次，亦可增加叩齿次数。

3. 唇部按摩

将口唇闭合，用右手四指并拢，轻轻在口唇外沿顺时针方向和逆时针方向揉搓，直至局部微热发红为止。其作用是促进口腔和牙龈的血液循环，健齿固齿，防治牙齿疾病，且有颜面美容保健作用。

4. 饮食保健

口腔、牙齿患病与营养不平衡有一定关系，应常食富含维生素C的新鲜蔬菜、水果；含维生素A、D、C的食品，如动物的肝、肾、蛋黄及牛奶等。

gestational period and lactation together with infants should pay particular attention to the supplementation of these foods to ensure the enamel development.

7.1.1.5　Health care with drugs

There exists an ancient secret recipe for consolidating the teeth which is composed of 30 g of Shengdahuang (*Radix et Rhizoma Rhei*), Shudahuang (*Radix et Rhizoma Rhei Preparata*), Shengshigao (*Gypsum Fibrosum*), Shushigao (*Gypsum Fibrosum Preparata*), Gusuibu (*Rhizoma Drynariae*), Duzhong (*Cortex Eucommiae*), Qingyan (crude salt) and table salt respectively, 15 g of Mingfan (*Alumen*), Kufan (*Alumen Exsiccatum*) and Danggui (*Radix Angelicae Sinensis*) respectively. All the above ingredients are ground into fine powder and applied as the dentifrice. The powder makes the teeth healthy and firm, and is especially applicable to toothache due to the lung heat.

7.1.2　Swallowing saliva

Swallowing the refluxed saliva was called "taishi" (fetal feeding) in ancient times and a method to strengthen health advocated by the ancients. Saliva is of special value in health preservation and health care. It not only helps digestion, protects digestive tract and removes toxic substances, but also promotes wound healing, delays ageing, prevents and fights cancer.

The method of refluxing and swallowing saliva: Assume the sitting, or lying, or standing posture. Keep calm and concentrate the mind. Then, lick the upper palate with the tongue, or rest the tongue on the maxillodental outside. Next, move the tongue upwards and downwards first. Afterwards, rest the tongue on the maxillodental inside and move the tongue upwards and downwards, from the left to the right. This method was

妊娠期、哺乳期妇女及婴幼儿尤应注意补充这类食品,以保证牙釉质的发育。

5. 药物保健

古代的健齿术中有固齿秘方,其方药为:生大黄、熟大黄、生石膏、熟石膏、骨碎补、杜仲、青盐、食盐各 30 g,明矾、枯矾、当归各 15 g,研成细末,做牙粉使用,可健齿、固齿。对胃热牙痛,尤为适用。

二、咽津

漱津咽唾,古称"胎食",是古人倡导的一种强身方法。唾液在养生保健中具有特殊价值,其作用如帮助消化、保护消化道、解毒,还能促使伤口愈合、延缓衰老、防癌抗癌。

漱津咽唾的方法:坐、卧、站姿势均可,平心静气,以舌舔上,或将舌伸到上颌牙齿外侧,上下搅动,然后伸向里侧,再上下左右搅动,古人称其为"赤龙搅海",待到唾液满口时,再分 3 次把津液咽下,并以意念送到丹田。或者与叩

termed as "The Red Dragon Stirring the Sea" by the ancients. Wait until there is a mouthful of saliva and swallow it in three divided times. Meanwhile, send the saliva down to Dantian with the mindwill. Or the method may be cooperated with tapping the teeth. Namely, first, tap the teeth; then, swallow the refluxed saliva. Do the exercise for three times and swallow the saliva in nine divided times. It is better to swallow the saliva in the morning and evening. Do it for more times if time permits.

7.2 Facial health care

Facial health care, called "zhu yan" (remaining young) by the ancients, actually refers to cosmetic health care. The face is rich in blood vessels and serves as a window to reflect the health status of the organism. Therefore, all the health preservation people attach much importance to the facial health care. The important sign of the ageing of the human body is the appearance of wrinkles on the face. Weak physique due to prolonged diseases and attack by the six exogenous pathogenic factors both may result in skin ageing and wrinkles. Besides, bad habitual actions are also a cause of premature skin ageing such as regular frowning, holding the cheeks with the hands, squinting, whistling, and resting the face on the pillow to sleep.

7.2.1 Massage and acumox

7.2.1.1 Massage

Cosmetological massage can be divided into two types. The first type refers to the direct massage on the face; the second one means achieving cosmetological effects by massaging the meridians and collaterals that are away from the face. For instance, Peng Zhu's Face-

Rubbing Method is the representative method of cosmetological massage. The method is as follows. After getting up in the early morning, rub the ears with both hands. Then, pull the ears gently. Afterwards, rub the scalp and comb the hair with the fingers. Finally, rub the hands against each other to get them warm and rub the face with the warm hands upwards and downwards for 14 times. The method can promote facial blood circulation, make the face lustrous, the hair free from grey hair and prevent cephalic diseases.

7.2.1.2 Acumox

Seven meridians have good cosmetological effects: the bladder meridian of foot-taiyang, the liver meridian of foot-shaoyin, the liver meridian of foot-jueyin, the stomach meridian of foot-yangming, the triple energizer meridian of hand-shaoyang, the small intestine meridian of hand-taiyang and the large intestine of hand-yangming. These meridians may be selected to form a prescription for the cosmetic purpose on the basis of syndrome differentiation according to the specific conditions. For instance, the health care of removing and preventing wrinkles may be realized by needling Sizhukong (TE 23), Zanzhu (BL 2), Taiyang (EX–HN 5), Yingxiang (LI 20), Jiache (ST 6) and Yifeng (TE 17); and Zhongwan (CV 12), Hegu (LI 4), Quchi (LI 11), Zusanli (ST 36), Weishu (BL 21), Guanyuan (CV 4) and Lougu (SP 7) may possibly be added to supplement qi, regulate blood, increase skin elasticity, remove and prevent wrinkles. Moxibustion has very marked cosmetic effects, too. The commonly-used acupoints for moxibustion include Shenque (CV 8), Guanyuan (CV 4), Qihai (CV 6), Zhongwan (CV 12), Mingmen (GV 4), Dazhui (GV 14), Shenzhu (GV 12), Gaohuang (BL 43), Shenshu (BL 23), Pishu (BL 20), Weishu (BL 21), Zusanli (ST 36), Sanyinjiao (SP 6), Quchi (LI 11)

按摩法,方法是:清晨起床用左右手摩擦耳朵,然后轻轻牵拉耳朵;再用手指摩擦头皮,梳理头发;最后把双手摩热,以热手擦面,从上向下14次。此法可使颜面气血流通,面有光泽,头发不白,且可预防头病。

2. 针灸

对美容有良效的经络有7条:足太阳膀胱经、足少阴肾经、足厥阴肝经、足阳明胃经、手少阳三焦经、手太阳小肠经、手阳明大肠经。可根据具体情况,辨证取穴组方进行调整。例如,除皱防皱保健,可针刺丝竹空、攒竹、太阳、迎香、颊车、翳风等,配中脘、合谷、曲池、足三里、胃俞、关元、漏谷等,其功用可益气和血,增加皮肤弹性,除皱防皱。灸法强身美容作用亦很显著,常用穴位主要有:神阙、关元、气海、中脘、命门、大椎、身柱、膏肓、肾俞、脾俞、胃俞、足三里、三阴交、曲池和下廉等。灸法美容简单易行,便于掌握使用。

and Xialian (LI 8). Moxibustion methods for cosmetic purpose are easy and simple in application, and can be easily handled.

7.2.2 Diet

TCM classics record many foods for "zhuyan" (remaining young), "nailao" (resisting ageing) and "fanlao" (rejuvenation) such as sesame, honey, Xianggu mushroom, human milk, milk, goat's milk, sea cucumber, pumpkin seed, lotus root, wax gourd, cherry and wheat. These foods can not only make the face tender, white, ruddy, moist and lustrous, but also prolong life.

7.2.3 Drugs

7.2.3.1 Cosmetological prescriptions and drugs for oral administration

7.2.3.1.1 Face-Whitening Powder of the Imperial Court of Emperor Yang Guang of the Sui Dynasty

30 g of Jupi (*Pericarpium Citri Reticulatae*), 50 g of Dongguaren (*Semen Benincasae*) and 40 g of Taohua (*Flos Persicae*). Grind the ingredients into fine powder. Take the powder 3 times a day, 2 g each time. It has the actions of drying dampness, resolving phlegm, promoting blood circulation and benefiting the complexion.

7.2.3.1.2 Pearl Powder Grind 2 g of the natural pearl into extremely fine powder and use it after it is dried. Take it orally 3 times a day, 0.5 g each time. It has the actions of clearing away heat, resolving phlegm, moistening the face and curing the facial black spots.

7.2.3.1.3 Gouqizi (*Fructus Lycii*) Wine Soak 50 g of Gouqizi (*Fructus Lycii*) in 500 ml of millet wine. Proper amount of the wine can be accordingly drunken. It strengthens the liver and stomach, makes people remain young and beautiful.

二、饮食

中医古籍中记载有很多"驻颜"、"耐老"、"返老"等食品,如芝麻、蜂蜜、香菇、人乳、牛乳、羊乳、海参、南瓜子、莲藕、冬瓜、樱桃、小麦等。这些食品不仅可使面色嫩白、红润光泽,而且还能延年益寿。

三、药物

1. 内服美容方药

隋炀帝后宫面白散 橘皮30 g、冬瓜仁50 g、桃花40 g,捣细为末即可,每次服用2 g,每日3次。有燥湿化痰,活血益颜的功效。

珍珠散 天然珍珠粉2 g,研成极细粉末,干燥后用。每次服用0.5 g,每日3次,有清热痰、润面容,治疗面部黑斑之作用。

枸杞子酒 枸杞子50 g,浸于500 ml黄酒中,酌量饮用。可补益肝胃,驻颜美容。

7.2.3.1.4 Cosmetic Wine with Taohua (*Flos Persicae*)
Soak 30 g of dry Taohua (*Flos Persicae*) in 500 ml of millet wine. Drink the wine. It moistens the face and makes the face look like the peach blossom.

The previous studies and practice believed that the following drugs have the actions of moistening the skin and increasing the skin elasticity: Baizhi (*Radix Angelicae Dahuricae*), Baifuzi (*Rhizoma Typhonii*), Yuzhu (*Rhizoma Polygonati Odorati*), Gouqizi (*Fructus Lycii*), Xingren (*Semen Armeniacae Amarum*), Taoren (*Semen Persicae*), Heizhima (*Semen Sesami*), Fangfeng (*Radix Ledebouriellae*), Zhuyi (*Pancreas Suis*), Taohua (*Flos Persicae*), and Xinyi (*Flos Magnoliae*), etc.

7.2.3.2 Cosmetic products for external application
These products include cosmetic powder, cosmetic lotion, cosmetic ointment, cosmetic paste, cosmetic facial film, etc.

7.2.3.2.1 Xi Shi's Cosmetic Powder
60 g of Lüdou (*Semen Phaseoli Radiati*) powder, 30 g of Baizhi (*Radix Angelicae Dahuricae*), Baiji (*Rhizoma Bletillae*), Bailian (*Radix Ampelopsis*), Baijiangcan (*Bombyx Batryticatus*), Baifuzi (*Rhizoma Typhonii*) and Tianhuafen (*Radix Trichosanthis*) respectively, 15 g of Gansong (*Rhizoma Nardostachyos*), Shannai (*Rhizoma Kaempferiae*) and Maoxiang (*Infloresoentia Hierochloes*) respectively, 6 g of Linglingxiang (*Herba Lysimachiae Foenigraeci*), Fangfeng (*Radix Ledebouriellae*) and Gaoben (*Rhizoma Ligustici*) respectively and Feizaojia (*Fructus Gymnocladi Chinensis*) (*two in number*). Grind all the above ingredients into fine powder and use it when washing the face. The powder expels wind, moistens the skin, dredges collaterals, makes the skin

桃花美容酒 干桃花30 g,浸黄酒500 ml,饮用。可润泽颜面,使人面如桃花。

根据历代研究和实践,认为下述药物有润泽皮肤,增加皮肤弹性的作用,如白芷、白附子、玉竹、枸杞子、杏仁、桃仁、黑芝麻、防风、猪胰、桃花、辛夷等。

2. 外用美容品

包括美容粉、美容液、美容软膏、美容糊剂、美容面膜等。

玉容西施散 绿豆粉60 g,白芷、白及、白蔹、白僵蚕、白附子、天花粉各30 g,甘松、山柰、茅香各15 g,零陵香、防风、藁本各6 g,肥皂荚2锭。诸药研为细末,每次洗面用之,其作用是,祛风润肤,通络香肌,令面色如玉。

fragrant and the face attractive.

7.2.3.2.2 Three-Blossom Lotion for Eliminating Wrinkles: A proper amount of peach blossom, lotus and Furonghua (*Flos Hibisci Mutabilis*) respectively. Decoct the three ingredients in snow water to wash the face frequently with the decoction. The lotion can promote blood circulation to remove blood stasis, moisten the skin and eliminate wrinkles.

7.3 Health care of the hair

Health care of the hair is also called beautification of hair. The healthy hair is black (or other natural hair colors), lustrous, thick, dense, long and beautiful.

The hair is closely related to the five zang organs. The state of the hair can directly reflect the states of the five zang organs, qi and blood. Extreme emotional activities may also cause the changes of the hair. For example, excessive worry and anxiety often give rise to premature grey hair and baldness.

7.3.1 Combing the hair and massaging the scalp

Combing the hair can promote qi flow and blood circulation, dispel wind, improve eye sight, tonify the brain, refresh people, make the hair lustrous and consolidated, relieve headache, prevent common cold, promote sleeping and reduce blood pressure. The correct method to comb the hair is as follows. Comb the hair from the front to the back, then from the back to the front, from the left to the right, then from the right to the left. Comb the hair this way for dozens of times or hundreds of times. The hair can be combed in the morning, during the lunch break and before bed time. Massage with the fingers may be cooperatively applied during combing the hair. The ten fingers of the both hands are apart from one another naturally. Knead circularly with the palmar sides or tips of the fingers from the anterior hairline to the posterior one. Then, knead and massage the scalp from the two sides to the vertex with even force. Repeat the process for 36 times until the scalp gets warm.

7.3.2　Diet

The diet should be various to maintain the balance between the acid and base inside the body. People may eat a proper amount of natural foods rich in protein, iodine, calcium, vitamins B, A, E, etc. such as fresh milk, fish, eggs, beans, green leafy vegetable, melon, fruit and coarse food grain. Simultaneously, people may select the nutritious foods to make the hair healthy.

7.3.2.1　The Immortal's Gruel
Decoct a proper amount of Heshouwu (*Radix Polygoni Multiflori*) and nonglutinous rice in an earthenware pot. Drink the gruel regularly. The gruel has the actions of tonifying the liver and kidney, benefiting qi and blood, making the hair black and people remain young.

7.3.2.2　Zhima Hetao Candy (Candy of Semen Sesami and Semen Juglandis)
500 g of Chishatang (*Saccharum Rubrum*), 250 g of Heizhima (*Semen Sesami*) and Hetaoren (*Semen Juglandis*) respectively. The three ingredients are made into candy. Eat several pieces a day. The candy can tonify the brain and the kidney, make the beard and hair black. Prolonged use can also prevent and cure neurasthenia, amnesia, premature grey hair, and baldness, etc.

从额前发际向后发际,做环状揉动,然后再由两侧向头顶揉动按摩,用力均匀一致,如此反复做 36 次,至头皮微热为度。

二、饮食

饮食宜多样化,可保持体内酸碱平衡。适量食用含蛋白质、碘、钙、维生素 B、A、E 等较丰富的天然食物,如:鲜奶、鱼、蛋类、豆类、绿色蔬菜、瓜果、粗粮等。同时,可根据情况适当选用健发营养食品。例如:

仙人粥　何首乌、粳米适量,用沙锅煮粥,常服。有补肝肾、益气血、乌发驻颜之效。

芝麻核桃糖块　赤砂糖 500 g,黑芝麻、核桃仁各 250 g,加工制作成糖块。日服数小块,可健脑补肾,乌须黑发。经常服用,又可防治神经衰弱、健忘、头发早白、脱发等症。

7.3.3 Drugs

7.3.3.1 Drugs for external application

These drugs have the actions of making the hair moist, clean, fragrant, dense and black, preventing and curing baldness.

7.3.3.1.1 Washing Method with the Pig's Bile

One pig's gallbladder. Take out the bile and pour it into water, or soak the gallbladder in the frankincense oil for more than seven days. Wash the hair with the water. When the hair is dry, apply a proper quantity of the pig's bile and the frankincense oil on the hair. This method has the actions of clearing away heat, expelling wind, making the hair moist and lustrous.

7.3.3.1.2 Hair-Aromatizing Powder

30 g of Linglingxiang (*Herba Lysimachiae Foenigraeci*), 15 g of Xinyi (*Flos Magnoliae*), 15 g of Meiguihua (*Flos Rosae Rugosae*), 18 g of Tanxiang (*Lignum Santali*), 12 g of Dahuang (*Radix et Rhizoma Rhei*), 12 g of Gancao (*Radix Glycyrrhizae*), 12 g of Mudanpi (*Cortex Moutan Radicis*), 9 g of Shannai (*Rhizoma Kaempferiae*), 9 g of Dingxiang (*Flos Caryophylli*), 9 g of Xixin (*Herba Asari*), 9 g of storax oil and 9 g of Baizhi (*Radix Angelicae Dahuricae*). Grind all the ingredients except storax oil into fine powder. Then, mix the powder with the storax oil evenly and dry it in the shade. Apply the powder on the hair and comb the hair with a double-edged fine-toothed comb. The prescription has the action of making the hair clean and fragrant. The prolonged application can make the exfoliated hair grow again and people free from grey hair for a lifetime.

7.3.3.1.3 Baldness-Preventing Prescription

Three Chinese torreyanuts, two walnuts and 30 g of Cebaiye (*Cacumen Biotae*). Pound the ingredients to

三、药物

1. 外用药

有润发、洁发、香发、茂发、乌发，防治脱发等作用。

猪胆汁洗法 猪胆一枚，取胆汁倾水中，或将猪胆置于乳香油中浸七日以上。用水洗头，待发干后适量抹猪胆汁及乳香油。本法有清热祛风，润发生辉之效。

香发散 零陵香30 g，辛夷15 g，玫瑰花15 g，檀香18 g，大黄12 g，甘草12 g，牡丹皮12 g，山奈9 g，丁香9 g，细辛9 g，苏合香油9 g，白芷9 g。研药为细末，用苏合香油搅匀，晾干。药面掺发上，篦去。本方有洁发香发作用，久用发落重生，至老不白。

令发不落方 榧子3个，胡桃2个，侧柏叶30 g，共捣烂，浸泡雪水内。用浸液洗

paste. Then, soak the paste in snow water. Wash the hair with the liquid. The prescription has the actions of preventing baldness, making the hair black and moist. It is especially very effective for baldness due to blood heat.

7.3.3.2　Drugs for oral administration

These drugs promote qi flow and blood circulation to make the hair healthy. Such commonly-used drugs are numerous like Huma (*Semen Sesami*), Youcaizi (rapeseed), Liuhua (*Flos Granati*), Hetao (*Semen Juglandis*), Yezijiang (*Succus Cocois Endospermatis*), Mihoutao (*Fructus Actinidiae Chinensis*), Huaishi (*Flos Sophorae Immaturus*), Sangshenzi (*Fructus Mori*) and Heidadou (*Semen Sojae Nigrum*). The prescriptions are as follows.

Guazi (*Semen Benincasae*) Powder　60 g of Guazi (*Semen Benincasae*), Baizhi (*Radix Angelicae Dahuricae*), Danggui (*Radix Angelicae Sinensis*), Chuanxiong (*Rhizoma Ligustici Chuanxiong*) and Zhigancao (*Radix Glycyrrhizae Praeparata*) respectively. Grind the ingredients into powder. Take the powder with the wine three times a day, 1 g or so each time. Regular administration of the powder promotes blood circulation, tonifies blood, nourishes the hair, makes the skin lustrous, prevents ageing and premature grey hair.

Besides, some Chinese patent medicines like Qibao Meiran Pill (Seven-Ingredient Beard-Beautifying Pill) and Shouwu Yanshou Pill (Life-Prolonging Pill with *Radix Polygoni Multiflori*) can strengthen the tendons and bones, consolidate essence and qi, make the beard and hair black. These medicines may be selected, too.

Finally, people should remain a cheerful frame of mind, avoid extreme emotional stimulation, actively participate in the physical training, prevent and cure general diseases, abstain from bad habits such as smoking, excessive drinking and craputence. All these points should be taken into account in the hair beautification.

7.4 Health care of the eyes

The eyes comprehensively reflect the spirit, qi and vitality of the human body. Whether the eyes are healthy or not is closely associated with the human daily life.

7.4.1 Exercising the eyes

7.4.1.1 Rotating the eyeballs

This can increase the luster of the eyeballs and the acuity of sight, remove cataract and nebula, remedy myopia and hyperopia. The method is as follows: After waking in the early morning, close the eyes first. Then, rotate the eyeballs from the right to the left and from the left to the right respectively for ten times. Next, sit with the eyes opening and look at the left and the right, the upper left corner, the upper right corner, the lower left corner and the lower right corner respectively and repeatedly for four to five times. Besides, open the eyes to rotate the eyeballs and then close the eyes to rotate the eyeballs respectively for about ten times before the bed time in the evening.

7.4.1.2 Looking far into the distance

This can regulate the function of the eyeballs and prevent hypopsia due to the distortion of the eyeballs. People may selectively look far into the mountain, trees, grassland, blue sky, white cloud, bright moon, starlit sky, etc. But they should not fix their eyes on one site. Otherwise, it is harmful conversely.

惯等,都是美发需要注意的问题。

第四节 眼睛保健

眼睛是人体精气神的综合反映。眼睛健康与否,与工作、学习,以及日常生活关系十分密切。

一、运目

1. 运睛

能增强眼珠光泽和灵敏性,祛除内障外翳,纠正近视和远视。做法是:早晨醒后,先闭目,眼球从右向左,从左向右,各旋转10次;然后睁目坐定,用眼睛依次看左右,左上角、右上角、左下角、右下角,反复四五次;晚上睡觉前,先睁目运睛,后闭目运睛各10次左右。

2. 远眺

能调节眼球功能,避免眼球变形而导致视力减退。可在清晨、休息或夜间,有选择地望远山、树木、草原、蓝天、白云、明月、星空等。但又不宜长时间专注一处,否则反而有害。

7.4.2 Massage

7.4.2.1 "Ironing" the eyes

Rub the palms against each other until the palms get warm. Then, open the eyes and place the palms on the eyes respectively. Let the warm palms "iron" the eyeballs. When the palms become cool, rub them against each other to "iron" the eyeballs again. Repeat the exercise for three to five times at a time. Do the exercise for several times a day. The exercise warms and activates yangqi, improves sight and refreshes people.

7.4.2.2 Kneading the canthi

After holding breathing, knead and press the four corners of the eyes with the hands until the feeling of being slightly warm and suffocating occurs. Then, take a breath and end the exercise. Do the exercise continuously for three to five times at a time. Do the exercise for many times a day. It improves sight.

7.4.2.3 Digitally pressing massage on the acupoints

Digitally press Sizhukong (TE 23), Yuyao (EX-HN 4), or Zanzhu (BL 2), Sibai (ST 2), Taiyang (EX-HN 5), etc. with the palmar side of the index finger or Qugu, the first joint of the back of the thumb. The manipulation varies gradually from the gentle one to the forceful one until there appears the feeling of being markedly sore and distending. Then, knead and stroke the acupoints gently for several times. The exercise makes the eyes healthy, improves sight and cures ocular diseases.

7.4.3 Sitting in repose with the eyes closed

Nourishing the eyes is closely associated with cultivating the mind. When asthenopia appears, get rid of all

二、按摩

1. 熨目

双手掌面摩擦至热,在睁目时,两手掌分别按在两目上,使其热气煦熨两目珠,稍冷再摩再熨,如此反复3~5遍,每天可做数次,有温通阳气,明目提神作用。

2. 捏眦

即闭气后用手捏按两目之四角,直至微感闷气时,即可换气结束。连续作3~5遍,每日可做多次,有提高视力作用。

3. 点穴

用食指指肚或大拇指背第一关节的曲骨,点按丝竹空、鱼腰,或攒竹、四白、太阳等穴,手法由轻到重,以有明显的酸胀感为准,然后再轻揉抚摩几次。有健目明目,治疗目疾的作用。

三、闭目养神

养目和养神密切相关。当视力出现疲劳时,可排除杂

stray thoughts, relax the whole body naturally. Then, sit quietly with the eyes closed for three to five minutes, or rest peacefully with the eyes closed at the fixed time for several times. The exercise has the actions of eliminating asthenopia and regulating the emotions. It is also an effective accessory method to cure ocular diseases.

7.4.4 Diet

Eat more vegetable, fruit, carrot, animal liver or a proper amount of cod liver oil. All these foods have the protective effect on sight. But do not eat excessive fat meat and fine grain as well as pungent and extremely hot-natured foods. Meanwhile, the dietary therapy may be co-operatively used as follows.

7.4.4.1 Caojueming Tugan Soup (Soup of *Semen Cassiae* and *Hepar Leporis*) Tugan (*Hepar Leporis*) (one to two in number) and 10 to 12 g of Caojueming (*Semen Cassiae*). Use the ingredients to cook soup and flavor the soup with salt. Drink the soup and eat the liver. The soup tonifies the liver, nourishes blood, clears away heat from the liver and improves sight.

7.4.4.2 Juhua Gruel (Gruel of *Flos Chrysanthemi*) 10 to 15 g of Juhua (*Flos Chrysanthemi*) and 30 g to 60 g of Jingmi (*Semen Oryzae Sativae*). Use Jingmi (*Semen Oryzae Sativae*) to make gruel first. Then, mix the gruel with the powder of Juhua (*Flos Chrysanthemi*). Afterwards, cook the gruel again until it boils for once or twice. The gruel tonifies the liver and improves the sight.

7.4.5 Drugs

The drugs are divided into the drugs for external application and the ones for oral administration.

7.4.5.1 Prescription for Clearing Away Heat

四、饮食

多吃蔬菜、水果、胡萝卜、动物的肝脏，或适当用些鱼肝油，对视力有一定保护作用，切忌贪食膏粱厚味及辛辣大热之品。同时，还可配合食疗，如：

草决明兔肝汤 兔肝1～2副，草决明 10～12 g。加工煲汤，食盐调味，饮汤食肝。可补肝养血，清肝明目。

菊花粥 菊花 10～15 g，粳米 30～60 g。先用粳米煮粥，粥成调入菊花末，再煮一二沸即可。有养肝明目之效。

五、药物

分外用和内服两类。

清目养阴洗眼方 甘菊

from the Eyes, Nourishing Yin and Washing the Eyes: 9 g of Ganju (*Flos Chrysanthemi*), 9 g of Shuangsangye (frosted *Folium Mori*), 3 g of Bohe (*Herba Menthae*), 0.5 g of Lingyangjiao (*Cornus Antelopis*) powder, 9 g of Shengdihuang (*Radix Rehmanniae*) and 9 g of Xiakucao (*Spica Prunellae*). Decoct the ingredients in water. Fumigate the eyes first and then wash them with the decoction. The method dispels wind, clears away heat from the liver, nourishes the liver and improves sight.

7.4.5.2 Sight-Improving Pillow The pillow is padded with Qiaomaipi (*Testa Fagopyri Esculenti*), Lüdoupi (*Testa Phaseoli Radiati*), Heidoupi (*Testa Sojae Nigrae*), Juemingzi (*Semen Cassiae*) and Juhua (*Flos Chrysanthemi*). The pillow dispels wind and heat, improves sight and removes nebula. Prolonged application keeps sight acute for lifetime.

7.4.5.3 Manjingzi (*Fructus Viticis*) Powder 500 g of Manjingzi (*Fructus Viticis*) and 1 000 g of Huangjing (*Rhizoma Polygonati*). Make the drugs into boluses and steam the boluses. Then, grind the boluses into fine powder. Take 9 g of the powder by mixing it with water after the meal every day. Prolonged administration of the powder tonifies the liver, improves sight and prolongs life.

7.4.5.4 Chinese patent medicines People may also select some Chinese patent medicines like Liuwei Dihuang Bolus (Bolus of Six Drugs Including Rehmannia), Qiju Dihuang Bolus (Bolus of Six Drugs, Rehmannia with Wolfberry and Chrysanthemum) and Shihu Yeguang Pill (Pill of *Herba Dendrobii* for Curing Night blindness).

7.5 Health care of the ears

The ears are the auditory organs closely related to

9 g,霜桑叶 9 g,薄荷 3 g,羚羊角 0.5 g,生地黄 9 g,夏枯草 9 g。水煎后,先薰后洗,有疏风清肝、养阴明目之作用。

明目枕 荞麦皮、绿豆皮、黑豆皮、决明子、菊花,有疏风散热、明目退翳之功,经常使用,至老目明。

蔓荆子散 蔓荆子 500 g,黄精 1 000 g,二药九蒸九曝干,研成细末,每日饭后调服 6 g,久服,补肝明目,延年益寿。

中成药 如六味地黄丸、杞菊地黄丸、石斛夜光丸等,亦可选择应用。

第五节 耳部保健

耳是人体的听觉器官,与

the five zang organs, especially the kidney. In modern society, environmental pollution, the side effects of drugs, etc. seriously harm hearing. Therefore, importance should be attached to health care of the ears.

7.5.1 Massage

7.5.1.1 Massaging the helix root

Massage the front and back of the two helix roots with the index fingers for 15 times respectively.

7.5.1.2 Pressing the helix

Press the helix with the both hands upwards and downwards for 15 times.

7.5.1.3 Shaking and pulling the ears

Shake and pull the both helixes for 15 times respectively with the thumb and index finger. But do not apply too much force.

7.5.1.4 Flicking the ears

Flick the ears with the middle fingers for 15 times.

7.5.1.5 Beating the drum

Cover the ear orifices with the hands. Put the five fingers of each hand at the back of the head with the index fingers placing on the middle fingers. Then, the index fingers slide downwards suddenly to beat the rear of the head for 24 times. Afterwards, open and close the palms continuously for ten times. The method makes the antrum auris filled with air and the tympanic membrane vibrate. This is called "ming tiangu" (beating the Heavenly drum).

Massaging the ear can promote qi flow and blood circulation of the auricular region, make the external auricular skin moist and lustrous, delay the ageing of the tympanic membrane, prevent frostbite, prevent and cure auricular diseases.

7.5.2 Avoiding the drug allergy

A considerably large percentage of deafness is caused by the improper use of drugs, especially the ototoxic antibiotics like streptomycin, gentamycin, neomycin, kanamycin, tobramycin, vancomycin and polymyxin. In addition, salts of salicylic acid, chloromycetin, quinine, chloroquine as well as the chemotherapeutic drugs for tumor like mustargen and vincristins have certain ototoxic effects. Accordingly, these drugs should be strictly controlled in clinic so as to avoid deafness due to auditory injury.

Apart from these medicines, correct the bad habits like picking the ears to prevent infection of antrum auris. Meanwhile, moderate sexual life and eat proper tonic products. These points are also beneficial to the prevention and treatment of tinnitus and deafness in middle-aged people.

7.6 Health care of the nose

The nose, the door of respiratory tract, is the important organ to perform metabolism in the human body as well as the first line of defense to prevent the viral invasion into the human body. Therefore, it is important to protect it.

7.6.1 Bathing the nose

Bath the nose with cold water and cold air. Persevering in bathing the nose can improve the blood circulation of the nasal mucosa effectively, enhance the nasal adaptive

二、避免药物过敏

使用药物不当而引起耳聋占有相当的比例，特别是耳毒性抗生素，如链霉素、庆大霉素、新霉素、卡那霉素、托布霉素、万古霉素、多粘霉素等。此外，还有柳酸盐类药、氯霉素、喹宁、氯喹，以及治疗肿瘤的化疗药物，如氮芥、长春碱类等，都有一定的耳毒作用。因此，临床使用应严格控制，避免引起听觉损伤而造成耳聋。

此外，纠正挖耳等不良习惯。防止刺伤耳道引起感染。注意节制房事，适当服食补肾之品，对防治中老年耳鸣耳聋亦有好处。

第六节 鼻部保健

鼻是呼吸道的门户，既是人体进行新陈代谢的重要器官之一，又是防止病菌侵入人体的第一道防线。应做好防护工作。

一、浴鼻

用冷水浴鼻和冷空气浴鼻。若能坚持不懈，可有效地改善鼻黏膜的血液循环，增强

capacity of weather changes and prevent common cold and other diseases of respiratory tract.

7.6.2 Massage

This includes three movements of rubbing the nose, scraping the nose and rubbing the apex of nose. Rub the middle joints of the thumbs against each other until they get warm. Then, rub the two sides of the nose bridge with the warm middle joints for 24 times. This is the first movement. Scrape the nose bridge from the upper part to the lower part for ten times. This is the second movement. Rub the apex of nose for 12 times respectively with the fingers of both hands. This is the third movement. This exercise promotes the local blood circulation, makes the nasal skin moist and lustrous, moistens the lung and prevents common cold.

7.6.3 Drugs

7.6.3.1 Nose-Moistening Decoction 9 g of Tianmendong (*Radix Asparagi*), 15 g of Heizhima (*Semen Sesami*), 9 g of Shashen (*Radix Adenophorae*), 9 g of Maimendong (*Radix Ophiopogonis*), 9 g of Huangjing (*Rhizoma Polygonati*), 9 g of Yuzhu (*Rhizoma Polygonati Odorati*), 9 g of Shengdihuang (*Radix Rehmanniae*) and 9 g of Chuanbeimu (*Bulbus Fritillariae Cirrhosae*). The prescription moistens the lung, nourishes the spleen, moistens and protects the nose.

7.6.3.2 Nose-Strengthening Decoction 27 g of Cang'erzi (*Fructus Xanthii*), 6 g of Chanyi (*Periostracum Cicadae*), 9 g of Baijili (*Fructus Tribuli*), 9 g of Yuzhu (*Rhizoma Polygonati Odorati*), 4.5 g of Zhigancao (*Radix Glycyrrhizae Praeparata*), 12 g of Yiyiren (*Semen Coicis*) and 9 g of Baihe (*Bulbus Lilii*). The prescription dispels wind and strengthens the nose mainly. It also moistens the lung, strengthens the spleen. The decoction has the actions of health care and prevention for the patients susceptible to running nose.

In addition, people should cultivate the good habit of blowing the nose. Namely, hold the nose between the thumb and index finger to discharge the nasal mucus forcefully. Do not press one side to blow the nose. This may make the nasal discharge in the nasal cavity of the other side inspired into the body.

7.7 Health care of the extremities

The extremities are the important organs of the human being in bodily movement. Whether the life force of the body is great or not is closely associated with the state of these organs. Accordingly, people should attach importance to the health care of the extremities.

7.7.1 Health care of the upper limbs

7.7.1.1 Swinging the hands

Clench the both fists gently and swing the upper limbs from the front to the back, first to the left side, then to the right side. Afterwards, drop the upper limbs at the two sides of the body and swing the hands. Repeat the above movements for 24 times respectively. The exercise has the actions of limbering up the muscles and joints, promoting qi flow and blood circulation of meridians and collaterals, making the upper limbs healthy. It may prevent the joint diseases of the shoulder, elbow and wrist, regulate qi and blood, prevent and cure hypertension.

7.7.1.2 Massage

Rub the palms against each other until they get warm. Then, place the palmar side of the fingers of one

另外，要养成正确擤鼻涕的习惯，即用拇指和食指捏住鼻子，用力排出鼻涕。不可压住一侧擤鼻涕，这样会使另一侧鼻腔内鼻涕吸入体内。

第七节 四肢保健

四肢、手足是人体运动的重要器官，机体生命力的强盛与否，与四肢手足的功能强弱密切相关。强身保健应重视四肢手足的摄养。

一、上肢保健

1. 甩手

双手轻握拳，由前而后，甩动上肢，先向左侧甩动，再向右侧甩动，然后两肢垂于身体两侧甩动，各 24 次。有舒展筋骨关节、流通经络气血、强健上肢的作用，可预防肩、肘、腕关节疾病，还可调节气血，防治高血压。

2. 按摩

双手合掌互相摩擦至热，一手五指掌面放在另一手五

hand on the back of the fingers of the other hand and rub to and fro from the tips of the fingers to the wrist until the local warm sensation appears. At this time, alternate the hand to do the exercise again. Afterwards, rub the medial upper limb with the palm from the wrist to the armpit, and again rub the lateral upper limb from the shoulder to the wrist. This is one cycle. Repeat the cycle for 24 times. Do the exercise once respectively before bed time in the evening and in the early morning after waking. This method may promote muscular blood circulation, increase metabolism and the absorption of nutrients, make the skin healthy, moist and free from wrinkles, the hand soft, moist and healthy, prevent and cure frostbite.

7.7.1.3 Tapping with the plum-blossom needle

Tap the skin of the back of the hand gently with the plum-blossom needle in a linear way from the fingertip to the wrist along the finger, once a day. The manipulation should not be too forceful. Tap the skin of the back of the hand until the skin turns warm each time. It is better to apply the hand-moistening paste on the skin. The exercise makes the skin moist, smooth and free from wrinkles, activates collaterals, promotes blood circulation and keeps the hands healthy and beautiful.

7.7.1.4 Drugs

7.7.1.4.1 Hand-Protecting Paste I 20 g of Taoren (*Semen Persicae*), 10 g of Xingren (*Semen Armeniacae Amarum with the tip removed*), 20 g of Juhe (*Semen Citri Reticulatae*), 20 g of Chishaoyao (*Radix Paeoniae Rubra*), 30 g of Xinyiren (*Semen Magnoliae*), Chuanxiong (*Rhizoma Ligustici Chuanxiong*) and Danggui (*Radix Angelicae Sinensis*) respectively, 60 g of Dazao (*Fructus Zizipi Jujubae*), Niunao (*Cerebrum Bovis*), Yangnao (*Cerebrum Caprae seu Ovis*) and Gounao (*Cerebrum Canis*) respectively. All the above ingredients are made into paste. Apply the paste on the hand evenly after washing it. Do not warm the hand by a fire. The product makes the skin lustrous and moist, protects the hands and prevents wrinkles.

7.7.1.4.2 Hand-Protecting Paste II: 60 g of Gualourang (*Fructus Trichosanthis*), 30 g of Xingren (*Semen Armeniacae Amarum*) and a proper quantity of Fengmi (*Mel*). The ingredients are made into paste. Apply the paste on the hands before bed time in the evening. The product prevents rhagadia, makes the skin white, clean, tender and elastic.

7.7.2 Health care of the lower limbs

7.7.2.1 Exercising the lower limbs

7.7.2.1.1 Swinging the leg in a standing position Put one hand against the wall or tree and stand with one leg. Swing the right leg forward with the toe tip sticking up. Then, swing the leg backward with the foot dorsum and leg straightening. Swing the legs in this way repeatedly and alternately for 20 times respectively.

7.7.2.1.2 Kicking in a sitting position Sit and keep the upper body erect. First, lift the left foot and extend it towards the anterosuperior direction slowly with the toe tip sticking up. When the leg is about to extend straightly, kick towards the anteroinferior direction with the great force applied on the heel. Do the exercise alternately with the both feet respectively for 20 times.

7.7.2.1.3 Twisting the knees Place the feet against each other parallelly. Then, flex the knees slightly to squat down with the palms placing on the knees. Afterwards, twist the knees forwards, backwards, leftwards and rightwards in a circular way. Twist the knees leftwards first, then rightwards for 20 times respectively.

The above methods may strengthen the function of

护手膏2 瓜蒌瓤60 g，杏仁30 g，蜂蜜适量。制作成膏，每夜睡前涂手。本品防止手部皲裂，使皮肤白净柔嫩，富有弹性。

二、下肢保健

1. 运腿

站立甩腿 一手扶墙或扶树，一脚站立，一脚甩动先向前甩动右腿，脚尖向上翘起，然后向后甩，脚面绷直，腿亦伸直，如此前后甩动，左右腿各甩动20次。

平坐蹬腿 平坐，上身保持正直，先提起左脚向前上方缓伸，脚尖向上，当要伸直时，脚跟稍用力向前下方蹬出，再换右脚做，双腿各做20次。

扭膝运动 两脚平行靠拢，屈膝微向下蹲，双手掌置于膝上，膝部向前后左右做圆周运动，先左转，后右转，各20次。

上述方法可增强下肢功

the lower limbs, promote flexible articular movement, prevent and cure hypodynamia of the lower limbs, arthralgia, spasm of the legs, hemiplegia, etc.

7.7.2.2 Massage

7.7.2.2.1 Rubbing the leg Assume the sitting position. Hold the root of one thigh between the hands. Then, rub from the upper part to the ankle and from the ankle to the root of the thigh. This is a cycle. Repeat the cycle for 20 times. Rub the other leg in the same way. This method enhances the force of the legs, promotes flexible aricular movements, prevents muscular atrophy and varix of lower limbs, etc.

7.7.2.2.2 Rubbing the sole After washing the feet before bed time every night, grasp the toes with one hand and rub the sole for 100 times until it becomes warm. Rub the soles alternately. The method has the actions of consolidating primordial qi, warming the kidney qi, regulating the heart and kidney, making the feet and legs healthy, preventing and curing foot diseases.

7.7.2.3 Soaking the feet

Soaking the feet in warm water promotes blood circulation and is beneficial to the heart, kidney and sleeping. Better effects may result from the combined use of soaking the feet and massaging the feet.

7.7.2.4 Drugs

7.7.2.4.1 Chu Wushi's Prescription Shengjiangzhi (*Succus Zingiberis Recentis*), alcohol, white salt and Layuezhugao (*Sebum Suis* in the twelfth month of the lunar year). Grind the ingredients into paste. Then, parch the paste until it is warm. Afterwards, apply the warm paste on the feet. The prescription dispels cold, warms meridians, moistens the skin and cures rhagadia.

7.7.2.4.2 Prescription for Moistening the Hands and Feet and Preventing Rhagadia in the

2. 按摩

干浴腿 平坐，两手先抱一侧大腿根，自上而下摩擦至足踝，然后再往回摩擦至大腿根，一上一下为1次，做20次，依同法再摩擦另一腿。其作用是：腿力增强，关节灵活，预防肌肉萎缩、下肢静脉曲张等病。

擦脚心 每夜洗脚后临睡之前，一手握脚趾，另一手摩擦足心100次，以热为度，两脚轮流摩擦。具有固真元，暖肾气，交通心肾，强足健步，防治足疾等作用。

3. 泡足

用温水泡脚，促进血液循环，对心脏、肾脏及睡眠都有益处。如果泡脚和按摩合在一起做，效果更好。

4. 药物

初虞世方 生姜汁、酒精、白盐、腊月猪膏。研烂炒热，擦于脚部。有散寒温经、润肤治裂之功效。

冬月润手足防裂方 猪脂油12 g，黄蜡60 g，白芷、升

Twelfth Moon 12 g of Zhuzhiyou (*Sebum Suis*), 60 g of Huangla (*Cera flava*), 3 g of Baizhi (*Radix Angelicae Dahuriae*), Shengma (*Rhizoma Cimicifugae*) and Zhuyazaojia (*Fructus Gleditsiae Abnormalis*) respectively, 1.5 g of Dingxiang (*Flos Caryophylli*) and 0.6 g of Shexiang (*Moschus*). Make the above ingredients into paste. Then, apply the paste on the feet after washing them. The prescription eliminates pathogenic factors, dredges collaterals, expels wind, relieves swelling, prevents rhagadia and frostbite.

7.8 Health care of the chest, back, waist and abdomen

7.8.1 Health care of the chest

Massage method Assume the sitting or the supine position. Push and rub the chest with the left palm from the left upper part to the right lower part and with the right hand from the right upper part to the left lower part. Push and rub the chest alternately with the both hands for 30 times. Then, knead the breast clockwise and anti-clockwise for 30 circles simultaneously with both hands. Afterwards, knead and press the breast with both hands for 30 times from the left to the right and from the upper part to the lower part. Besides, women may grasp the breast for health care. The method is as follows. Cross the lower arms. Then, hold the left breast with the right hand and the right breast with the left hand. Next, grasp the breast with the fingers. One cycle is composed of grasping and releasing the breast once respectively. Repeat the cycle for 30 times. Massaging the chest may invigorate yangqi, promote qi flow and blood circulation and enhance the functions of the heart and lung.

7.8.2 Health care of the back

7.8.2.1 Keeping the back warm

The back is the place where the acupoints of viscera of the human body are located. Pathogenic cold may invade viscera directly. Therefore, pay attention to keeping the back warm at all times. People may protect the back with clothes, warm the back in the sun, avoid exposure to cold, etc. to achieve health care of the back.

7.8.2.2 Pounding the back

7.8.2.2.1 Pounding the back People may pound the back by themselves or ask others to pound the back for them. This has the actions of dredging meridians, promoting blood circulation, invigorating yangqi, strengthening the heart and benefiting the kidney.

7.8.2.2.2 Rubbing the back People may rub the back by themselves or ask others to rub the back for them. People can rub the back by themselves while taking a bath. Place a wet towel on the shoulder. Then, pull the two ends of the towel tightly with the both hands and rub the back forcefully until it turns warm. When asking someone to rub the back, assume the prone position with the naked back. Ask the person to press and rub the back upwards and downwards along the spine until the back gets warm. Do not apply the force too violently to avoid hurting the skin. Rubbing the back prevents and cures common cold, aching pain of the waist and back, chest tightness and abdominal distension.

7.8.2.2.3 Kneading the spine Assume the prone position with the naked back. Ask someone to lift up the muscle of the middle of the spine with the both hands (the thumb and index finger) and hold-twist it continuously from Dazhui (GV14) to the sacrum for three times. The method is applicable to adults and children. It regulates

二、背部保健

1. 保暖

背部是人体五脏六腑腧穴之所在,受寒会直接侵犯脏腑,故应时刻注意保暖。可用衣服护背、晒背取暖、避免受寒等措施来保暖护背。

2. 捶背

捶背 可自我捶打,也可他人捶打。有舒经活血,振奋阳气,强心益肾作用。

搓背 搓背也分自搓和他人搓。自搓方法,可在洗浴时进行。以湿毛巾搭于背后,双手扯紧毛巾两端,用力搓背,直至背部发热为止。他人搓法:取俯卧位,裸背。请他人以手掌沿脊柱上下按搓,至发热为止。注意用力不宜过猛,以免搓伤皮肤。搓背法有防治感冒、腰背酸痛、胸闷腹胀之功效。

捏脊 取俯卧位,裸背。请他人用双手(拇指与食指合作)将脊柱中间的皮肤捏拿起来,自大椎开始,自上而下,连续捻动,直至骶部。可连续捏拿3次。此法对成人、小儿皆

viscera, promotes qi flow and blood circulation, and strengthens the spleen, regulates the stomach and also has certain effects on the regulation of blood pressure. Do not apply very strong force too violently and quickly while the movements should be in harmony with one another.

7.8.3 Health care of the waist

7.8.3.1 Exercising the waist

7.8.3.1.1 Swinging the hip and waist Assume the standing posture with arms akimbo. The thumb is on the front and the other four fingers are on the back. Use the middle finger to press Shenshu (BL 23). When inhaling the air, swing the hip from the left to the right; when exhaling the air, from the right to the left. This is one cycle. Repeat the cycle for eight to thirty-two times continuously.

7.8.3.1.2 Bending down and lifting the waist Assume the standing position. When inhaling air, raise the both hands from the front of the body overhead with the palms facing downwards and the fingertips upwards; when exhaling air, bend down with the both hands touching the ground or feet. Do the exercise continuously for eight to thirty-two times.

7.8.3.1.3 Twisting the waist and spine Assume the standing posture. Raise the both hands beside the two sides of the head with the shoulder-width apart, the thumb tip as high as the eyebrow and the palms against each other. When inhaling air, twist the upper body from the left to the right and twist the head with the body towards the right posterior direction; when exhaling air, from the right to left. This is a cycle. Repeat the cycle continuously for eight to thirty-two times.

7.8.3.2 Massage

Massaging the waist strengthens the waist and the

宜,可调和脏腑、疏通气血、健脾和胃,对调整血压也有一定作用。注意用力不宜过大、过猛、速度不宜太快,动作要协调。

三、腰部保健

1. 摇腰

转胯运腰 取站立姿势,双手叉腰,拇指在前其余四指在后,中指按在肾俞穴上,吸气时,将胯由左向右摆动,呼气时,由右向左摆动,一呼一吸为一次,可连续做8～32次。

俯仰健腰 取站立姿势,吸气时,两手从体前上举,手心向下,一直举到头上方,手指尖朝上,呼气时,弯腰两手触地或脚。如此连续做8～32次。

旋腰转脊 取站立姿势,两手上举至头两侧与肩同宽,拇指尖与眉同高,手心相对,吸气时,上体由左向右扭转,头也随着向右后方扭动,呼气时,由右向左扭动,一呼一吸为一次,可连续做8～32次。

2. 按摩

经常按摩腰部有壮腰强

kidney. The method is as follows. Rub the both hands against each other to make them warm. Inhale air with the nose and exhale it slowly. Rub the two Shenshu (BL23) acupoints with the warm hands for 120 times respectively.

7.8.4 Health care of the abdomen

7.8.4.1 Keeping the abdomen warm

In addition to keeping the abdomen warm in daily life, old and weak people may use the "abdominal wrapper" or the "abdominal band" for health care.

7.8.4.1.1 The abdominal wrapper Beat moxa to make it soft. Then, spread it evenly. Put silk floss (or cotton) on it. Place the moxa and silk floss or cotton into a two-layer abdominal wrapper. Finally, tie the abdominal wrapper around the abdomen.

7.8.4.1.2 The abdominal band Tie the seven-to eight-cun-wide band around the lumboabdominal region.

Both the abdominal wrapper and abdominal band can be padded with medicinal powder with the warming action to make the abdomen warmer.

7.8.4.2 Massage

Massaging the abdomen is actually massaging the stomach and intestine. It is especially advisable to massage the part after the meal. The specific method is as follows. Rub the hands against each other to make them warm. Then, put one hand on the top of another and place the overlapped hands on the abdomen. At this time, rub the abdomen with the palm around the navel clockwise and anticlockwise from the small cycle to the large one for 36 cycles respectively. The method increases enterokinesia and gastric peristalsis, regulates qi, removes food retention, enhances the digestive function, prevents and cures gastrointestinal diseases.

8 Rehabilitation Examples of Commonly-Seen Diseases

8.1 Rehabilitation for Sequelae

After the basic recovery, certain diseases still leave over or occur in some people. Therefore, they cannot restore health for a long time. This is caused by deficiency of healthy qi, the residual pathogenic factors or repeated attack by exogenous pathogenic factors. Accordingly, various methods of rehabilitation should be adopted to strengthen healthy qi and eliminate the residual pathogenic factors on the basis of syndrome differentiation.

8.1.1 Low fever

Low fever below 38℃ is a commonly-seen symptom after the recovery from the febrile disease. This low fever is often lingering and prolonged and consumes essence and qi, manifested as a certain degree of physical and psychological disturbances like mental fatigue, poor appetite and feeble pulse.

8.1.1.1 Syndrome differentiation and treatment

8.1.1.1.1 Fever due to yin deficiency

This is mostly seen in febrile diseases at the late stage with the manifestations of hectic fever in the afternoon and at night, feverish palms and soles, dysphoria,

第八章 常见病证的康复实例举隅

第一节 疾病后遗症状的康复

疾病基本痊愈后,有些人仍会遗留或发生某种病证,久久不能康复,这是由于正气亏损、余邪未尽或复感外邪所致。应在辨证的前提下,采用各种康复方法,扶正固本,清除余邪。

一、低热

病后低热,体温一般不超过38℃,是热病瘥后一种常见病证。这种低热往往病程缠绵,迁延日久,耗伤精气,表现出一定程度的体力、心理方面的障碍,如精神疲乏、食欲不振、脉虚无力等症。

【辨证施治】

1. 阴虚发热

多见于发热性疾病后期,午后或夜间潮热,手足心热,烦躁盗汗,失眠多梦,口干咽

night sweat, dream-disturbed sleep, dry mouth and throat, red and dry tongue with a little or no fur, thready and rapid pulse. It is advisable to nourish yin and clear away heat. The prescription used is the modified Qinghao Biejia Decoction (Decoction of Herba Artemisiae and Carapax Trioncis) or Powder for Clearing away Heat from the Bone. Shashen Maidong Decoction (Decoction of Radix Adenophorae and Radix Ophiopogonis) or Stomach-Strengthening Decoction is advisable in the case of pneumogastric yin impairment with residual heat and dry cough, scanty sputum or retching and anorexia; the modified Pulsation-Promoting Decoction is advisable in the case of hepatorenal yin deficiency with palms and soles warmer than the dorsa of the hand and foot, mental fatigue, sleepiness, feeble and thready or knotted and intermittent pulse; the modified Sanjia Powder is advisable in the case of yin deficiency with residual heat intermingled with phlegm stagnating collaterals concurrently manifested as palpitation, dysphoria, vibration of the hand and foot and dull expression.

8.1.1.1.2　Fever due to qi deficiency

It manifests low or high fever often occurring or aggravated after over strain, mental fatigue, hypodynamia, short breath, disinclination to speaking, poor appetite, loose stool, spontaneous sweating, pale tongue with thin and white fur, and weak pulse. It is advisable to supplement qi, strengthen the spleen and remove heat with sweet and warm-natured drugs. The prescription used is the modified Decoction for Tonifying the Middle Energizer and Supplementing Qi. For the patients with profuse sweat, Muli (*Concha Ostreae*) and Fuxiaomai (*Fructus Tritici Levis*) may be added; for the patients with alternative cold and fever, sweat and aversion to cold, Guizhi (*Ramulus Cinnamomi*) and Shaoyao (*Radix Paeoniae*

燥,舌质红干,苔少或无苔,脉细数。宜滋阴清热。青蒿鳖甲汤或清骨散加减。若肺胃阴伤,而余热未净,兼见干咳少痰或干呕纳差,宜用沙参麦冬汤或益胃汤。若肝肾阴亏而见手足心热甚于手足背,神倦欲眠,脉虚细或结代,宜用加减复脉汤。若阴虚兼余热夹痰,瘀滞络脉,而伴见心悸烦躁,手足颤动,神情呆钝,可用三甲散加减。

2. 气虚发热

发热,热势或低或高,常在劳累后发作或加剧,神疲乏力,短气懒言,食少便溏,自汗,舌质淡,苔薄白,脉弱。宜益气健脾,甘温除热。补中益气汤加减。自汗多者,可加牡蛎、浮小麦;时冷时热、汗出恶风者,可加桂枝、芍药;大便稀溏、手足欠温者,可酌加干姜、肉桂;胸脘痞闷、呕恶苔腻者,可加苍术、厚朴、藿香。

Alba) are added; for the patients with loose stool, cold hands and feet, Ganjiang (*Rhizoma Zingiberis*) and Rougui (*Cortex Cinnamomi*) are added; for the patients with stuffiness and tightness of the chest and stomach, vomiting, nausea and greasy fur, Cangzhu (*Rhizoma Atractylodis*), Houpo (*Cortex Magnoliae Officinalis*) and Huoxiang (*Herba Agastachis*) are added.

8.1.1.1.3 Fever due to the residual pathogenic factors

It manifests lingering low fever without remission, or lingering alternate cold and fever, vexation, bitter taste, thirst, inclination to vomiting, red tongue with thin and yellow fur, thready and rapid or taut and rapid pulse. It is advisable to clear away the residual heat and take healthy qi and pathogenic factors into consideration simultaneously. The prescription used is the modified Minor Decoction of Bupleurum; Zhuye Shigao Decoction (Decoction of *Folium Phyllostachydis Nigrae* and *Gypsum Fibrosum*) may be used for the patients with consumption of both qi and body fluids due to the residual heat.

8.1.1.2 Rehabilitation methods

8.1.1.2.1 Regulating emotions and musical therapy

The low fever patients with psychological disturbances like mental fatigue, dysphoria and anxiety should overcome their misgivings, tranquilize their mind to recuperate, enhance their vigor and cooperate in the treatment. They may be properly treated with the musical therapy; for those with dysphoria and anxiety, soft and peaceful music should be selected; for those with mental fatigue and listlessness, inspiring, bold and unrestrained music should be selected.

8.1.1.2.2 Acumox and massage

Acumox: Select Feishu (BL 13), Dazhu (BL 11),

3. 余邪发热

低热不退，或见往来寒热，缠绵不解，心烦，口苦，口渴，欲呕，舌红，苔薄黄，脉细数或弦数。宜清解余热，正邪兼顾。小柴胡汤加减。若余热未尽而气液两伤者，可用竹叶石膏汤。

【康复方法】
1. 调节情志和音乐疗法

低热患者有精神疲乏，烦躁焦虑的心理障碍，必须使之消除顾虑，静心调养，振作精神，配合治疗。可适当配合音乐疗法，对心情烦躁焦虑者，选择幽雅、恬静的乐曲；对精神疲乏或委靡者，选择激昂、奔放的乐曲。

2. 针灸、推拿疗法

针灸 可取肺俞、大杼、

Hegu (LI 4), etc. for acumox. For the patients with yin deficiency, Shenmen (HT 7), Shenshu (GV 12) and Sanyinjiao (SP 6) are added; for the patients with qi deficiency, Qihai (CV 6), Guanyuan (CV 4) and Zusanli (ST 36) are added and moxibustion applied; for the patients with fever due to the residual pathogenic factors, Dazhui (GV 14), Quchi (LI 11) and Xingjian (LR 2) are added. The filiform needles are generally used for shallow puncturing, with the uniform reinforcing-reducing method.

Massage: Acupoint massage is mainly used. Digitally press Dazhui (GV 14), Quchi (LI 11), Hegu (LI 4), Sanyinjiao (SP 6), etc; lift and grasp Jianjing (GB 21); pull finger joints; pinch the nail roots, and again knead finger joints as well as finger tips. This is one cycle. Repeat the cycle for five times.

8.1.1.2.3 Dietary therapy

In the case of fever due to yin deficiency, select Maidong Gruel (Gruel of Radix Ophiopogonis); in the case of fever due to qi deficiency, select Huangqin Dazao Gruel (Gruel of *Radix Scutellariae* and *Fructus Ziziphi Jujubae*); in the case of fever due to residual heat, select Gefen Gruel (Gruel of Powder of *Radix Puerariae*). The diet should be bland, tasty, refreshing, nutritious and digestible. Eat more fresh vegetables, fruits, soup and gruel. But abstain from greasy, fried and pungent foods. In the case of yin deficiency, regularly ingest Thick Soup of Baihe (*Bulbus Lilii*), Soup of Soft-Shelled Turtle and Soup of Yin'er (*Tremella*); in the case of qi deficiency, eat the foods for tonifying the spleen and stomach like Lianzi (*Semen Nelumbinis*), Chinese dates (*Fructus Ziziphi Jujubae*) and Guiyuan (*Arillus Longan*); in the case of lingering residual heat, drink fruit juice, wax gourd soup and mung bean soup.

8.1.2 Cough

Cough after the recovery from a disease is mostly related to deficiency of qi and yin as well as lingering residual pathogenic factors. Delayed treatment may bring about endogenous cough which occurs repeatedly and worsens increasingly.

8.1.2.1 Syndrome differentiation and treatment

8.1.2.1.1 Residual heat haunting the lung

It manifests severe dry cough in the daytime, scanty and sticky sputum, dry mouth and throat, dysphoria, thirst, or low fever, red tongue with scanty body fluid, thready and rapid pulse. It is advisable to nourish the lung yin and clear away the residual heat simultaneously. The prescription used is Shashen Maidong Decoction (Decoction of *Adenophorae* and *Ophiopogonis*) with additional Chuanbeimu (*Bulbus Fritillariae Cirrhosae*), Tianxingren (*Semen Armeniacae*), Sangbaipi (*Cortex Mori Radicis*) and Digupi (*Cortex Lycil Radicis*).

8.1.2.1.2 Deficiency of qi and yin

It manifests cough, short breath, unsmooth expectoration, or sputum with blood, dry throat and mouth, flushing of zygomatic region, pale complexion, hectic fever, night sweat, emaciation, mental fatigue, hypodynamia, red and dry tongue and feeble pulse. It is suitable to supplement qi, nourish yin, moisten the lung and check cough. The prescriptions used include Ziwan Powder (Powder of *Radix Asteris*) with additional Xingren (*Semen Armeniacae Amarum*), Kuandonghua (*Flos Farfarae*) and Maimendong (*Radix Ophipogonis*), as well as the modified Baihe Gujin Decoction (Lily Decoction for Strengthening the Lung).

二、咳嗽

病后咳嗽多与肺之气阴亏虚及余邪未尽有关。若久延失治，可转化为内伤性咳嗽，反复发作，日益加重。

【辨证施治】

1. 余热恋肺

干咳日间较甚，痰少而黏，口燥咽干，心烦口渴，或有低热，舌红少津，脉细数。宜滋养肺阴，兼清余热。沙参麦冬汤加川贝母、甜杏仁、桑白皮、地骨皮。

2. 气阴亏损

咳嗽气短，咯痰不爽，或痰中带血，咽燥口干，颧红面白，潮热盗汗，形体消瘦，神疲乏力，舌红质干，脉虚数。宜益气养阴，润肺止咳。紫菀散加杏仁、沙参、款冬花、麦门冬之类，也可用百合固金汤加减。

8.1.2.1.3 Residual wind and cold

It manifests lingering exogenous cough, vomiting with white sputum, nasal obstruction, itching throat, or slight aversion to cold and fever, red lingual edge and tip, white and thin fur, floating and slippery pulse. It is advisable to check cough, resolve sputum, disperse the lung and relieve the exterior syndrome. The prescription used is the modified Cough Powder. In the case of phlegm intermingled with dampness manifested as sticky and thick sputum and saliva, chest tightness and greasy fur, add Banxia (*Rhizoma Pinelliae*), Houpo (*Cortex Magnoliae Officinalis*) and Fuling (*Poria*); in the case of concurrent dysphoria due to stagnated heat, add Sangbaipi (*Cortex Mori Radicis*), Huangqin (*Radix Scutellariae*) and Tianhuafen (*Radix Trichosanthis*); in the case of pulmonary dryness and dry cough, add Gualou (*Fructus Trichosanthis*), Beimu (*Flos Fritillariae Thunbergii*) and Zhimu (*Rhizoma Anemarrhenae*).

8.1.2.2 Rehabilitation methods

8.1.2.2.1 Regulating emotions and recreation therapy

Checking one emotion with another, musical therapy, recreation therapy and color therapy may be applied in the case of grief and depression.

8.1.2.2.2 Acumox and massage

Acumox: Select Feishu (BL 13), Hegu (LI 4), Qihai (CV 6), Zusanli (ST 36), etc. in acumox. In the case of profuse sputum, add Fenglong (ST 40); in the case of inching throat, add Tiantu (CV 22); in the case of chest tightness, add Neiguan (PC 6) and Danzhong (CV 17); in the case of prolonged cough and weakness, moxibustion with the warming needle may be applied on Feishu (BL 13), Shenshu (BL 23) and Pishu (BL 20). The uniform reinforcing-reducing manipulation is advisable. The shal-

3. 风寒未尽

外感咳嗽迁延不愈,咳吐白痰,鼻塞咽痒,或微有恶寒发热,舌边尖红,苔薄白,脉浮滑。宜止咳化痰,宣肺疏表。止嗽散加减。若夹痰湿而见痰涎黏稠、胸闷苔腻者,加半夏、厚朴、茯苓;若兼郁热而烦渴苔黄者,加桑白皮、黄芩、天花粉;若见肺燥而干咳无痰者,加瓜蒌、贝母、知母。

【康复方法】

1. 调节情志和娱乐疗法

若情志悲郁不舒,可应用情志相胜、音乐、娱乐、色彩等疗法。

2. 针灸、推拿疗法

针灸　取肺俞、合谷、气海、足三里等穴。痰多加丰隆;咽痒加天突;胸闷加内关、膻中;久咳体弱可温灸肺俞、肾俞、脾俞。针法宜平补平泻,若兼外感宜浅刺用泻法。

low puncturing with the reducing method is simultaneously applied in the case of concurrent exopathy.

Massage: The digital pressing method is used in massage with the selection of Shaoshang (LU 11), Lieque (LU 7), Taiyuan (LU 9), Fengmen (BL 12), Feishu (BL 13) and Xuanji (CV 21). Press Tiantu (CV 22) for two minutes until it turns sore and distending. Besides, tap Dingchuan (EX‑B 1) with the fingertip, or pat Fenglong (ST 40) and Zusanli (ST 36). Lift and grasp the back and spine, digitally press Feishu (BL 13) and knead Mingmen (GV 4). Afterward, pat the back repeatedly to promote free respiration; press and knead Danzhong (CV 17) to promote expectoration.

8.1.2.2.3 Dietary therapy

In the case of residual heat haunting the lung, select snow Pear Paste or ingest Shashen Gruel (Gruel of *Radix Adenophorae*); in the case of deficiency of qi and yin, ingest Baihe Gruel (Gruel of *Bulbus Lilii*); in the case of residual wind and cold, ingest Zisu Gruel (Gruel of *Fructus Perillae*). The diet should avoid pungent, aromatic, dry-natured, hot-natured, fat, greasy and extremely cold- and cool-natured foods. In the case of fever due to yin deficiency, take decoction for more times, a bit each time. Simultaneously, eat Baihe (*Bulbus Lilii*), Lianzi (*Semen Nelumbinis*) and Yin'er (*Tremella*); in the case of residual wind and cold, take warm decoction and add more clothing and quilts. Meanwhile, drink warm beverage and gruel to strengthen the body resistance and dispel pathogenic factors.

8.1.2.2.4 Nursing in daily life

Avoid smoke, dust as well as abnormal odor stimulation. Smokers should abstain from smoking. Prevent cold and keep the body warm. People with susceptibility due to weakness of the body may take Yupingfeng Powder (Jade

8 Rehabilitation Examples of Commonly Seen Diseases

Screen Powder) and the like to supplement qi and strengthen the superficial body resistance. All those with prolonged cough should abstain from sexual life to preserve essence and qi.

8.1.3 Edema

Edema is a disorder of muscular tumefaction. In this section, edema refers to mild tumefaction, in which urinary test shows no marked abnormal changes and nephrotic edema is not included.

8.1.3.1 Syndrome differentiation and treatment

8.1.3.1.1 Edema due to dampness and heat

It manifests sublumbar edema, abdominal fullness, dyspnea, dysphoria with thirst, unsmooth urination and defecation, yellowish and greasy fur, deep and rapid pulse. It is advisable to dispel water and clear away heat. The prescription used is Muli Zexie Powder (Powder of *Concha Ostreae* and *Rhizoma Alismatis*). Take the powder by mixing it in rice soup three times a day, five to ten grams. After smooth urination, reduce the dosage accordingly or stop the administration. The modified Sanren Decoction (Decoction of Three Kinds of Kernels) may be applied in the case of the mild symptoms of dampness-heat stagnation.

8.1.3.1.2 Edema due to qi deficiency

It manifests edema of the face and limbs which happens and vanishes alternately, lassitude, hypodynamia, pale and lustreless complexion, short breath, anorexia, pale tongue with a little fur, slow and weak pulse. In the case of yang deficiency of the spleen and stomach, edema is marked, especially on the lower limbs, with the concurrent manifestations of epigastric and abdominal distension, loose stool, scanty urine, sallow complexion, cold

凡久嗽不愈者,均应戒房事以保精气。

三、浮肿

浮肿,是指肌肤肿胀的一种病证。本节所指,是肿势不甚,尿液化验无明显异常,排除肾病者。

【辨证施治】

1. 湿热水肿

腰以下浮肿,腹胀满,喘逆烦渴,小便不利,大便不爽,苔黄腻,脉沉数。宜逐水清热。方用牡蛎泽泻散,每次5～10 g,以米汤调服,每日3次,见小便通利后,可酌减或停服。若为湿热郁滞轻证,可用三仁汤加减。

2. 气虚水肿

头面或四肢浮肿,时肿时消,倦怠乏力,面白不华,少气纳差,舌淡苔少,脉缓弱。若脾胃阳虚,则浮肿明显,以下肢为甚,并见脘腹胀闷,便溏尿少,面黄肢冷,苔白滑,脉沉缓。宜健脾化湿。轻证可用冬瓜汤泡白术一宿,去白术加

limbs, pale and slippery fur, deep and slow pulse. It is suitable to strengthen the spleen and eliminate dampness. In the case of mild symptoms, after soaking Baizhu (*Rhizoma Atractylodis Macorcephalae*) in waxgourd decoction for a night, remove Baizhu (*Rhizoma Atractylodis Macrocephalae*) and add Yiyiren (*Semen Coicis*) to the decoction to be decocted for oral administration; in the case of severe symptoms, use the modified Shenling Baizhu Powder (Powder of Ginseng, Poria and Bighead Atractylodes); in the case of severe edema due to yang deficiency of the spleen and stomach, it is suitable to warm the spleen and promote diuresis with the modified Shipi Decoction (Decoction for Reinforcing the Spleen).

8.1.3.1.3 Edema due to yang deficiency

It manifests general edema which is particularly severe below the waist, soreness and flaccidity of the waist and knees, aversion to cold, cold limbs, reduced amount of urine, pale tongue with white fur, deep and weak pulse. In the case of prolonged renal yang deficiency, yang impairment involving yin, symptoms mainly due to renal yin deficiency may occur as well which manifest as repeated onset of edema, mental fatigue, soreness of the waist, seminal emission, dry mouth and throat, dysphoria with feverish sensation of the chest, palms and soles, red tongue, thready and rapid pulse. It is advisable to warm the kidney to promote diuresis. The prescription used is the modified Jisheng Shenqi Pill (Life-Preserving Pill for Replenishing the Kidney Qi) in combination with Zhenwu Decoction (Decoction for Strengthening the Spleen Yang).

8.1.3.1.4 Edema due to qi stagnation

It manifests marked edema of the abdomen and limbs with normal skin color, bulging abdomen like a drum when tapped, oppressed sensation and distension of the

薏苡仁煎服；重证可用参苓白术散加减。若证属脾胃阳虚而浮肿较甚者，宜温脾利水，方用实脾饮加减。

3. 阳虚水肿

全身浮肿，腰以下尤甚，腰膝酸软，畏寒肢冷，尿量减少，舌淡苔白，脉沉弱。若肾阳久衰，阳损及阴，也可出现以肾阴亏虚为主的病证，表现为浮肿反复发作，精神疲惫，腰酸遗精，口咽干燥，五心烦热，舌红，脉细数等。宜温肾行水。济生肾气丸合真武汤加减。

4. 气滞浮肿

浮肿以腹部和四肢明显，皮色不变，按之即起，腹虽大叩之如鼓，胸闷胀，喜嗳气，小

chest, susceptibility to eructation, smooth urination, white fur and taut pulse. It is advisable to activate qi flow, remove qi stagnation and promote diuresis. The prescription used is Kuanzhong Decoction with additional Muxiang (*Radix Aucklandiae*), Xiangfu (*Rhizoma Cyperi*) and Qingpi (*Pericarpium Citri Reticulatae Viride*). In the case of gastric fullness, belching, loose stool, greasy fur and slippery pulse, it is advisable to dry dampness, activate the spleen, remove food retention and regulate the stomach with the modified prescription of Pingwei Powder (Peptic Powder) in combination with Baohe Pill (Lenitive Pill).

8.1.3.1.5 Edema due to yin deficiency

This is commonly seen in the patients who have not recovered from deficiency of yin and blood following the febrile disease, with the manifestations of mild edema of limbs, or low fever, flushed complexion, feverish palms and soles, dry mouth and throat, mental fatigue, deep red tongue with a little fur, feeble and thready or knotted and intermittent pulse. It is suitable to nourish and tonify the kidney yin and promote diuresis simultaneously. The prescription used is Zuogui Pill with additional Fuling (*Poria*) and Zexie (*Rhizoma Alismatis*), or the modified Fumai Decoction (Decoction of Prepared *Licorice*) with large dosage of Gancao (*Radix Glycyrrhizae*).

8.1.3.2 Rehabilitation methods

8.1.3.2.1 Sports

Proper sports activities promote qi flow and blood circulation and relief of edema. The patients may take a walk, jog and practice qigong and Taijiquan.

8.1.3.2.2 Acumox and massage

Acumox: Select Shuifen (CV 9), Qihai (CV 6), Sanjiaoshu (BL 22), Zusanli (ST 36) and Yinlingquan (SP

9) for accumox. In the case of yang syndrome with dampness and heat, add Feishu (BL 13) and Hegu (LI 4); in the case of yin syndrome with deficiency and cold, add Pishu (BL 20) and Shenshu (BL 23), with the reinforcing method and moxibustion with the warming needle; in the case of edema due to qi stagnation, add Zhongwan (CV 12) and Tianshu (ST 25), with the reducing method and moxibustion; in the case of edema due to yin deficiency, add Xuehai (SP 10) and Sanyinjiao (SP 6), with the uniform reinforcing-reducing method.

Massage: Massage the underbelly clockwise. Meanwhile, press and knead Zhongwan (CV 12), Qihai (CV 6) and Guanyuan (CV 4). In the case of dampness and heat, press and knead Sanyinjiao (SP 6), Yinlingquan (SP 9) and Pangguangshu (BL 28); in the case of splenic asthenia, press and rub Weishu (BL 21) and Pishu (BL 20); in the case of renal asthenia, push and rub Shenshu (BL 23) and Mingmen (GV 4); in the case of yin deficiency, press and knead Xuehai (SP 10), Sanyinjiao (SP 6) and Zusanli (ST 36). The manipulations should be gentle, slow and mild.

8.1.3.2.3 Dietary therapy

In the case of edema due to dampness and heat, select Maogen Chidou Gruel (Gruel of *Radix Rubi Parvifolii* and *Semen Phaseoli*); in the case of edema due to splenorenal asthenia, select Fuling Yiyiren Gruel (Gruel of *Poria* and *Semen Coicis*); in the case of edema due to qi stagnation, select Jupi Gruel (Gruel of *Pericarpium Citri Reticulatae*); in the case of edema due to yin deficiency, select Yali Pear Gruel.

TCM has always emphasized that the patients with edema should abstain from salt. They may be given the low salt diet or the salt-free diet. The patients with edema have the weak splenogastric function in transportation

湿热阳证者,加肺俞、合谷;虚寒阴证者,加脾俞、肾俞,针刺用补法,并可温灸;气滞肿胀者,加中脘、天枢,针刺用泻法,可灸;阴亏浮肿者,加血海、三阴交,用平补平泻法。

推拿 以顺时针方向摩小腹,并按揉中脘、气海、关元等穴。湿热者,加按、揉三阴交、阴陵泉、膀胱俞;脾虚者,按擦胃俞、脾俞;肾虚者,推擦肾俞、命门;阴亏者,按、揉血海、三阴交、足三里。手法要轻柔、缓和。

3. 食疗

湿热水肿者,可选用茅根赤豆粥。脾肾虚肿者,可选用茯苓薏苡仁粥。气滞肿胀者,可选用橘皮粥。阴虚浮肿者,可选用鸭粥。

中医历来强调水肿忌盐,可给予低盐或无盐饮食。浮肿患者脾胃运化无力,故要求饮食宜细软而清淡,营养丰富

and transformation. Therefore, their diet should be fine, soft, bland, nutritious and readily digestible. They should abstain from pungent, fat and sweet foods and drink. They should avoid craputence completely, particularly at the time of recovery.

8.1.3.2.4 Nursing in daily life

The patients with edema should attach importance to rest and abstinence from sexual life so as to prevent the relapse of edema due to overstrain. Common cold may aggravate the illness. Accordingly, they should pay attention to climatic changes to prevent repeated attack by exogenous pathogenic factors. Simultaneously, they should keep the skin clean and avoid skin injury. Otherwise, it may cause infection easily and the resultant deterioration. However, the patients with edema are not advisable to take more showers in order to prevent the internal invasion by water and dampness from influencing the removal of edema.

8.1.4 Hypodynamia

Hypodynamia, a disease of weakness, refers to physical and mental tiredness as well as short breath with concurrent low fever, sweat, vexation, thirst, poor appetite, anorexia, red tongue with a little fur, feeble and rapid pulse.

8.1.4.1 Syndrome differentiation and treatment

8.1.4.1.1 Impairment of both qi and yin

It manifests lingering residual heat, emaciation, short breath, mental fatigue, anorexia, nausea with the inclination to vomiting, or concurrent low fever, vexation, thirst, dark urine, constipation, red tongue with yellowish and scanty fur, thready and rapid pulse. It is advisable to supplement qi, nourish yin and clear away the

而易于消化。忌食辛辣、醇酒、肥甘之品，尤其在康复好转之际，切忌暴饮暴食。

4. 起居护理

浮肿患者要注意休息，戒房事，以防劳复。感冒可使病情加重，故应注意寒温变化，以防再感外邪。同时要保持皮肤清洁，避免皮肤破损，否则容易引起感染，发生变证。但水肿患者一般不宜多沐浴，以免水湿内侵，影响水肿消退。

四、乏力

乏力是指身体无力，精神困倦，少气不足以息的一种虚弱不足的病证，可伴见低热汗出，心烦口渴，食少纳呆，舌红苔少，脉虚数等症。

【辨证施治】

1. 气阴两伤，余热未清

形体消瘦，少气神疲，食少纳呆，呕恶欲吐，或伴有低热，心烦口渴，尿黄便干，舌红苔少而黄，脉细数。宜益气养阴，兼清余热。竹叶石膏汤加减。若为暑伤气津而见低热

residual heat simultaneously. The prescription used is the modified Zhuye Shigao Decoction (Decoction of Lophatherum and Gypsum). The modified Wang's Qingshu Yiqi Decoction (Wang's Summer-heat-Removing and Qi-Supplementing Decoction) is advisable for the patients with low fever and profuse sweat due to summer-heat consuming qi and body fluids.

8.1.4.1.2　Asthenia of the spleen and stomach

It manifests emaciation, sallow complexion, short breath with disinclination to speak, poor appetite, epigastric oppression, anorexia, flaccidity of limbs, loose stool, pale and tender tongue, feeble and weak pulse. It is suitable to strengthen the spleen and supplement qi. The prescription used is Shenling Baizhu Powder (Powder of Ginseng, Poria and Bighead Atractylodes). In the case of concurrent thoracic and epigastric fullness and oppression due to food retention, add Shenqu (*Massa Fermentata Medicinalis*), Shanzha (*Fructus Crataegi*), Maiya (*Fructus Hordei Germinatus*) and Houpo (*Cortex Magnoliae Officinalis*) accordingly; in the case of concurrent cold body with aversion to cold belonging to yang deficiency of the spleen and stomach, it is suitable to select Huangqi Jianzhong Decoction (Decoction of Astragalus for Tonifying Middle Energizer).

8.1.4.1.3　Deficiency of qi and blood

It manifests emaciation, short breath, hypodynamia, lustreless complexion, wrinkly skin, light-headedness, palpitation, insomnia, or sluggish expression, poor sleep, pale tongue with thin fur, thready and weak pulse. It is advisable to supplement qi and nourish blood. The prescription used is Renshen Yangrong Decoction (Ginseng Nutrition Decoction) with Zhimu (*Rhizoma Anemarrhenae*) removed and Huangjing (*Rhizoma Polygonati*) and Gouqizi (*Fructus Lycii*) added. In the case of dull ex-

多汗者，宜用王氏清暑益气汤加减。

2. 脾胃虚弱

形体消瘦，面色萎黄，少气懒言，食欲不振，脘闷纳呆，肢软便溏，舌淡嫩，脉虚弱。宜健脾益气。参苓白术散加减。兼有饮食不消而胸脘满闷者，可酌加神曲、山楂、麦芽、厚朴等；若兼见形寒畏冷，证属脾胃阳虚者，宜用黄芪建中汤。

3. 气血亏虚

身体瘦削，少气无力，面色不华，皮肤皱缩，头晕目眩，心悸失眠，甚或神志呆滞，似寐非寐，舌淡苔薄，脉细弱。宜补气养血。人参养营汤去知母，加黄精、枸杞子等。兼见神志呆滞者，可酌加菖蒲、木香等芳香醒神之品，也可服用集灵膏。

pression, add aromatic mind-refreshing drugs like Changpu (*Rhizoma Acori Graminei*) and Muxiang (*Radix Aucklandiae*) accordingly, or take Jiling Paste.

8.1.4.2 Rehabilitation methods

8.1.4.2.1 Regulating emotions and recreation therapy

Participate in recreational activities like appreciating music, playing a musical instrument, practicing calligraphy and painting, cultivating flowers and raising birds.

8.1.4.2.2 Acumox and massage

Acumox: Rectifying deficiency is mainly advisable in acumox. In the case of impairment of both qi and yin, and lingering residual heat, it is advisable to regulate the lung and stomach, nourish yin and clear away heat by selecting Feishu (BL 13), Weishu (BL 21), Qihai (CV 6) and Zusanli (ST 36); in the case of deficiency of qi and blood as well as asthenia of the spleen and stomach, it is mainly advisable to strengthen both the spleen and stomach by selecting Pishu (BL 20), Zusanli (ST 36), Zhongwan (CV 12) and Qihai (CV 6). Puncturing with the filiform needle is applied in all the above cases in general, with the reinforcing method and moxibustion; in the case of lingering residual heat, the uniform reinforcing-reducing method is applied.

Massage: Moreover, health care massage is mainly adopted, the acupoints are selected in the light of acupoint selection in acumox.

8.1.4.2.3 Dietary therapy

In the case of impairment of both qi and body fluids as well as lingering residual heat, select Zhuye Gruel (Gruel of *Folium Phyllostachydis Nigrae*); in the case of splenogastric asthenia, select Shenling Gruel (Gruel of *Radix Ginseng* and *Poria*); in the case of deficiency of qi and blood, select Buxu Zhengqi Gruel (Deficiency-Rectifying

【康复方法】

1. 调节情志和娱乐疗法

参加娱乐活动，诸如欣赏音乐、琴棋书画、种花养鸟等。

2. 针灸、推拿疗法

针灸 宜以补虚为主。气阴两伤、余热未清证，从调理肺胃、养阴清热入手，取肺俞、胃俞、气海、足三里等穴；气血亏虚证和脾胃虚弱证，均以培补脾胃为主，取脾俞、足三里、中脘、气海等穴。一般均以毫针刺，用补法，并灸；余热未清者用平补平泻法。

推拿 以保健按摩法为主。参照针灸取穴点揉穴位。

3. 食疗

气液两伤、余热未清证，可选用竹叶粥。脾胃虚弱证，可选用参苓粥。气血亏虚证，可选用补虚正气粥。

and Qi-Strengthening Gruel).

8.1.5 Polyhidrosis

Polyhidrosis refers to excessive perspiration of the body. It can be divided into spontaneous sweating, night sweat, sweating in shock, chilly sweating, yellowish sweating, etc. Polyhidrosis after recovery from a disease mainly belongs to spontaneous sweating and night sweat. Excessive and prolonged sweating inevitably consumes yin, yang, qi and blood of the human body.

8.1.5.1 Syndrome differentiation and treatment

8.1.5.1.1 Unconsolidation due to qi deficiency

It manifests spontaneous sweating, aversion to cold aggravated by slight strain, susceptibility to common cold, tiredness, hypodynamia, lustreless complexion, pale tongue with white and thin fur and weak pulse. It is advisable to supplement qi and consolidate the superficial body resistance. The prescription used is the modified Yupingfeng Powder (Jade Screen Powder). In the case of profuse sweat, add Fuxiaomai (*Fructus Fritici Levis*), Nuodaogen (*Radix Oryzae Glutinosae*) and Muli (*Concha Ostreae*); in the case of severe qi deficiency, add Dangshen (*Radix Codonopsis Pilosulae*), Huangjing (*Rhizoma Polygonati*) and Zhigancao (*Radix Glycyrrhizae Praeparata*); in the case of cold body and aversion to cold due to concurrent yang deficiency, Huangqi Jianzhong Decoction (Decoction of Astragalus for Tonifying Middle Energizer) is used in combination with Yupingfeng Powder (Jade Screen Powder); in the case of concurrent general aching pain, alternate cold and fever and slow pulse pertaining to incoordination between nutrient qi and defensive qi or with concurrent slight exopathy, the modified Guizhi Decoction (Cinnamon Twig Decoction) is

五、多汗

多汗，即身体出汗过多，可分为自汗、盗汗、脱汗、战汗、黄汗等。病后多汗则以自汗、盗汗为主。若汗出过多过久，势必进一步耗损人体的阴阳气血。

【辨证施治】

1. 气虚不固

自汗恶风，稍劳尤甚，易于感冒，体倦乏力，面色少华，舌淡苔薄白，脉弱。宜益气固表。玉屏风散加味。汗出多者，加浮小麦、糯稻根、牡蛎；气虚甚者，加党参、黄精、炙甘草；兼阳虚而形寒畏冷者，可与黄芪建中汤合用；兼见周身酸楚，时寒时热，脉缓，证属营卫不和或微兼外感，则宜用桂枝汤加减调和营卫。

used to regulate nutrient qi and defensive qi.

8.1.5.1.2 Internal heat due to yin deficiency

It manifests night sweat, dysphoria with less sleep, feverish chest, palms and soles, or osteopyrexia and hectic fever, flushing of zygomatic region, dry mouth, red tongue with a little fur, thready and rapid pulse. It is suitable to nourish yin and remove fire. The prescription used is the modified Liuhuang Decoction. In the case of profuse sweat, add Muli (*Concha Ostreae*), Fuxiaomai (*Fructus Tritici Levis*) and Noudaogen (*Radix Oryzae Glutinosae*); in the case of severe hectic fever, add Qinjiao (*Radix Gentianae Macrophyllae*), Yinchaihu (*Radix Stellariae*) and Baiwei (*Radix Cynanchi Atrati*); in the case of yin deficiency of the lung and kidney with less fire and heat, it is advisable to use the modified Maiwei Dihuang Bolus (Eight-Immortal Longevity Bolus).

8.1.5.1.3 Deficiency of both yin and yang

It manifests spontaneous sweating, endless night sweat, emaciation, weakness of limbs, cold body, aversion to cold, palpitation with less sleep, pale complexion with flushing of cheeks, feverish palms and soles, reddish tongue, thready and weak pulse. It is advisable to warm yang and strengthen yin. The prescription used is the modified Biejia Powder (Powder of *Carapax Trionycis*). In the case of deficiency of qi and blood with concurrent short breath and palpitation, use Renshen Yangrong Decoction (Gingseng Nutrition Decoction); in the case of deficiency of both qi and yin with concurrent dysphoria, fever and short breath, select Xiyangshen (*Radix Panacis Quinguefolii*), Shengdihuang (*Radix Rehmanniae*), Maimendong (*Radix Ophiopogonis*), Huanglian (*Rhizoma Coptidis*), Gancao (*Radix Glycyrrhizae*), Xiaomai (*Fructus Trtiici Levis*), Baihe (*Bulbus Lilii*), Zhuye (*Folium Phyllistachydis Nigrae*), Lianzixin (*Plumula*

2. 阴虚内热

夜寐盗汗,虚烦少眠,五心烦热,或骨蒸潮热,颧红口干,舌红少苔,脉细数。宜滋阴降火。当归六黄汤加减。汗出多者,加牡蛎、浮小麦、糯稻根;潮热甚者,加秦艽、银柴胡、白薇;证属肺肾阴虚,而火热不甚者,则宜用麦味地黄丸加减。

3. 阴阳两虚

自汗、盗汗不止,身体消瘦,四肢无力,形寒畏冷,心悸少眠,面白颧红,手足心热,舌质淡红,脉细弱。宜温阳益阴。鳖甲散加减。证属气血两虚而兼少气惊悸者,可用人参养荣汤;若属气阴两虚而兼烦热气短者,可用西洋参、生地黄、麦门冬、黄连、甘草、小麦、百合、竹叶、莲子心之类。

Nelumbinis) and the like.

8.1.5.2 Rehabilitation methods

8.1.5.2.1 Regulating emotions and recreation therapy

Avoid emotional anxiety, impetuosity and excitement to remain a sound and stable mental state. Besides, participate in recreational activities like balls and appreciating music under the guidance of a doctor. When dancing, select the social dance with slow rhythm; when appreciating music, select lively music.

8.1.5.2.2 Acumox and massage

Acumox: In the case of spontaneous sweating, select Daheng (SP 15), Hegu (LI 4), Yuji (LU 10), Fuliu (KI 7) and Neiting (ST 44); in the case of night sweat, Jianshi (PC 5), Hegu (LI 4), Yuji (LU 10), Fuliu (KI 7) and Yinxi (HT 6). Generally, use the reinforcing method with additional moxibustion; in the case of internal heat due to yin deficiency, adopt the uniform reinforcing-reducing method.

Massage: Adopt the methods of health care massage and digitally knead acupoints in the light of acupoint selection in acupuncture.

8.1.5.2.3 Dietary therapy

In the case of unconsolidation due to qi deficiency, select Huangqi Dazao Gruel (Gruel of *Radix Astragali seu Hedysari* and *Fructus Ziziphi Jujubae*); in the case of internal heat due to yin deficiency, select Dihuang Zaoren Gruel (Gruel of *Radix Rehmanniae* and *Semen Ziziphi Jujubae*); in the case of deficiency of both yin and yang, select Gouqi Gruel (Gruel of *Fructus Lycii*); in the case of spontaneous sweating or night sweat, select wheat gruel.

8.1.5.2.4 External therapy

In the case of night sweat, grind Wubeizi (*Galla*

【康复方法】

1. 调节情志和娱乐疗法

避免情绪紧张、急躁和激动,以保持良好稳定的精神状态,并指导其参加娱乐活动,如舞会、欣赏音乐等。跳舞宜选择慢节奏的交谊舞,音乐宜选择轻松欢快的乐曲。

2. 针灸、推拿疗法

针灸 自汗者,可取大横、合谷、鱼际、复溜、内庭等穴;盗汗者,可取间使、合谷、鱼际、复溜、阴郄等穴。一般针刺用补法,并可加灸,阴虚内热者用平补平泻法。

推拿 可采用保健按摩法,并参照针灸取穴点揉穴位。

3. 食疗

气虚不固证,可选用黄芪大枣粥。阴虚内热证,可选用地黄枣仁粥。阴阳两虚证,可选用枸杞粥。自汗或盗汗,均可食用小麦粥。

4. 外治

盗汗,可用五倍子研末,

Chinensis) into powder and mix the powder with vinegar to make cake-shaped paste. Then, apply the drug on the navel and fix it with gauze externally. In the case of spontaneous sweating, grind Heshouwu (*Radix Polygoni Mulfiflori*) into powder and mix the powder with water. Then, apply the drug on the navel.

8.1.6 Insomnia

Insomnia refers to the disease marked by the constant inability to have normal sleep, or difficulty in falling asleep, even lying awake all night in severe cases. Insomnia after recovery mostly results from deficiency of yin and body fluids, or asthenia of the heart and spleen, or residual heat intermingled with phlegm disturbing the mind.

8.1.6.1 Syndrome differentiation and treatment

8.1.6.1.1 Asthenia of the heart and spleen

In manifests dream-disturbed sleep, light sleep, palpitation, susceptibility to fright, amnesia, light-headedness, tiredness of limbs, mental fatigue, poor appetite, lustreless complexion, pale tongue with thin fur, thready and week pulse. It is suitable to tonify the heart, strengthen the spleen, nourish blood and tranquilize the mind. The prescription used is the modified Guipi Decoction (Decoction for Invigorating the Spleen and Nourishing the Heart). In the case of the cardiac blood deficiency, add Shudihuang (*Radix Rehmanniae Preaparata*), Baishaoyao (*Radix Paeoniae Alba*) and Ejiao (*Colla Corii Asini*); in the case of light sleep, add Wuweizi (*Fructus Schisandrae*), Baiziren (*Semen Biotae*), Hehuanhua (*Flos Albiziae*), Yejiaoteng (*Caulis et Folium Polygoni Multiflori*), Longgu (*Os Draconis*) and Muli (*Concha Ostreae*) accordingly.

8.1.6.1.2 Excessive fire due to yin deficiency

In manifests dysphoria, sleeplessness, palpitation, dizziness, tinnitus, amnesia, soreness of the waist, nocturnal emission, dysphoria with feverish chest, palms and soles, dry mouth, red tongue with a little fur or cracked fur, thready and rapid pulse. It is suitable to nourish yin and remove fire, nourish the heart and tranquilize the mind. The prescription used is the modified Huanglian Ejiao Decoction (Decoction of *Rhizoma Coptidis* and *Colla Corii Asini*), or Zhusha Anshen Bolus (Sedative Bouls of Cinnabaris). In the case of feverish and reddish complexion, vertigo, tinnitus, add Muli (*Concha Ostreae*), add Guiban (*Plastrum Testudinis*) and Cishi (*Magnetitum*).

8.1.6.1.3 Residual heat intermingled with phlegm

It manifests sleeplessness, headache, heavy sensation of the head, or light sleep, profuse sputum, chest tightness, aversion to food, eructation, acid regurgitation, nausea, vexation, bitter taste, dizziness, yellowish and greasy fur, slippery and rapid pulse. It is advisable to clear away heat, resolve phlegm, regulate the middle energizer and tranquilize the mind. The prescription used is Huanglian Wendan Decoction (Decoction of *Rhizoma Coptidis* for Clearing away Gallbladder Heat) with additional Shanzhi (*Radix Pittospori*). In the case of palpitation and restlessness, add Zhenzhumu (*Concha Margaritifera Uista*), Longchi (*Dens Draconis*) and Cishi (*Magnetitum*); in the case of stagnation of phlegm and food, incoordination between the spleen and stomach, this prescription is used in combination with Banxia Shumi Decoction (Decoction of *Rhizoma Pinelliae* and *Husked Sorghum*) with additional Shenqu (*Massa Fermentata Medicinalis*), Shanzha (*Fructus Crataegi*) and Laifuzi

2. 阴虚火旺

心烦不寐,心悸不安,头晕耳鸣,健忘,腰酸梦遗,五心烦热,口干津少,舌红苔少或中有裂纹,脉细数。宜滋阴降火,养心安神。黄连阿胶汤或朱砂安神丸加减。若见面热微红、眩晕耳鸣,可加牡蛎、龟版、磁石等。

3. 余热夹痰

不寐,头痛或头重,或时寐时醒,痰多胸闷,恶食嗳气,吞酸恶心,心烦口苦,目眩,苔腻而黄,脉滑数。宜清热化痰,和中安神。黄连温胆汤加山栀。心悸惊惕不安者,可加珍珠母、龙齿、磁石;痰食阻滞,胃中不和者,可合半夏秫米汤加神曲、山楂、莱菔子等;若证属余热扰心者,则宜用栀子乌梅汤加减。

(*Semen Raphani*); in the case of residual heat disturbing the heart, use the modified Zhizi Wumei Decoction (Decoction of *Fructus Gardeniae* and *Fructus Mume*).

8.1.6.2 Rehabilitation methods
8.1.6.2.1 Regulating emotions

Insomnia is a psychosomatic disease. Regulating emotions can achieve better therapeutic effects. The doctor may remove the patient's psychogenic stimulation by means of diverting his emotions, clearing up his suspicion, doing as he wishes, pleasing him and suggestion. Besides, the doctor may use hypnotherapy as well.

8.1.6.2.2 Recreation therapy

Recreation may regulate the mind, mould the temperament and is the effective therapy for insomnia. For instance, as far as musical therapy is concerned, the doctor can select the gentle and sweet, slow and light music.

8.1.6.2.3 Physical training and bathing

The patient may have the endurance training events such as running, ball games and setting-up exercises to radio music according to the differences of the patient's psychological features, musical accomplishment and personality. Besides, the patient may practice Taijiquan. When practicing it, tranquilize and concentrate the mind and seek for tranquility from activity. Practice it once or twice a day, 20 minutes each time. It is better to practice it until the body is tired before bed time.

Adopt the hot spring bath or lukewarm bath once a day, 30 minutes each time. In the case of good constitution, the patient may select the cold water bath as well. The patient with severe insomnia may take an additional bath before bed time.

【康复方法】
1. 调节情志

失眠是一种心身疾病，用调节情志法进行康复，有较好疗效。可根据患者的心理状态，通过移情、释疑、顺意、怡悦、暗示等方式，消除其心因性刺激。亦可采用催眠疗法。

2. 娱乐疗法

娱乐可调摄心理，陶冶情志，为失眠康复的有效方法，如音乐疗法，可根据患者的心理特点、音乐修养和个性差异等，选用情调柔绵婉转、旋律缓慢轻悠的乐曲。

3. 体育和沐浴疗法

可进行跑步、球类、广播操、游泳等耐力性锻炼，亦可练简化太极拳，练拳时要求心静神敛，动中求静。每日练1～2次，每次约20分钟，最好在临睡前练习，使形体稍感劳累为佳。

采用温泉或温水沐浴，每日1次，每次约30分钟。体质较好者，也可选用冷水浴。失眠严重者，睡前可加浴1次。

8.1.6.2.4 Acumox and massage

Acumox: Select Shenmen (HT 7), Sanyinjiao (SP 6) and Neiguan (PC 6) in acumox. In the case of asthenia of both the heart and spleen, add Xinshu (BL 15), Pishu (BL 20) and Jueyinshu (BL 14), with the reducing method and additional moxibustion; in the case of excessive fire due to yin deficiency, add Ganshu (BL 18), Jianshi (PC 5), Taichong (LR 3) and Taixi (KI 3), with the uniform reinforcing-reducing method; in the case of residual heat intermingled with phlegm, add Feishu (BL 13), Fenglong (ST 40) and Chize (LU 5), with the uniform reinforcing-reducing method.

Massage: After digitally pressing Yintang (EX - HN 3) for half a minute, wipe the part from the supercilliary arch to Taiyang (EX - HN 5) to and fro for five to six times; press the part around the orbit, digitally press Ermen (TE 21), Tinghui (GB 2) and Yifeng (TE 17), knead the anterior ear and posterior ear for three to four times and wipe the forehead for ten times; digitally press Baihui (GV 20) and knead the head for four to five times, press and grasp Fengchi (GB 20) and the bilateral Jianjing (GB 21) acupoints. In the case of asthenia of the heart and spleen, press and knead Xinshu (BL 15), Weishu (BL 21) and Ganshu (BL 18); in the case of excessive fire due to yin deficiency, horizontally rub Shenshu (BL 23) and Mingmen (GV 4) until the acupoints are completely warm before rubbing the bilateral Yongquan (KI 1) acupoints; in the case of residual heat intermingled with phlegm, press Zhongwan (CV 12), Zusanli (ST 36) and Fenglong (ST 40).

8.1.6.2.5 Dietary therapy

In the case of asthenia of the heart and spleen, select Suanzaoren Gruel (Gruel of *Semen Ziziphi Spinosae*); in the case of excessive fire due to yin deficiency, select

4. 针灸、推拿疗法

针灸 取神门、三阴交、内关等穴。心脾两虚证，加心俞、脾俞、厥阴俞，针用补法，并可灸；阴虚火旺证，加肝俞、间使、太冲、太溪，针用平补平泻法；余热夹痰证，加肺俞、丰隆、尺泽，针用平补平泻法。

推拿 先点按印堂穴半分钟后，用抹法沿眉弓至太阳穴往返5～6次；按压眼眶周围，点压耳门、听会、翳风穴，揉耳前、耳后3～4次，抹前额10遍；点按百会，揉头部4～5遍，按拿风池穴、两侧肩井。心脾两虚，可按揉心俞、胃俞、肝俞；阴虚火旺，可横擦肾俞、命门穴，以透热为度，再擦两侧涌泉穴；余热夹痰，可按揉中脘、足三里、丰隆穴。

5. 食疗

心脾两虚证，可选用酸枣仁粥。阴虚火旺证，可选用地黄枣仁粥。余热夹痰证，可选

Dihuang Zaoren Gruel (Gruel of *Radix Rehmanniae* and *Semen Ziziphi Spinosae*); in the case of residual heat intermingled with phlegm, select Baihe Xingren Gruel (Gruel of *Bulbus Lilii* and *Semen Armeniacae Amarum*).

8.1.7 Anorexia

8.1.7.1 Syndrome differentiation and treatment

8.1.7.1.1 Deficiency of stomach yin

It manifests loss of appetite, thirst with inclination to drink, red and dry lips, constipation, scanty urine, or nocturnal low fever, reddish complexion, red tongue with a little fur, thready and slightly rapid pulse. It is advisable to nourish yin and regulate the stomach. The prescription used is Yiwei Decoction (Stomach-Benefiting Decoction) or Wuzhi Beverage (Five-juice Drink). In the case of adverse qi flow with the desire for vomiting due to gastric heat, select Zhuye Shigao Decoction (Lophatherum and Gypsum Decoction); in the case of deficiency of qi and yin and concurrent short breath, palpitation and listlessness, select Xue's Shenmai Decoction (Xue's Decoction of *Radix Ginseng* and *Radix Ophiopogonis*).

8.1.7.1.2 Residual dampness and turbidity

It manifests removal of fever, no appetite or anorexia, slight thoracic and epigastric oppression, mild lightheadedness, mental fatigue, thin and greasy fur, soft and slow pulse. It is advisable to remove the residual dampness and turbidity with light-natured and aromatic-flavored drugs. The prescription used is the modified Xue's Wuye Lugen Decoction (Xue's Five-Leaf and Reed Rhizome Decoction).

8.1.7.1.3 Asthenia of the spleen and stomach

It manifests freedom from starvation feeling, loss of appetite, constant abdominal distension after meals, or

用百合杏仁粥。

七、食少

【辨证施治】

1. 胃阴不足

饥不欲食,口渴喜饮,唇红干燥,大便干结,小便短少,或夜间低热,面微赤,舌红苔少,脉细略数。宜养阴和胃。方用益胃汤或五汁饮。胃热甚而气逆欲吐者,可用竹叶石膏汤;气阴两亏而兼气短心悸、精神委顿者,可用薛氏参麦汤。

2. 湿浊未净

身热已退,不思饮食或知饥不食,胸脘稍闷,头目微觉昏蒙,精神困倦,苔薄腻,脉濡缓。宜轻清芳化,涤除余邪。薛氏五叶芦根汤加减。

3. 脾虚胃弱

不知饥饿,不思饮食,食后腹胀不消,或泛泛欲吐,四

inclination to vomiting, lassitude of limbs, loose stool, or edema of limbs in severe cases, pale tongue with white fur, feeble and weak pulse. It is suitable to strengthen the spleen and regulate the middle energizer, regulate qi and remove dampness. The prescription used is Yigong Powder with additional ingredients (Highly Effective Powder with Additional Ingredients) or the modified Shenling Baizhu Powder (Powder of Ginseng, Poria and Bighead Atractylodes). Xiao Jianzhong Decoction (Minor Decoction for Strengthening Middle Energizer) may be used in the case of loss of appetite due to yang deficiency of the spleen and stomach, sallow complexion, feeble and taut pulse.

8.1.7.2 Rehabilitation methods

8.1.7.2.1 Regulating emotions and recreation therapy

Emotional activities are closely related to the splenogastric functions in transportation and transformation, and thus directly affect appetite. Accordingly, encourage the patient to be free from worries and vexation, and remain a cheerful frame of mind and a sanguine disposition. Before taking a meal, do not think of difficult problems and avoid adverse mental stimulation. Besides, stabilize the mood, avoid noises and do not eat while talking during the meal. It is advisable to appreciate music while taking a meal.

8.1.7.2.2 Physical training

Physical training can promote the splenogastric function. In addition to taking a walk, jogging, setting-up exercises and Taijiquan, practice deep abdominal breathing to promote gastrointestinal peristalsis, increase digestive juice and improve appetite.

8.1.7.2.3 Acumox and massage

Acumox: Select Zhongwan (CV 12), Pishu (BL 20), Weishu (BL 21), Zusanli (ST 36) and Rangu (KI 2)

肢乏力，大便溏薄，甚或肢体浮肿，舌淡苔白，脉虚弱。宜健脾和中，理气化湿。加味异功散或参苓白术散加减。若脾胃阳虚而不思饮食，面色萎黄，脉虚弦者，可用小建中汤。

【康复方法】

1. 调节情志和娱乐疗法

情志活动与脾胃运化功能密切相关，可直接影响食欲，故应鼓励病人少忧愁、少烦恼，保持心境的愉快、开朗。就餐前不要思考疑难棘手的问题，接触不良的精神刺激；用餐时要安定情绪，避免噪音，不要边谈边吃。进餐时可用佐餐音乐。

2. 体育疗法

可促进脾胃的功能。除散步、慢跑、体操、太极拳等活动外，还可练习腹式深呼吸，以促进胃肠蠕动，使消化液增多，增强食欲。

3. 针灸、推拿疗法

针灸 可取中脘、脾俞、胃俞、足三里、然谷等穴，针刺

in acumox, with the reinforcing method or the uniform reinforcing-reducing method. In the case of qi deficiency or yang deficiency, add moxibustion.

Massage: Assume the supine position. First, knead the upper abdomen, mainly on Jiuwei (CV 15) and Zhongwan (CV 12). Then, proceed downwards to the lower abdomen, chiefly on the part around the navel as well as Tianshu (ST 25) and Qihai (CV 6). Meanwhile, vibrate Zhongwan (CV 12) and the upper abdomen with the fingers, and rub the two parts clockwise and anticlockwise respectively for 100 times. Next, ask the patient to assume the prone position and massage the bilateral urinary bladder meridians with the gentle rolling manipulation, mainly on the bilateral acupoints of the sixth to the twelfth thoracic vertebrae. Finally, massage Feishu (BL 13), Weishu (BL 21) and Ganshu (BL 18) with the gentle manipulation.

8.1.7.2.4 Dietary therapy

In the case of deficiency of the kidney yin, select Maidong Gruel (Gruel of *Radix Ophiopogonis*); in the case of residual dampness, select Heye Gruel (Gruel of *Folium Nelumbinis*); in the case of asthenia of the spleen and stomach, select Huaishanyao and Biandou Gruel (Gruel of *Rhizoma Dioscoreae* and *Semen Dolichoris*); in the case of yang deficiency of the spleen and stomach, select Shanyao Yangrou Gruel (Gruel of *Rhizoma Dioscoreae* and *Caro Caprae seu Ovis*).

8.1.8 Palpitation due to fright

Palpitation due to fright means that the patient has the subjective symptoms of violent heart beat, fright, even loss of autonomy in severe cases. The disease is mostly caused by consumption of qi and blood, cardiac loss of nourishment after recovery from a disease, or concur-

用补法或平补平泻法,气虚或阳虚者可加灸。

推拿 取仰卧位,先揉上腹部,以鸠尾、中脘为重点,然后循序往下至少腹部,以脐周围及天枢、气海为重点,同时用指振法在中脘穴和掌振法在上腹部振动,再用摩法顺时针和逆时针方向各摩100次。再令患者俯卧位,沿脊柱两侧膀胱经用轻揉的滚法,重点在胸椎6~12两旁腧穴,然后在脾俞、胃俞、肝俞用较轻手法按摩。

4. 食疗

胃阴不足证,可选用麦门冬粥。湿浊未净证,可选用荷叶粥。脾虚胃弱证,可选用怀山药扁豆粥。若脾胃阳虚者,可选用怀山药羊肉粥。

八、惊悸

惊悸,是指患者自觉心中急剧跳动,惊惕不安,甚则不能自主的症状。多因病后气血耗伤,心失所养,或兼痰浊内扰所导致。

rent phlegm disturbing the interior.

8.1.8.1 Syndrome differentiation and treatment

8.1.8.1.1 Qi deficiency of the heart and gallbladder

It manifests palpitation, susceptibility to fright, timidness and overcautiousness, short breath, hypodynamia, low voice, poor and dream-disturbed sleep, pale tongue with thin fur and weak pulse. It is advisable to supplement qi and nourish the heart. The prescription used is the modified Fushen Powder (Powder of *Poria cum Ligno Hospite*). In the case of fright and restlessness due to asthenia of the heart and timidness, add Longchi (*Dens Draconis*), Hupo (*Succinum*), Cishi (*Magnetitum*) and Zhusha (*Cinnabaris*); in the case of deficiency of cardiac qi and yin, this prescription is used in combination with Shengmai Powder (Pulsation-Promoting Powder), or select the modified Wuweizi Decoction (Decoction of *Fructus Schisandrae*); in the case of deficiency of the heart yang and concurrent thoracic oppression, short breath, cold body and limbs, use Guizhi Gancao Longgu Muli Decoction (Decoction of *Ramulus Cinnamomi, Radix Glycyrrhizae, Os Draconis* and *Concha Ostreae*) with additional ingredients.

8.1.8.1.2 Deficiency of yin and blood

It manifests palpitation, insomnia, vertigo, amnesia, fatigue, short breath, dysphoria with smothery sensation, night sweat, lustreless complexion, red tongue with a little fur, thready or knotted and intermittent pulse. It is suitable to nourish and tonify yin and blood. The prescription used is the modified Tianwang Buxin Pill (Cardiotonic Pill). In the case of marked heat manifestations like concurrent restlessness, dry throat and mouth and bitter taste, use Zhusha Anshen Bolus (Sedative Bolus); in the

【辨证施治】

1. 心胆气虚

心悸易惊,胆怯怕事,气短乏力,语言低微,少寐多梦,舌淡苔薄,脉弱。宜益气养心。茯神散加减。心虚胆怯而惊恐不安者,加龙齿、琥珀、磁石、朱砂等;心之气阴亏虚者,可合用生脉散,或用五味子汤加减;心阳不振而兼胸闷气短,形寒肢冷者,则宜用桂枝甘草龙骨牡蛎汤加味。

2. 阴血不足

心悸失眠,眩晕健忘,神疲少气,烦热盗汗,面色不华,舌红少苔,脉细或结代。宜滋养阴血。天王补心丹加减。兼虚烦咽燥、口干口苦等明显热象者,用朱砂安神丸;气血两亏而见心动悸,脉结代者,可用炙甘草汤;心脾两虚而兼食少体倦者,可选用归脾汤或

case of severe palpitation, knotted and intermittent pulse due to deficiency of qi and blood, use Zhigancao Decoction (Decoction of *Radix Glycyrrhizae Praeparata*); in the case of concurrent anorexia and tiredness due to deficiency of both the heart and spleen, use Guipi Decoction (Decoction for Invigorating the Spleen and Nourishing the Heart) or the modified Xiao Jianzhong Decoction (Minor Decoction for Strengthening Middle Energizer).

8.1.8.1.3 Phlegm disturbing the interior

It manifests palpitation due to fright, vexation, restless nocturnal sleep, profuse sputum, nausea, anorexia, or edema of limbs, white and greasy fur, taut and slippery pulse. It is advisable to resolve phlegm and tranquilize the mind. The prescription used is the modified Shiwei Wendan Decoction (Ten-Ingredient Gallbladder-Heat-Clearing Decoction). In the case of concurrent bitter taste, dry mouth, yellowish and greasy fur, slippery and rapid pulse due to phlegm and heat disturbing the interior, use the modified Huanglian Wendan Decoction (Gallbladder-Heat-Clearing Decoction with *Rhizoma Coptidis*).

8.1.8.2 Rehabilitation methods

8.1.8.2.1 Regulating emotions and recreation therapy

Most patients have the psychological disturbances of fright and fear which are induced or aggravated by emotional changes. Therefore, it is of vital importance to regulate emotions.

(1) **Checking one emotion with another** Guide the patient to think about the relevant questions to remove or divert the patient's fear in the light of "checking fear with pensiveness".

(2) **Removing suspicion** Most patients suspect that they suffer from "heart disease". The doctor may rule out the organic cardiac diseases diagnostically, and

小建中汤加减。

3. 痰浊内扰

惊悸烦闷，夜寐不安，痰多泛恶，食少无味，或四肢浮肿，苔白腻，脉弦滑。宜化痰宁心。十味温胆汤加减。若痰热内扰而兼口苦口干、舌苔黄腻、脉滑数者，则宜用黄连温胆汤加减。

【康复方法】

1. 调节情志和娱乐疗法

患者大多存在惊慌和恐惧的心理障碍，每因情志波动所诱发或加重，因而调节情志尤为重要。

（1）情志相胜　按"思胜恐"之意，可引导患者思考有关问题，以解除或分散其恐惧心情。

（2）释疑　患者多怀疑自己患"心脏病"，采用释疑疗法，通过心脏专科的必要检

remove their nervousness and fear psychologically with the affirmative tone by means of removing their suspicion and the necessary examinations of cardiac special department.

(3) **The recreation therapy**　Guide the patient to have recreational activities. The activities like enjoying the sight of scenery with hills and waters, flower and grass, appreciating music, calligraphy and painting, playing a musical instrument, playing chess and attending a ball can make the patient happy, divert his emotions and achieve mental relaxation.

8.1.8.2.2　Physical training

Taking a walk, jogging, setting-up exercises, Wushu (martial arts), five mimic-animal games, Taijiquan, eight-section brocade, etc, are all advisable. But, abstain from sudden excitement or overfatigue so as to avoid increasing the cardiac burden. The amount of exercise is suitable if the heart rate is less than 110 beats per minute, and thoracic tightness, palpitation and short breath are not caused after the training.

8.1.8.2.3　Acumox and massage

Acumox: Select Xinshu (BL 15), Juque (CV 14), Shenmen (HT 7), Neiguan (PC 6) and Ximen (PC 4) in acumox. In the case of qi deficiency of the heart and gallbladder, add Qihai (CV 6), Danshu (BL 19) and Pishu (BL 20); in the case of deficiency of yin and blood, add Pishu (BL 20), Geshu (BL 17) and Zusanli (ST 36); in the case of phlegm disturbing the interior, add Chize (LU 5), Danzhong (CV 17) and Fenglong (ST 40). The uniform reinforcing-reducing method is advisable.

Ear acupuncture: Select the points of Xin, Nao, Ershenmen (MA-TF 1) and Xiaochang (MA-SC 2) in ear acupuncture therapy. Each time, select two or three of these points. Puncture the points gently with the twirling-

查，以肯定的语气加以解释，可从诊断上排除心脏器质性病变，从心理上消除其紧张恐惧的心理。

（3）娱乐　指导患者进行娱乐活动。如观赏山水花草，欣赏音乐书画，弹琴弈棋，参加舞会等，怡情移志，松弛精神。

2. 体育疗法

散步、慢跑、体操、武术、五禽戏、太极拳、八段锦等均为相宜。但应避免情绪突然激动或过分疲劳，以免增加心脏负担。一般以活动后心率不超过110次/分，不引起胸闷、心慌、气短等症状为度。

3. 针灸、推拿疗法

针灸　可取心俞、巨阙、神门、内关、郄门等穴。心胆气虚证，加气海、胆俞、脾俞；阴血不足证，加脾俞、膈俞、足三里；痰浊内扰证，加尺泽、膻中、丰隆。针法宜平补平泻。

耳针　可取心、脑、神门、小肠等，每次选择2～3穴，捻转轻刺激，留针20～30分钟。也可用王不留行子贴压法。

rotating method. Retain the needle for twenty to thirty minutes. Or use the pressing method with Wangbuliuxingzi (*Semen Vaccariae*) applied on these points.

Massage: Health care massage is mainly applied. First, massage the head and face. Then, massage the back, waist and limbs with the soft and relaxing manipulation. Meanwhile, better therapeutic effects may be achieved by the combined use of digitally kneading the acupoints like Neiguan (PC 6), Shenmen (HT 7), Tongli (HT 5) and Danzhong (CV 17) with the gentle, slow and even digital acupoints-pressing manipulation. Besides, massage the chest and precordial region clockwise or from the upper part to the lower part with the palm.

8.1.8.2.4 Dietary therapy

In the case of qi deficiency of the heart and gallbladder, select Cishi Gruel (Gruel of Magnetitum); in the case of deficiency of yin and blood, select Baiziren Gruel (Gruel of *Semen Biotae*); in the case of phlegm disturbing the interior, select Fuling Yiyiren Gruel (Gruel of *Poria* and *Semen Coicis*). The patient may eat heart-tonifying food at ordinary times such as Zhuxin (*Cor Suis*), Dazao (*Fructus Ziziphi Jujubae*) and Lianzi (*Semen Nelumbinis*). However, do not overeat them. Abstain from smoking, drinking, strong tea, pungent, irritating, fatty and sweat foods. The patient with concurrent edema should be given the low salt diet or salt-free diet.

8.1.8.2.5 Nursing in daily life

The living surroundings should be free from various noises and adverse irritations so as to prevent the induced palpitation due to fright.

8.1.9 Constipation

Constipation is caused by deficiency of qi, blood and body fluids as well as internal accumulation of dryness and heat after the recovery from a disease.

8.1.9.1 Syndrome differentiation and treatment

8.1.9.1.1 Intestinal dryness due to deficiency of body fluids

Dry stool, difficult defecation, dry lips and mouth, dry throat, thirst, scanty urine, red tongue with a little fur and without fluid, thready and unsmooth pulse. In the case of concurrent residual dryness and heat, it manifests flushed face, dysphoria, abdominal distension or abdominalgia, dry mouth, foul breath, red tongue with yellowish fur and rapid pulse. It is advisable to nourish body fluids and moisten the intestine. The prescription used is Wuren Pill (Five-Kernel Pill) with additional Shengdihuang (*Radix Rehmanniae*), Xuanshen (*Radix Scrophulariae*) and Maimendong (*Radix Ophiopogonis*). In the case of concurrent enterogastric dryness and heat manifested by abdominal distension or abdominalgia, foul breath and yellowish fur, use the modified Maziren Pill (Hemp Seed Pill).

8.1.9.1.2 Deficiency of qi and blood

Constipation, lustreless complexion, light-headedness, palpitation, or no dry and hard stool, strain in defecation, sweating, short breath, mental fatigue, lassitude of limbs, pale lips and tongue, thin fur, thready and weak pulse. It is advisable to supplement qi, nourish blood, moisten the intestine to promote defecation. The prescription used is Danggui Buxue Decoction (Chinese Angelica Decoction for Replenishing blood) with additional Shengheshouwu (unprepared *Radix Polygoni Multiflori*), Zhike (*Fructus Aurantii*) and Digupi (*Cortex Lycii Radicis*). In the case of marked qi deficiency, use Huangqi Decoction (Decoction of *Radix Astragali seu Hedysari*); in the case of marked blood deficiency, use Runchang

【辨证施治】

1. 津亏肠燥

大便干结,坚硬难排,唇燥口干,咽干欲饮,小便短少,舌红苔少无津,脉细涩。若兼燥热未清,可见面红心烦,腹胀或痛,口干口臭,舌红苔黄,脉数。宜滋液润肠。五仁丸加生地黄、玄参、麦门冬等。若兼肠胃燥热而见腹胀或痛、口臭苔黄者,可用麻子仁丸加减。

2. 气血亏虚

大便秘结,面色无华,头晕目眩,心悸,或大便并不干硬,虽有便意,但临厕努挣乏力,汗出短气,神疲肢倦,唇舌淡,苔薄,脉细弱。宜益气养血、润肠通便。当归补血汤加生何首乌、枳壳、地骨皮等。偏气虚者,用黄芪汤;偏血虚者,用润肠丸。

Pill (Intestine-Moistening Pill).

8.1.9.1.3 Accumulation of cold due to yang deficiency

Possible dry stool, difficult defecation, slight abdominal cold and pain, cold hands and feet, or soreness and cold of waist and spine, pale complexion, clear and profuse urine, pale tongue with white fur, deep and slow pulse. It is advisable to relax the bowels with warm- and moist-natured drugs. The prescription used is the modified Jichuan Decoction, or Banliu Pill or Congrong Runchang Pill (Pill of *Herba Cistanchis* for Moistening the Bowels).

8.1.9.2 Rehabilitation methods
8.1.9.2.1 Physical training

Physical training increases gastrointestinal peristalsis and promotes defecation. Walking with rapid steps and fitness running are more suitable. Do it in the morning every day, fifteen to twenty minutes each time. The distance is determined by personal conditions and the amount of exercise by the fact that mild short breath and sweating appear. After training, take a lukewarm bath or hot hip bath for five to ten minutes. Then, go to number two. Besides, practice the abdominal breathing for thirty to forty minutes each time. It has the actions of massaging the stomach and bowels, and promoting gastrointestinal peristalsis due to the obvious rhythmical upward and downward movements of the diaphragm.

8.1.9.2.2 Acumox and massage

Acumox: Select the Back-shu point, Front Mu-point and Lower-He (sea) point of the large intestine meridian, specifically, Dachangshu (BL 25), Tianshu (ST 25) and Shangjuxu (ST 37) in acumox. In the case of intestinal dryness due to deficiency of body fluids, add Hegu (LI 4) and Quchi (LI 11), with the reducing method or the

3. 阳虚积冷

大便干或不干,排出困难,腹微冷痛,手足欠温,或腰脊酸冷,面色㿠白,小便清长,舌淡苔白,脉沉迟。宜温润通便。济川煎加减,也可用半硫丸或苁蓉润肠丸等。

【康复方法】
1. 体育疗法

可增强胃肠蠕动,促进排便。快步行走及健身跑较为适宜。可在每天早上进行,每次15~20分钟。距离的长短因人而异,以微有气急出汗为宜。运动后作温水浴或温水坐浴5~10分钟,再去解大便。还可以练习深腹式呼吸,每次30~40分钟,因膈肌有节律上下明显移动,可对胃肠起按摩的作用,促进胃肠蠕动。

2. 针灸、推拿疗法

针灸 取大肠经俞、募穴及下合穴,如大肠俞、天枢、上巨虚。津亏肠燥证,加合谷、曲池,针用泻法或平补平泻法;气血亏虚证,加脾俞、胃俞,针用补法;阳虚冷秘证,加

uniform reinforcing-reducing method; in the case of deficiency of qi and blood, add Pishu (BL 20) and Weishu (BL 21), with the reinforcing method; in the case of cold constipation due to yang deficiency, apply moxibustion on Shenque (CV 8) and Qihai (CV 6) additionally. As for the ear acupuncture therapy, select Zhichang (MA - H 2), Dachang (MA - SC 4) and Nao with the moderate or forceful stimulation and the twirling-rotating manipulation. Retain the needle for twenty to thirty minutes.

Massage: First, press and knead Zhongwan (CV12), Tianshu (ST 25) and Guanyuan (CV 4). Then, massage the abdomen clockwise, press and knead Pishu (BL 20), Weishu (BL 21), Shenshu (BL 23) and Zusanli (ST 36). After that, massage Chengshan (BL 57) and Fenglong (ST 40). Simultaneously, press and rub the waist until the part is completely warm for fifteen to twenty minutes each time respectively in the morning and evening.

Besides, self-massage of the abdomen may be applied as follows.

(1) **Pressing with the palm** Assume the supine position and unfasten the trouser belt. Then, flex the knees. After rubbing the palms against each other to make them warm, place the left hand flat on the right side of the lower abdomen and the right hand on the back of the left hand. At this time, push the hands upward to the lower part of the right costal region. Next, proceed to pass the abdomen horizontally along the part above the navel to the left side of the lower abdomen. Knead and press this part deep and slowly. Finally, press the above regions in the opposite direction to the original site. This is one cycle. Repeat the cycle for ten to dozens of times, or press the regions for ten to fifteen minutes.

(2) **Digital pressing** After finishing the above

灸神阙、气海。耳针取直肠下段、大肠、脑，捻转中强刺激，留针20~30分钟。

推拿　先按揉中脘、天枢、关元等穴，然后顺时针方向摩腹，并按揉脾俞、胃俞、肾俞、足三里，推拿承山、丰隆穴，按擦腰部，以透热为度。每次推拿15~20分钟，一般早晚各1次。

也可用腹部自我按摩，主要方法是：

掌按　仰卧松开裤带，屈曲双膝，两掌搓热后，左手平放在右下腹部，右手放在左手背上，向上推至右肋下部，顺着脐上方横过腹部，至左下腹，在该处作深而慢的揉按，然后推到原处即是一圈。次数从10次至数10次或历时10~15分钟。

点按　在完成掌按后，改

pressing with the palm, change the palm into one finger to press digitally and slowly alone the above-mentioned course. Press one point digitally for three to five times with a total duration of five to ten minutes. Massage the abdomen with the even force until mild abdominal soreness and distension or the sound of "cooing, cooing" appear. Practice it once or twice a day. After the massage, shift to the sitting position and pat the sacral part gently with the hand for one minute.

(3) **Pounding-tapping** Bend the upper body forward. Then, clench the fists. Next, pound and tap Zusanli (ST 36) with the fist bottoms until soreness and distension appear locally.

8.1.9.2.3　Diet therapy

In the case of intestinal dryness due to deficiency of body fluids, select Baiziren Gruel (Gruel of Semen Biotae); in the case of deficiency of qi and blood, select Heshouwu Gruel (Gruel of *Radix Polygoli Multiflori*); in the case of cold constipation due to yang deficiency, select Congrong Yangrou Gruel (Gruel of *Herba Cistanchis* and *Caro Caprae seu Ovis*). Eat more vegetables and fruits usually such as spinach, Chinese cabbage, celery, banana and peach to increase the stimulation of plant fiber on intestinal peristalsis; drink more boiled water usually, or light salty boiled water in the morning; abstain from irritating things like pungent food and alcohol, and do not overeat cold, cool and uncooked food, either.

8.1.9.2.4　External therapy

Put the honey suppository, or pig's bile enema, or glycerin suppository into the anus to relax the bowels.

8.1.10　Diarrhea

Diarrhea after the recovery from a disease is mostly chronic and of repeated recurrence.

8.1.10.1 Syndrome differentiation and treatment

8.1.10.1.1 Asthenia of the spleen and stomach

It manifests loose stool with undigested food, increased frequency of defecation in the case of ingestion of slight greasy food, poor appetite, epigastric and abdominal distension and oppression, sallow complexion, lassitude, hypodynamia, pale tongue with white fur, thready and weak pulse. It is advisable to strengthen the spleen and stomach. The prescription used is the modified Shenling Baizhu Powder (Powder of Ginseng, Poria and Bighead Atractylodes). In the case of concurrent food stagnation, add Shenqu (*Massa Fermentata Medicinalis*), Maiya (*Fructus Hordei Germinatus*) and Shanzha (*Fructus Crataegi*); in the case of splenogastric yang deficiency, complicated by abdominal cold and pain, cold hands and feet, use Fuzi Lizhong Decoction (Decoction of *Radix Aconiti* for Regulating Middle Energizer) with additional ingredients; in the case of lingering chronic diarrhea, sunken qi of the middle energizer and concurrent proctoptosis, use Buzhong Yiqi Decoction (Decoction for Reinforcing Middle Energizer and Replenishing Qi).

8.1.10.1.2 Residual dampness and heat

It manifests diarrhea accompanied by abdominalgia, simultaneous onset of pain and diarrhea with scanty amount of stool and urgent defecation, perianal calor aggravated by depression and anger with concurrent thoracic and hypochondriac distension and tightness, eructation, poor appetite, yellowish and thin fur, taut, thready and slightly rapid pulse. It is advisable to eliminate the residual pathogenic factors, strengthen the spleen and check the liver. The prescription used is the combined application of Gegen Qinlian Decoction (Decoction of Pueraria, Scutellaria and Coptis) with Tongxie Yaofang Prescription (Im-

【辨证施治】

1. 脾胃虚弱

大便时溏时泻,水谷不化,稍进油腻之物,则大便次数增多,饮食减少,脘腹胀闷不舒,面色萎黄,体倦乏力,舌淡苔白,脉细弱。宜健脾益胃。参苓白术散加减。夹食滞者,加神曲、麦芽、山楂;脾胃阳虚而兼腹中冷痛、手足不温者,宜用附子理中汤加味;久泻不愈,中气下陷,而兼有脱肛者,用补中益气汤。

2. 湿热未尽

泄泻伴腹痛,痛时即泻,量少而急,肛门灼热,或每因情志郁怒而增剧,可并见胸胁胀闷不舒,嗳气食少,苔薄黄,脉弦细略数。宜清解余邪而扶土抑木。葛根芩连汤合痛泻要方,可加茯苓、木香等。兼胃阴虚而舌尖红无苔,或中心有斑剥,加怀山药、玉竹、石斛。

portant Prescription for Diarrhea with Pain). Fuling (*Poria*) and Muxiang (*Radix Aucklandiae*) may be added. In the case of red tongue tip without fur due to concurrent gastric yin deficiency, add Huaishanyao (*Rhizoma Dioscoreae*), Yuzhu (*Rhizoma Polygonati Odorati*) and Shihu (*Herba Dendrobii*).

8.1.10.1.3 Deficiency of the kidney yang

It manifests occasional diarrhea with undigested food, abdominal cold and pain relieved by warming and pressing, or diarrhea immediately after abdominalgia and borborygmus before dawn relieved by defecation, cold body and limbs, soreness and flaccidity of the waist and knees, pale tongue with white fur, deep and thready pulse. It is advisable to warm and strengthen the spleen and kidney, stop diarrhea with astringents. The prescription used is Sishen Pill (Pill of Four Miraculous Drugs) with additional ingredients. Besides, Fuzi (*Radix Aconiti Praeparata*) and Paojiang (baked ginger) may be accordingly added. In the case of old age and weak constitution, chronic diarrhea and sunken qi of the middle energizer, add Renshen (*Radix Ginseng*), Huangqi (*Radix Astragali seu Hedysari*) and Baizhu (*Rhizoma Atractylodis Macrocephalae*), or the prescription is used in combination with Taohua Decoction (Pink Decoction).

8.1.10.2 Rehabilitation methods

8.1.10.2.1 Regulating emotions and recreation therapy

The disease is mostly due to asthenia of the spleen and dysfunctional activities of qi which cause the abnormal emotional changes like melancholy and anxiety. Regulating emotions should be adopted to regulate the functions of the spleen and stomach and promote rehabilitation. The doctor can not only adopt the methods of straightening out the patient, checking one emotion with another, but also

3. 肾阳虚衰

泄泻时发时止,完谷不化,腹中冷痛,喜温喜按,或黎明前腹痛肠鸣即泻,泻后则安,形寒肢冷,腰膝酸软,舌淡苔白,脉沉细。宜温补脾肾,固涩止泻。四神丸加味,可酌加附子、炮姜。若年老体衰,久泻不止,中气下陷,宜加人参、黄芪、白术,或合桃花汤。

【康复方法】

1. 调节情志和娱乐疗法

本证多为脾虚,气机不畅,使人产生忧思和焦虑的异常情志,应通过调节情志,以调整脾胃功能,促进康复。既可采用说理开导、情志相胜等方法舒畅患者情志,也可指导其参加娱乐活动,如听音乐、

guide him to take part in recreational activities such as listening to music, appreciating calligraphy and painting and playing a musical instrument and chess.

8.1.10.2.2 Physical training

The movements like taking a walk, jogging, doing setting-up exercises to radio music and practicing Taijiquan can strengthen constitution, promote the recovery of the splenogastric functions. Besides, the patient may take a sun bath locally to solarize the abdomen.

8.1.10.2.3 Acumox and massage

Acumox: Select Pishu (BL 20), Zhongwan (CV 12), Zhangmen (LR 13), Tianshu (ST 25) and Zusanli (ST 36). In the case of deficiency of the kidney yang, add Mingmen (GV 4) and Guanyuan (CV 4), with the reinforcing method and additional moxibustion; in the case of residual dampness and heat, it is advisable to remove dampness and heat by selecting Zhongwan (CV 12), Tianshu (ST 25), Zusanli (ST 36) and Yinglingquan (SP 9) with the reducing method or the uniform reinforcing-reducing method.

Massage: Select Zhongwan (CV 12), Tianshu (ST 25), Qihai (CV 6) and Guanyuan (CV 4) of the abdomen with the pushing manipulation with one-finger meditation and rubbing manipulation; select Pishu (BL 20), Weishu (BL 21), Shenshu (BL 23), Dachangshu (BL 25) and Changqiang (GV 1) of the back with the rolling, pressing, kneading and scrubbing manipulations. In the case of asthenia of the spleen and stomach, press and knead Zusanli (ST 36) and rub the epigastric region; in the case of deficiency of the kidney yang, horizontally scrub Shenshu (BL 23), Mingmen (GV 4) and Baliao; in the case of residual dampness and heat, press and knead Ganshu (BL 18), Danshu (BL 19), Geshu (BL 17), Taichong (LR 3) and Xingjian (LR 2), and obliquely scrub the bilateral hypochondriac regions additionally.

Self-massage: Persist in kneading the abdomen after getting up in the morning and before bed time in the evening. The method is as follows: Press the region around the navel slowly and forcefully with the alternate hands while rubbing and scrubbing the part for over one hundred circles without the directional limitation. Apply the force increasingly strongly and knead slowly.

8.1.10.2.4 Dietary therapy

In the case of splenogastric asthenia, select Huaishanyao Biandou Gruel (Gruel of *Rhizoma Dioscoreae* and *Semen Dolichoris*); in the case of residual dampness and heat, select Gegenfen Gruel (Gruel of the Powder of *Radix Puerariae*); in the case of deficiency of the kidney yang, select Lianzi Qianshi Gruel (Gruel of *Semen Nelumbinis* and *Semen Euryales*) or Huaishanyao Yangrou Gruel (Gruel of Rhizoma Dioscoreae and *Caro Caprae seu Ovis*). Select the bland, thin, soft and light diet with less lipid and fibre as the principle in daily life. Take meals at the regular time and quantity, and avoid craputence so as to lessen the gastrointestinal burden and promote the absorption of nutrients. Abstain from the uncooked, cold, greasy, thick, hard and unhygienic food and the food which has more dregs and easily produces air.

8.2 Rehabilitation for senile diseases

Senile patients mostly manifest various degrees of deficiency of yin, yang, qi and blood because their visceral functions decline increasingly. The pathological basis of senile diseases is the deficiency of healthy qi, of which the main manifestations include deficiency of qi and blood in the case of asthenia as well as blood stasis and phlegm stagnation in the case of sthenia.

The rehabilitation of senile diseases should concentrate on strengthening healthy qi, with the simultaneous method of eliminating pathogenic factors. Regulating the mind focuses on regulation of emotions and recreational rehabilitation methods; regulating the physique focuses on the rehabilitation methods of traditional sports activities and bathing; acumox, massage, diet and drugs should be applied on the basis of syndrome differentiation; other rehabilitation methods are adopted according to the patient's conditions.

8.2.1 Hypertension

The patients manifest persistent high blood pressure, accompanied by general symptoms like vertigo and headache. Some senile patients have high blood pressure, but are free from marked subjective symptoms. In this case, diagnosis should be made on the basis of the lab examinations.

8.2.1.1 Syndrome differentiation and treatment

8.2.1.1.1 Hyperactive yang due to yin deficiency

It manifests headache, dizziness, tinnitus, blurred vision, insomnia, dream-disturbed sleep, soreness and flaccidity of the waist and knees, occasional flushed face, numbness of limbs, red tongue with thin fur or without fur, taut, thready and rapid pulse. It is advisable to nourish yin and suppress yang. The prescription used is the modified Tianma Gouteng Decoction (Decoction of Gastrodia and Uncaria). As for the traditional Chinese patent medicine, select Zhibai Dihuang Pill (Pill of Anemarrhena, Phellodendrono and Rehmannia).

老年病证的康复医疗当以扶助正气为主，兼以祛邪。调神，以调节情志和娱乐康复法为主；调形，以传统体育、沐浴康复法为主；针灸、推拿、饮食、药物诸法，须在辨证的基础上予以施行；根据病情采用其他康复法。

一、高血压病

患者表现为血压持续增高，伴有眩晕、头痛等全身症状。部分老年人血压高而无明显自觉症状，应结合实验室检查的结果加以诊断。

【辨证施治】

1. 阴虚阳亢

头痛头晕，耳鸣眼花，失眠多梦，腰膝酸软，面时潮红，四肢麻木，舌质红，苔薄或无苔，脉弦细数。宜滋阴潜阳。天麻钩藤饮加减。中成药可选知柏地黄丸。

8.2.1.1.2 Yin deficiency of the liver and kidney

It manifests light-headedness, unsmooth and dry eyes, tinnitus, deafness, lumbar soreness, flaccidity of legs, pain of heels, red tongue without fur, deep, thready and slow pulse. It is suitable to nourish and tonify the liver and kidney. The prescription used is the modified Qiju Dihuang Decoction (Bolus of Six Drugs, *Rehmannia* with *Wolfberry* and *Chrysanthemum*). It is also advisable to select its patent.

8.2.1.1.3 Deficiency of both yin and yang

It manifests light-headedness with the sensation of walking like sitting in a boat, lusterless complexion, occasional fever, palpitation, short breath, soreness and flaccidity of the waist and knees, frequent and profuse nocturnal urine, or edema, pale and tender tongue, deep and thready or tense pulse. It is advisable to regulate and strengthen yin and yang. The prescription used is the modified Erxian Decoction. As for the traditional Chinese patent medicine, select Jinkui Shenqi Pill.

8.2.1.2 Rehabilitation methods
8.2.1.2.1 Regulating emotions

Emotional dissatisfaction, excessive joy and anger often affect the hepatic function of regulating qi and blood, the renal function of nourishment, giving rise to continuous high blood pressure. Therefore, regulating emotions is of great importance for the rehabilitation of the disease.

(1) **Enlightening method** Adopt the methods of interpretation, consolation, encouragement and assurance to lessen and eliminate abnormal emotional reactions and pathogenic emotional factors.

(2) **Behavior therapy** Adopt mostly biofeedback therapies, apply the continuous value-displaying electronic manometer, dermothermometer and electromyograph to

2. 肝肾阴虚

头晕眼花,目涩而干,耳鸣耳聋,腰酸腿软,足跟痛,舌质红,无苔,脉沉细尺弱。宜滋补肝肾。杞菊地黄汤加减。也可选用同名中成药。

3. 阴阳两虚

头目昏花,行走如坐舟船,面白少华,间有烘热,心悸气促,腰膝酸软,夜尿频多,或有水肿,舌质淡嫩,脉沉细或紧。宜调补阴阳。二仙汤加减。中成药可选金匮肾气丸。

【康复方法】
1. 调节情志

情志不遂,喜怒太过,常可影响肝木之疏泄、肾水之涵养而致血压升高不降。因此调节情志在本病康复过程中具有重要的地位。

(1) 说理开导法 采用解释、安慰鼓励、保证等方法,减轻和消除异常情志反应和致病性情志因素。

(2) 行为疗法 多采用生物反馈疗法,使用连续显示数值的电子血压仪、皮肤温度

instruct patients in judging the effect of lowering blood pressure from the readings of these instruments or other visible and audible signals. Besides, train the patients to practice muscular relaxation and normal respiration. Synthesize the results displayed in the instruments to adjust the training methods constantly. Maintain the self control over blood pressure by means of repeated self somatopsychic training.

8.2.1.2.2 Recreation therapy

Participate in recreational activities like gardening, fishing, practicing calligraphy and painting, playing a musical instrument and appreciating music. As for the musical therapy, select the type of music of "expressing emotions" and "removing depression" alternately.

8.2.1.2.3 Physical training

Physical training can lower blood pressure to a certain extent. Practicing Taijiquan is very suitable. The patients with good constitution may play the whole set of simplified Taijiquan while the patients with poor constitution may play half, or several postures of it. Besides, the patients can have other activities like jogging to increase the amount of exercise, extend the distance and quicken the speed gradually.

The patients should not have the activities with the movement of the head below the horizontal position so as to avoid aggravating the symptom of discomfort of the head due to the gravitational influence no matter whatever sports events are selected; it is not advisable to have competitive activities to prevent emotional excitement; do not have weight-carrying activities to avoid breath holding which conversely and reflexively elevates blood pressure.

8.2.1.2.4 Acumox and massage

Acumox The commonly-used acupoints include Fengchi (GB 20), Baihui (GV 20), Quchi (LI 11),

计、肌电图仪,指导患者从仪器的读数或其他可视、听的信号中,判断降压效果。训练患者练习肌肉放松和平静呼吸方法,结合仪器的效果显示,随时调整练习方法。经过反复地自我身心训练,保持血压的自我控制。

2. 娱乐疗法

参加园艺、钓鱼、书画、弹琴赏乐等娱乐活动,音乐疗法可交替选听"抒情解郁"和"宁心安神"类乐曲。

3. 体育疗法

可起到一定的降压效果,练习太极拳颇为合适。体质较好者,可打全套简化太极拳,体力较差者可打半套,或选练几手招式。还可结合进行慢跑等活动,逐渐增加运动量,延长距离并加快速度。

不论何种体育运动,均不应作头低于心脏水平位的活动,以免由于重力性影响而加重头部不适症状;不宜进行带有竞赛性的活动,以免情绪激动,不作负重性活动,以免引起屏气,而反射性引起血压升高等。

4. 针灸、推拿疗法

针灸 常用穴位有风池、百会、曲池、足三里、三阴交

Zusanli (ST 36), Sanyinjiao (SP 6), etc. In the case of marked hyperactive hepatic yang, add Xingjian (LR 2), Xiaxi (GB 43) and Taichong (LR 3); in the case of hepatorenal yin deficiency, add Ganshu (BL 18) and Shenshu (BL 23); in the case of excessive phlegm, add Fenglong (ST 40), Zhongwan (CV 12) and Jiexi (ST 41). Puncture the acupoints once every other day and 7 days constitute one course of treatment. Besides, the acupoint injection may be alternately applied on the above-mentioned acupoints. Select two acupoints each time with the acupoint injection of 1 ml of 0.25% procaine hydrochloride for each acupoint, once a day; or select Chimai (TE 18) with the acupoint injection of 1 ml of vitamin B_{12}, once a day and seven days constitute one course of treatment.

The commonly-used auricular acupoints include Pizhixia (MA‐AT 1), Jiangyagou, Naogan, Neifenmi (MA‐IC 3), Ershenmen (MA‐TF 1), Xin, etc. Select one or two acupoints every day or every other day and retain the needle for 30 minutes. Besides, the needle-embedding therapy may be adopted, or apply Wangbuliuxingzi (*Semen Vaccariae*) on the auricular acupoints instead of the needle-embedding therapy.

Cupping therapy: Select the acupoints of the first lateral line of the dorsal gallbladder meridian and Jianyu (LI 15), Quchi (LI 11), Shousanli (LI 10), Weizhong (BL 40), Chengjin (BL 56), Zusanli (ST 36), Fenglong (ST 40), Fengchi (GB 20), etc. Cup ten acupoints or so each time for ten to fifteen minutes.

Massage: Apply self-massage mainly. The commonly-used methods include kneading Zanzhu (BL 2), scrubbing the nose, beating the Heavenly drum (Tiangu), combing the hair with the hand, kneading Taiyang (EX-HN 5), wiping the forehead, pressing-kneading Naohou, rubbing the hands to bathe the face, kneading

Yaoyan (EX - BT) and scrubbing Yongquan (KI 1). Simultaneously, pat the relevant regions with the fist and palm.

8.2.1.2.5 Dietary therapy

In the case of hepatorenal yin deficiency, select Haizhe Biqi Soup (Soup of Cavum Rhopilemae and Bulbus Heleocharis Dulcis). If the conditions permit, select Fengru (*Lac Apis Melliferum*) to eat. In the case of hyperactive yang due to yin deficiency, select cold celery in sauce. Meanwhile, it is also advisable to decoct 5 to 10 g of Juhua (*Flos Chrysanthemi*) or Yejuhua (*Flos Chrysanthemi Indici*) in water until the water boils for three to five minutes. Drink the decoction as tea. In the case of deficiency of yin and yang, select 20 g of Heizhima (*Semen Sesami*), Gouqizi (*Fructus Lycii*) and Hutaorou (*Semen Juglandis*) respectively to be decocted in water. Take the dregs and the decoction simultaneously, once a day.

The commonly-used dietary prescriptions for lowering blood pressure are as follows.

Stewed Sea Cucumber Stew 30 g of sea cucumber (soaked in water) in a proper amount of water with slow fire until it is thoroughly cooked. Then, add a proper quantity of crystal sugar to be dissolved. Eat it.

Stewed Edible Fungus Soak 10 g of tremella or black fungus in water. Then, wash it clean and add a proper amount of water to it. Next, stew it with slow fire until it is thoroughly cooked. Finally, add a proper quantity of crystal sugar to it. Take it in the evening.

Shelled Peanut Pickled in Vinegar Soak 250g of shelled peanut (with the red coating) in a proper amount of vinegar for five to seven days. Eat it three times a day, a proper amount each time.

Fermented Juhua (*Flos Chrysanthemi*) Cook

5. 食疗

肝肾阴虚证,可用海蜇荸荠汤。有条件者,则可选食蜂乳。阴虚阳亢证,可加用凉拌芹菜。同时,亦可取菊花(或野菊花)5～10 g,加沸水煮3～5分钟成菊花饮,代茶喝。阴阳两虚证,可取黑芝麻、枸杞子、胡桃肉各20 g水煎,每日1次,渣汤同服。

常用降血压食疗方剂:

炖海参 水发海参30 g,加水适量,文火炖烂,加入适量冰糖融化,即可食用。

炖木耳 白木耳或黑木耳10 g,水发后洗净,加水适量,文火炖烂,加适量冰糖,晚上服。

醋泡花生米 花生米(带红衣)250 g,加醋适量,浸泡5～7天,每日食3次,每次适量。

菊花醪 甘菊花10 g,元

10 g of Ganjuhua (*Flos Chrysanthemi*) and a proper amount of glutinous rice wine in a pot until the wine boils. Take it at a draught, twice a day.

Egg Stewed with Tianma (*Rhizoma Gastrodiae*)

Decoct 9 g of Tianma (*Rhizoma Gastrodiae*) in water for one hour. Then, remove the dregs and stew two eggs in the decoction. Take it orally.

The patients should eat more melon, fruit and vegetable usually, of which celery and water melon have the action of lowering blood pressure to a certain extent. Do not overeat fat meat and fine grain and do not eat the vegetarian diet all the time, either. They should eat the low salt diet with a daily intake of less than 5 g of salt.

8.2.1.2.6 Drugs for external treatment

Mix a proper amount of the minced Wuzhuyu (*Folium Evodiae*) with vinegar. Then, apply the drug on Yongquan (KI1) on the sole. Conduct the dressing change once a day.

Decoct 6g of Cishi (*Magnetitum*), Shijueming (*Semen Cassiae*), Dangshen (*Radix Angelicae Sinensis*), Huangqi (*Radix Astragali seu Hedysari*), Danggui (*Radix Angelicae Sinensis*), Sangzhi (*Ramulus Mori*), Zhike (*Fructus Aurantii*), Wuyao (*Radix Linderae*), Manjingzi (*Fructus Viticis*), Baijili (*Fructus Tribuli*), Baishaoyao (*Radix Paeoniae Alba*), Chaoduzhong (parched *Cortex Eucommiae*) and Niuxi (*Radix Achyranthis Bidentatae*) respectively and 18 g of Duhuo (*Radix Angelicae Pubescentis*). Soak the feet in the decoction for an hour once a day.

Make a medicinal pillow with Yejuhua (*Flos Chrysanthemi Indici*), Danzhuye (*Herba Lophatheri*), Dongsangye (*Folium Mori* collected in winter), Shengshigao (*Gypsum Fibrosum*), Baishaoyao (*Radix Paedoniae Alba*), Chuanxiong (*Rhizoma Ligustici Chuan-*

xiong), Cishi (*Magnetitum*), Manjingzi (*Fructus Viticis*) and Cansha (*Excrementa Bombycum*). Use it for more than six hours a day. It is applicable to the patients with hyperactive yang due to yin deficiency. Besides, Lüdouke (*Testa Phaseoli Radiati*) can be used to make the medicinal pillow as well.

8.2.2 Sequelae of apoplexy

Apoplexy is divided into the two types of "apoplexy involving meridians and collaterals" and "apoplexy involving viscera" in TCM. The former generally refers to freedom from changes of mentality and the latter often to the more serious state of illness with unconsciousness. The main clinical manifestation is hemiplegia, namely paralysis of unilateral limbs. Therefore, the disease is also called "ban shen bu sui" (hemiplegia), "pian ku" (hemilateral withering) and "pian fei" (unilateral disuse) in TCM. The patients are often accompanied by facial distortion. If the disease lasts long, the affected limbs are skinny and numb.

8.2.2.1 Syndrome differentiation and treatment

8.2.2.1.1 Blood stasis due to qi deficiency

It manifests hemiplegia of limbs, pale and lusterless complexion, emaciation, spontaneous sweating, numbness of skin, or swelling of hands and feet, spasm of muscle or with stabbing pain of unilateral body, squamous and dry skin, enlarged tongue with dental marks or dim and sluggish tongue with ecchymosis and petechiae, taut and thready or unsmooth and intermittent pulse. It is advisable to benefit qi and activate blood circulation, and dredge meridians and collaterls. The prescription used is the modified Buyang Huanwu Decoction (Yang-Strengthening Decoction for Recuperation). In the case of severe numb

二、中风后遗症

中医将中风分为"中经络"和"中脏腑"两大类，前者一般无神志改变，后者常有神志不清，病情较重。中风后遗症的主要临床表现为偏瘫，即一侧肢体瘫痪，故又称"半身不遂"、"偏枯"、"偏废"。常伴口眼歪斜，久则患肢枯瘦，麻木不仁。

【辨证施治】

1. 气虚血瘀

肢体偏瘫，面白无华，形瘦自汗，肌肤不仁，或手足肿胀，筋脉拘急，或有半身刺疼，肌肤甲错，舌体胖大有齿痕，或舌晦滞、有瘀斑瘀点，脉弦细或涩结。宜益气活血，疏通经络。补阳还五汤加减。肢体麻木甚者加桑寄生、蜈蚣、鸡血藤；上肢瘫痪加桑枝、桂枝、威灵仙；下肢瘫痪加川牛膝。

limbs and body, add Sangjisheng (*Ramulus Loranthi*), Wugong (*Scolopendra*) and Jixueteng (*Caulis Spatholobi*); in the case of paralysis of upper limbs, add Sangzhi (*Ramulus Mori*), Guizhi (*Ramulus Cinnamomi*) and Weilingxian (*Radix Clematidis*); in the case of paralysis of lower limbs, add Chuanniuxi (*Radix Cyathulae*).

8.2.2.1.2 Asthenia of the liver and kidney

It manifests hemiplegia, numbness and trembling of limbs and body, aching pain and flaccidity of the waist and legs, or odontoseisis and baldness, tinnitus, amnesia, light-headedness, stiff tongue with non-fluent speech, dull expression, red tongue with a little fur, taut and thready pulse. It is advisable to strengthen the liver and kidney. The prescription used is the modified Qiju Dihuang Decoction (Decoction of Six Drugs, Rehmannia with Wolberry and Chrysanthemum). In the case of palpitation and insomnia, add parched Zaoren (*Semen Ziziphi Jujubae*), Baiziren (*Semen Biotae*), Fuling (*Poria*) and Yejiaoteng (*Caulis Polygoni Multiflori*); in the case of dry mouth and red tongue, add Tainmendong (*Radix Asparagi*) and Ejiao (*Colla Corii Asini*). As for the Chinese patent drug, it is suitable to use Qiju Dihuang Bolus(Bolus of Six Drugs, Rehmannia with Wolfberry and Chrysanthemum).

8.2.2.1.3 Phlegm and dampness due to asthenia of the spleen

It manifests paralysis and numbness of the limbs and body, cold limbs, facial edema, chest tightness with abdominal distension, poor appetite, lassitude without physical strength, loose stool, fat body, yellowish complexion with pale lips, or cough with short breath, profuse sputum, pale tongue with white and greasy fur, taut and slippery pulse. It is advisable to strengthen the spleen, resolve phlegm and remove dampness. The prescriptions used are the Xiangsha Liujunzi Decoction (Decoction of

2. 肝肾亏虚

肢体偏瘫、麻木、颤抖,腰酸腿软,或齿摇发脱,耳鸣健忘,头晕目眩,舌强语謇,神情呆滞,舌质红,舌苔少,脉弦细。宜补益肝肾。杞菊地黄汤加减。心悸失眠加炒枣仁、柏子仁、茯神、夜交藤;口干舌红加天门冬、阿胶。成药可用杞菊地黄丸。

3. 脾虚痰湿

肢体偏瘫,麻木,四肢不温,面浮,胸闷腹胀,食欲不振,倦怠乏力,大便溏,形体肥胖,面黄唇淡,或有咳嗽气短,痰多,舌淡,苔白腻,脉弦滑。宜健脾,化痰,祛湿。香砂六君子汤合二陈汤,再加石菖蒲、远志、郁金、白僵蚕。

Cyperus and Amomum with Six Noble Ingredients) in combination with Erchen Decoction (Two Old Drugs Decoction) with the additional ingredients of Shichangpu (*Rhizoma Acori Graminei*), Yuanzhi (*Radix Polygalae*), Yujin (*Radix Curcumae*) and Baijiangcan (*Bombyx Batryticatus*).

8.2.2.2 Rehabilitation methods

8.2.2.2.1 Functional training

When the patients gradually restore their functions of limbs and the body, they may be supported to practice some simple free activities in bed such as getting up, raising arms, lifting legs and lifting feet. The patients should leave the bed as early as possible to practice standing and slow walking. At the beginning, the patients should be supported by the medical and nursing staff to practice these activities. Then gradually increase the amount of exercise from the moment the patients use the walking stick to the moment the patients stop using it. Or the patients may do some knitting by hand to have functional training. The patients with stiff tongue and non-fluent speech may say simple words during the training. Then practice saying longer sentences gradually.

As for the keep-fit patting method, please refer to the relevant content in Chapter 5.8.4.

As for functional training of fingers and upper limbs, it is advisable to adopt the method of playing games. As for the relevant detailed content, please refer to Chapter 5.3.4.

8.2.2.2.2 Acumox

Acupuncture: Select Qihai (CV 6), Guanyuan (CV 4), Zusanli (ST 36), Shenshu (BL 23), Taixi (KI 3) and Xuehai (SP 10) as the main acupoints; Jianyu (LI 15), Shousanli (LI 10), Quchi (LI 11), Waiguan (TE 5), Hegu (LI 4), Huantiao (GB 30), Fengshi (GB 31), Yan-

【康复方法】

1. 功能锻炼

当患者肢体功能逐渐恢复时,可在扶持之下,在床上做一些简单的自由活动,如坐起、举臂、抬腿、抬脚等。尽早下床练习站立、慢走。开始须在医护人员搀扶下进行,由扶杖到弃杖,逐渐增加活动量。或作手工编织进行功能训练。对舌强语謇病人,先训练说简单的话,逐步说较长的话。

拍打健身法 见本书第五章第八节相关内容。

关于手指、上肢功能锻炼,可采用游戏的方法,详见本书第五章第三节相关内容。

2. 针灸疗法

针灸 取气海、关元、命门、足三里、肾俞、太溪、血海,配穴取肩髃、手三里、曲池、外关、合谷、环跳、风市、阳陵泉、飞扬、绝骨、悬钟。每次主穴、

glingquan (GB 34), Feiyang (BL 58), Juegu (LI 16) and Xuanzhong (GB 39) as the adjunct acupoints. Select 3 to 4 main acupoints and adjunct acupoints respectively. Adopt the reinforcing method when needling Qihai (CV 6), Guanyuan (CV 4), Shenshu (BL 23), Zusanli (ST 36) and Mingmen (GV 4); apply the reducing manipulation while puncturing Taixi (KI 3) and Xuehai (SP 10) as well as the acupoints of limbs. Add Fenglong (ST 40) and Yinlingquan (SP 9) in the case of phlegm and dampness due to splenic asthenia.

It is advisable to apply moxibustion on every acupoint of the above with moxa sticks for 10 to 15 minutes in patients with asthenia.

Acupoint injection: Inject 4ml of magnesium sulfate injection or injection of compound Danggui (*Radix Angelicae Sinensis*), 1 ml each acupoint. As for the upper limbs, select Neiguan (PC 6), Quchi (LI 11) and Shousanli (LI 10); as for the lower limbs, select Sanyinjiao (SP 6), Zusanli (ST 37), Yanglingquan (GB 34) and Chengshan (BL 57). Select two acupoints from the upper and lower limbs respectively each time. First, puncture the acupoints with the syringe needle while injecting the medicine to enhance the stimulation until there appears the sensation of soreness and distension. Then inject the drug. Inject the drug once every other day, and five times in succession constitute one course of treatment. Assume the second course of treatment after three-day rest. Stop the treatment when the muscular strength of the affected limbs reaches degree four during the treatment.

Scalp acupuncture Select the motor area and sensory area of the healthy side of the head and the adjunct foot motor sensory area of the two sides of the head. Add the speech area in the case of stiff tongue and difficult speech. Insert the filiform needle with the size of 1.5 to 2

配穴各取3～4穴。气海、关元、肾俞、足三里、命门等用补法,太溪、血海及四肢穴位用泻法。脾虚痰湿证加丰隆、阴陵泉。

虚证患者可加艾条灸各穴10～15分钟。

穴位注射 硫酸镁注射液或复方当归注射液4 ml,每穴注射1 ml。上肢取穴内关、曲池、手三里。下肢取穴三阴交、足三里、阳陵泉、承山。每次上下肢各选两穴。注射时先用针头在穴位内提插,增强刺激,有酸胀感后推药。隔日1次,连用5次为1疗程。休息三天后进行第二疗程。在治疗中患肢肌力达到4级即可停止治疗。

头针 选健侧头部运动区、感觉区配双侧足运感区。有舌强语謇者加语言区。用1.5～2寸毫针沿皮分段快速刺入,进针1～1.5寸。以每分

cun quickly beneath the skin section by section with the depth of 1 to 1.5 cun. First twirl the needle for 5 minutes at the frequency of 200 times per minute. Then twirl the needle for 5 minutes again after a ten-minute rest. Repeat the acupuncture for three times. Afterward, withdraw the needle. Puncture the scalp once a day, and five times in succession make up one course of treatment. It is also advisable to replace the manual twirling with electric impulses. Besides, it is also suitable to penetrate Qubin (GB 7) (the healthy or affected side) from Baihui (GV 20), or penetrate Xuanlu (GB 5) (motor area) from Qianding (GV 21), which is very effective as well.

Ear acupuncture: Alternately puncture all the acupoints of Shen, Naogan, Ershenmen (MA-TF 1), Xin, Zhen and Pizhixia (MA-AT 1). It is also advisable to use needle-embedding method.

8.2.2.2.3 Massage

Shift the manipulations from gentle ones to heavy ones, and increase the strength gradually as the patients adapt to the methods until no muscular spasmodic contraction is caused. Generally, use the rubbing method first. Then gradually shift to kneading method, proceeding from the distal end to the proximal end of the limbs for five minutes. The massage points of the upper limbs include Quepen (ST 12), Jianyu (LI 15), Jianzhen (SI 19), Quchi (LI 11), Chize (LU 5), Shaohai (HT 3), Daling (PC 7), Yangchi (TE 4), Yangxi (LI 5), Yanggu (SI 5), Shousanli (LI 10) and Hegu (LI 4); the massage points of lower limbs include Qichong (ST 30), Huantiao (GB 30), Juliao (GB 29), Fengshi (GB 31), Zusanli (ST 36), Yanglingquan (GB 34), Xuehai (SP 10), Weizhong (BL 40), Chengshan (BL 57), Taixi (KI 3), Kunlun (BL 60) and Jiexi (ST 41). Passive activities may be adopted at the same time in combination with massage. The doctors may

钟200次的速度捻转5分钟,休息10分钟后,再捻转5分钟,重复3次后起针。每日1次,10次为1疗程。亦可用头针通脉冲电取代手捻转刺激。此外,还可选百会透曲鬓(健侧或患侧),或前顶透悬颅(运动区),亦有良效。

耳针 交替针刺肾、脑干、耳神门、心、枕、皮质下诸穴,亦可埋针。

3. 推拿疗法

推拿 手法由轻而重,随患者逐渐适应而加大力量,以不引起肌肉痉挛性收缩为好。一般先用摩法,逐渐改用揉法,从肢体远心端推到近心端,约5分钟左右,上肢推拿穴位:缺盆、肩髃、肩贞、曲池、尺泽、少海、大陵、阳池、阳溪、阳谷、手三里、合谷等;下肢推拿穴位:气冲、环跳、居髎、风市、足三里、阳陵泉、血海、委中、承山、太溪、昆仑、解溪等。在推拿的同时可结合被动运动。可指导患者用健肢帮助患肢作各种被动运动。

guide the patients to have various passive activities for the affected limbs with the help of the healthy limbs.

When the muscle has slight autonomic activities, use forceful manipulations with kneading and pinching the muscle as the main manipulations. Reduce acupoint massage, but still massage more on the acupoints of the yangming meridians such as Shousanli (LI 10) and Zusanli (ST 36). The patients should mainly have sports events and medical training after the adjunct massage when the limbs restore autonomic activities, but resistance still exists in the muscle. It is advisable to knead and pinch the muscle, strike and pat the whole limbs to promote the excitability of tissues. At the end of the activities, it is suitable to massage with the kneading, rolling and palm-pushing manipulations from the distal end to the proximal end. The manipulations may promote muscular relaxation and venous return.

8.2.2.2.4 Dietary therapy

For the patients with blood stasis due to qi deficiency, cook gruel with 30 g of Huangqi (*Radix Astragali seu Hedysari*), 30 g of Shanzha (*Fructus Crataegi*) and a proper amount of Jingmi (*Fructus Oryzae Sativae*). Eat the gruel in the morning and evening, one dose a day.

For the patients with asthenia of the liver and kidney, cook 15 g of Huaishanyao (*Rhizoma Dioscoreae*), 30 g of Guiban (*Carapax et Plastrum Testudinis*) (to be decocted first) and 60 g of lean meat until the ingredients are done. Eat the food in different times of a day for 10 days in succession, one dose a day.

For the patients with phlegm and dampness due to splenic asthenia, cook 30 g of Yiyiren (*Semen Coicis*), 30 g of Baibiandou (*Semen Dolichoris Album*), 30 g of Huaishanyao (*Rhizoma Dioscoreae*), 60 g of radish and 60 g of Jingmi (*Fructus Oryzae Sativae*). Eat the food

当肌肉有轻微的自主活动时,推拿手法可渐重,以揉捏肌肉的手法为主,穴位推拿可减少,但对手三里、足三里等阳明经穴仍需多推拿。当肢体已能自主活动,但肌肉仍存在抗阻力时,应以体育运动、医疗练功为主,在运动前辅以推拿。可揉捏肌肉和捶拍整个肢体,以提高组织的兴奋性。在活动结束后,可做揉、搓、掌推等手法,由远端到近端,以使肌肉放松,促进静脉血回流。

4. 食疗

气虚血瘀者,用黄芪30 g,山楂30 g,粳米适量同煮粥,每日1剂,早晚餐服用。

肝肾亏虚者,用怀山药15 g、龟版30 g(先煎),瘦猪肉60 g,煮熟服食。每日1剂,分食。连服10日。

脾虚痰湿者,用薏苡仁30 g,白扁豆30 g,怀山药30 g、白萝卜60 g,粳米60 g,煮粥服用。每日1剂,连服7~10天。

for 7 to 10 days in succession, one dose a day.

Sangzhi Tea (Tea of *Ramulus Mori*)　　Add 600 ml of water to 20 g of Sangzhi (*Ramulus Mori*), and decoct it until there is 200 ml of water left. Use the decoction as tea to drink. It is applicable to hemiplegia, swelling and distension of unilateral limbs and body with pain and numbness, unsmooth flexion and extension after apoplexy. It is also applicable to hypertension, numbness of limbs and the body as well as underlying apoplexy.

Immortals' Food　　Grind 1,000 g of Tianmendong (*Radix Asparagi*) and 100 g of Xingren (*Semen Armeniacae Amarum*) into powder. Soak the powder in honey. Take the powder twice a day, 5 g each time. It is applicable to sequelae of apoplexy, numbness of limbs and the body, pain and contracture as well as constipation.

8.2.2.2.5　Nursing in daily life

Keep defecation unobstructed. The patients should eat bland foods, and avoid greasy and fine foods. Abstain from drinking and smoking. Strengthen the nursing of the affected limbs, and take care to keep the local part warm. If the conditions permit, the patients may jointly play a musical instrument, play chess and practice calligraphy and painting to cultivate the mind. At the late stage of rehabilitation, the patients may jointly have traditional sports therapies like five mimic-animal games and Taijiquan.

8.2.3　Hypotension

The pathological region of senile hypotension involves the heart, spleen and kidney. The disease is mostly caused by old age, weak constitution, improper diet, physical and sexual overstrain. The pathogenesis mainly includes deficiency of healthy qi, or deficiency of healthy qi occasionally intermingled with pathogenic sthenia.

桑枝茶　桑枝20 g,加水600 ml,煎取200 ml,当茶饮。适用于中风后偏瘫,半侧肢体肿胀、疼痛麻木,屈伸不利。也可用于高血压,肢体麻木,有中风倾向者。

仙人粮　天门冬1 000 g,杏仁100 g。上为末,蜜渍。每服5克,每日2次。适用于中风后遗症,肢体麻木不仁,疼痛拘急,大便干结者。

5. 起居护理

保持大便通畅。饮食宜清淡,避免油腻厚味。忌烟酒。加强患肢护理,注意局部保暖。有条件者可配合琴棋书画、音乐疗法等陶冶性情。后期康复亦可配合五禽戏、太极拳等传统体育疗法。

三、低血压症

老年低血压症,病位涉及心、脾、肾诸脏。病因多为年老体虚、饮食失调、劳欲过度等。病机主要是正气亏损,时可兼挟实邪。

8.2.3.1 Syndrome differentiation and treatment

8.2.3.1.1 Asthenia of the heart and spleen

Vertigo and palpitation aggravated by moving and easily induced by overstrain, short breath, low voice, pale and lustreless complexion, or sallow complexion, pale tongue, thready pulse without force. It is advisable to tonify the heart, strengthen the spleen, promote qi flow and blood production. The prescription used is the modified Guipi Decoction (Decoction for Invigorating the Spleen and Nourishing the Heart) or Renshen Yangrong Decoction (Ginseng Nutrition Decoction).

8.2.3.1.2 Deficiency of the middle energizer qi

Occasional vertigo, mental fatigue, disinclination to speak, poor apetite, lassitude of limbs, loose stool, even down-bearing sensation of the lower abdomen in severe cases, pale tongue, slow or soft and thready pulse. It is advisable to supplement qi, strengthen the middle energizer and raise the pure yang. The prescription used is the modified Buzhong Yiqi Decoction (Decoction for Reinforcing Middle Energizer and Replenishing Qi).

8.2.3.1.3 Deficiency of the kidney yang

Dizziness, tinnitus, listlessness, soreness of the waist and flaccidity of legs, amnesia, pale or darkish complexion, cold body and limbs, pale tongue, deep and thready pulse particularly in the chi region. It is suitable to warm and strengthen the kidney yang. The prescription used is the modified Yougui Bolus (the Kidney Yang-Reinforcing Bolus) or Jinkui Shenqi Bolus.

8.2.3.1.4 Phlegm stagnation in the middle energizer

Dizziness with a heavy sensation, chest tightness, nausea, even vomiting of phlegm and saliva in severe

【辨证施治】

1. 心脾两虚

眩晕、心悸,动则加剧,劳累易发,气短声低,面白少华,或萎黄,舌质淡,脉细无力。宜补益心脾,助气生血。归脾汤或人参养荣汤加减。

2. 中气不足

时时眩晕,神倦懒言,纳食减少,四肢乏力,大便溏薄,甚则少腹下坠,舌质淡,脉缓或濡细。宜益气补中,升举清阳。补中益气汤加减。

3. 肾阳亏虚

头昏耳鸣,精神萎靡,腰酸腿软,健忘,面色㿠白或黧黑,形寒肢冷,舌淡白,脉沉细而尺部尤弱。宜温补肾阳。右归丸或金匮肾气丸加减。

4. 痰浊中阻

头晕作重,胸闷泛恶,甚则呕吐痰涎,舌苔白腻,脉濡

cases, white and greasy fur, soft and slippery pulse. It is advisable to resolve phlegm, strengthen the spleen and regulate the stomach. The prescriptions used include the modified Banxia Tianma Baizhu Decoction (Decoction of Pinellia, Gastrodia and Bighead Atractylodes) and Zexie Decoction (Decoction of *Rhizoma Alismatis*).

8.2.3.2 Rehabilitation methods

8.2.3.2.1 Physical training

Playing Taijiquan can make qi and blood sufficient, blood vessels full, pulsation harmonious, slow and forceful and is effective for hypotension. The patient with this disease has a poor adaptive capacity for physical training and is susceptible to fatigue. Therefore, it is advisable to select the walking activities with easily controllable amount of exercise and which can enhance the physical strength. At the beginning, walk for 1 km once, in the second week 1.5 km, in the third week 2 km, in one month 3 km, and maintain this final distance. Persisting in walking for 3 km a day is very beneficial to the improvement of the symptoms of hypotension.

8.2.3.2.2 Acumox

Acumox: In the case of asthenia of the heart and spleen, select Xinshu (BL 15), Pishu (BL 20), Zusanli (ST 36), Qihai (CV 6), Baihui (GV 20) and Neiguan (PC 6) and needle them with the reinforcing manipulation; in the case of deficiency of the middle energizer qi, select Baihui (GV 20), Qihai (CV 6), Pishu (BL 20), Zusanli (ST 36) and Guanyuan (CV 4) and needle (them) with the reinforcing method; in the case of deficiency of the kidney yang, select Shenshu (BL 23), Yingu (KI 10), Mingmen (GV 4), Baihui (GV 20) and Qihai (CV 6) and needle them with the reinforcing method; in the case of phlegm stagnation in the middle energizer, select Fenglong (ST 40), Zhongwan (CV 12), Touwei (ST 8),

Neiguan (PC 6) and Jiexi (ST 41) and needle them with the uniform reinforcing-reducing method. Moxibustion can be coordinatively applied in all the above cases so as to enhance the therapeutic effects. Besides, it is advisable to select Fengchi (GB 20), Yiming (EX - HN 14) and Neiguan (PC 6) with the acupoint injection of 3 ml to 5ml of 5% or 10% glucose solution, or 0.5 ml of vitamin B_{12} in each acupoint once every other day.

Ear acupuncture: Insert a one-cun-long filiform needle into Shengyagou and twirl the needle towards one direction endlessly until the patient feels slightly warm in the body, distending and painful on the auricle. Then, retain the needle for 20 minutes and twirl the needle again during this period of time. Five to ten times constitute one course of treatment. Or insert a five-fen-long needle into Jiaogan (MA - AH 7), Shenshangxian, Xin and Ershenmen (MA - TF 1) with the brief and forceful stimulation method without retaining the needle once a day.

8.2.3.2.3 Dietary therapy

In the case of cardiosplenic asthenia, eat three to nine grams of Guiyuanrou (*Cortex Cinnamomi*) every day, or Guiyuan Shenmi Paste (Paste of *Cortex Cortex Cinnamomi*, *Radix Ginseng* and *Mel*), Stewed Chicken with Danggui (*Radix Angelicae Sinensis*), or Stewed Chicken with Tianma (*Rhizoma Gastrodiae*), Gouqizi (*Fructus Lycii*), Huaishanyao (*Rhizoma Dioscoreae*) and Dangshen (*Radix Codonopsis Pilosulae*); in the case of deficiency of middle energizer qi, it is advisable to add Shengma (*Rhizoma Cimicifugae*) and Gegen (*Radix Puerariae*); in the case of renal yang deficiency, drink three to five milliliters of Lurong Wine (Wine of *Cornu Cervi Pantotrichum*) three times a day. It is also advisable to cook gruel with polished glutinous rice and one or two ingredients from the following drugs: Renshen

液3~5 ml,或维生素B_{12}注射液0.5 ml,隔日1次。

耳针　取升压沟,以1寸毫针刺入后向一个方向捻转,以捻不动为止。患者感到身体稍发热、耳郭作胀、疼痛后,留针20分钟,中间再捻针一次,5~10次为一疗程。或取交感、肾上腺、心、神门等穴,用5分毫针刺入耳穴后,行短促强刺激法,不留针,每日1次。

3. 食疗

心脾两虚证,可每日食桂圆肉3~9 g,或用桂圆参蜜膏、当归炖母鸡,亦可用天麻、枸杞子、怀山药、党参炖鸡食。若系中气不足证,还可加入升麻、葛根等。肾阳亏虚证,可饮用鹿茸酒,每日3次,每次3~5 ml。亦可在人参、党参、黄芪、怀山药、胡桃肉、葛根、红枣中任选一二种,与元米煮粥食,也有较好效果。若低血压症由缺铁性贫血引起者,还可加用铁强化酱油。

(*Radix Ginseng*), Dangshen (*Radix Codonopsis Pilosulae*), Huangqi (*Radix Astragali seu Hedysari*), Huaishanyao (*Rhizoma Dioscoreae*), Hutaorou (*Semen Juglandis*), Gegen (*Radix Puerariae*) and Chinese dates (*Fructus Ziziphi Jujubae*). This has better therapeutic effects, too. In the case of hypotension due to iron-deficiency anemia, it is advisable to use iron-enriched soy sauce.

In daily life, eat for more times with less amount at a time; for in the case of overeating, blood accumulates in blood vessels of the abdominal cavity, which reduces the cerebral blood supply, consequently inducing the occurrence of symptoms of hypotension.

8.2.3.2.4　Nursing in daily life

Avoid sitting and standing long. It is advisable to wear the tight elastic socks. This can prevent the onset and aggravation of varix of the lower limbs. The patients with postural hypotension are not advisable to change the posture too quickly and make the head too low during sleeping. They should wait for a while and then leave the bed when getting up at night and in the morning. Or they may exercise the hands and legs in the bed before getting up, with a transitional period of five to ten minutes. After leaving the bed, wait for a moment and then step forward.

8.2.4　Coronary heart disease

The pathological region of the disease lies in the heart, but is related to the spleen, stomach, etc. The commonly-seen causes of the disease include internal invasion of pathogenic cold, improper diet, emotional disorder, old age, and weak constitution, etc. It is advisable to nourish yin and promote blood circulation.

日常饮食宜少食多餐，因为进食过饱，血液会集聚于腹腔血管，使大脑的供血减少而诱发低血压症状的发生。

4. 起居护理

避免久坐、久站，可穿贴身的弹力袜，以防止下肢静脉曲张的发生和加重。体位性低血压症者，体位变化时不宜动作过快，睡眠时头部不宜过低，夜间和清晨起床应稍待片刻再下地。或先在床上作一些手脚活动，有5~10分钟的过渡期再起床。下地后亦应稍等片刻再起步。

四、冠心病

本病病位在心，但与脾、胃等脏有关。病因常见有寒邪内侵、饮食不当、情志失调、年老体弱等。宜养阴活血。

8.2.4.1 Syndrome differentiation and treatment

8.2.4.1.1 Yin deficiency intermingled with blood stasis

It manifests thoracic oppression and calor with intermittent stabbing pain, palpitation, night sweat, soreness of the waist and flaccidity of knees, dizziness, tinnitus, red tongue with a little fur and concurrent ecchymoses, thready and unsmooth pulse. The prescription used is the modified Zuogui Decoction in combination with Danshen Decoction (Red Sage Decoction). In the case of concurrent qi stagnation, add Gualou (*Fructus Trichosanthis*), Lü'emei (*Flos Mume Albus*) and Hehuanhua (*Flos Albiziae*).

8.2.4.1.2 Yang deficiency intermingled with blood stasis

It manifests thoracic oppression and discomfort, or with oppressed pain, palpitation, short breath, aversion to cold, cold limbs, lumbar soreness, hypodynamia, whitish or cyanotic lips and nails, pale tongue with ecchymoses, deep, thready and unsmooth pulse. It is advisable to warm yang and remove blood stasis. The prescription used is the modified Yougui Decoction (the Kidney Yang-Reinforcing Decoction) in combination with CHD Prescription Ⅱ. In the case of concurrent phlegm stagnation, add Gualou (*Fructus Trichosanthis*), Xiebai (*Bulbus Allii Macrostemi*) and Banxia (*Rhizoma Pinelliae*) to remove phlegm and blood stasis.

8.2.4.1.3 Deficiency of qi and yin

It manifests dull and occasional precordial and thoracic pain and oppression, palpitation, short breath, lassitude, disinclination to speak, lustreless complexion, lightheadedness worsened by overstrain, relatively red tongue with dental marks, thready and weak or knotted and in-

【辨证施治】

1. 阴虚挟瘀

胸闷灼痛,间有刺痛,心悸盗汗,腰酸膝软,头晕耳鸣,舌红苔少,兼有瘀斑,脉细涩。左归饮合丹参饮加减。兼有气郁者,加瓜蒌、绿萼梅、合欢花等。

2. 阳虚挟瘀

胸闷不适,或感闷痛,心悸气短,畏寒肢冷,腰酸乏力,唇甲淡白或青紫,舌淡有瘀斑,脉沉细而涩。当温阳化瘀。右归饮合冠心Ⅱ号方加减。若兼有痰阻,可加瓜蒌、薤白、半夏豁痰开结。

3. 气阴两虚

心胸隐痛而闷,时作时止,心悸气短,倦怠懒言,面色少华,头晕目眩,遇劳则甚,舌偏红或有齿印,脉细弱或结代。宜益气养阴,活血通络。

termittent pulse. It is advisable to supplement qi, nourish yin, promote blood circulation and dredge collaterals. The prescription used is the modified Shengmai Powder (Pulsation-Promoting Powder) in combination with CHD Prescription Ⅱ.

8.2.4.2 Rehabilitation methods
8.2.4.2.1 Regulating emotions

Use the enlightening method to remove the patients' misgivings, inspire their enthusiasm and establish their self confidence. It is also advisable to adopt the color therapy to make them exposed to the cold color environment. The patients with depression may place the fresh depression-removing flowers indoors. Besides, it is also advisable to combine the above methods with suggestion and behavior therapies.

8.2.4.2.2 Recreation therapy

Take part in the recreational activities like appreciating music, calligraphy and painting, raising flowers and birds, visiting a park and fishing to increase joys of life and eliminate adverse emotional reactions. Musically, select the tunes of the musical prescriptions of "tranquilizing the mind" if the patients mainly suffer from anxiety; the tunes of the musical prescriptions of "expressing the emotions and removing depression" if the patients chiefly have depression.

8.2.4.2.3 Physical training

Please refer to the relevant part of "Hypotension". In the case of overfatigue or worsened precordial discomfort after the training, reduce the amount of exercise properly or stop the training for a period of time.

8.2.4.2.4 Acumox and massage

Acumox: In the case of yin deficiency intermingled with blood stasis, select the acupoints of the heart meridian,

生脉散合冠心Ⅱ号方加减。

【康复方法】
1. 调节情志

以说理开导法使患者消除顾虑，振作精神，树立信心。亦可用色彩疗法，使患者处于冷色环境中。抑郁者则可在室内放置具有解郁作用的鲜花。必要时也可结合暗示及行为疗法。

2. 娱乐疗法

欣赏音乐、观赏书画、种花养鸟、游园钓鱼等娱乐活动，可以增加生活乐趣，消除不良情志反应。在选择音乐时，如患者以精神焦虑为主，可选"宁心安神"类乐曲；若患者以抑郁为主，则可选"抒情开郁"类乐曲。

3. 体育疗法

参照"低血压症"。如运动后出现过度疲劳或心前区不适感加重等现象，即应适当减轻运动量或暂停一段时间的锻炼。

4. 针灸、推拿疗法

针灸 阴虚挟瘀证，取手足少阴、任脉经穴，如阴郄、神

kidney meridian and gallbladder meridian and conception vessel like Yinxi (HT 6), Shenmen (HT 7), Taixi (KI 3) and Danzhong (CV 17). In the case of vertigo, add Fengchi (GB 20); in the case of tinnitus, add Tinggong (SI 19). It is advisable to use the reinforcing manipulation and reducing manipulation simultaneously. In the case of yang deficiency intermingled with blood stasis, select the Back-Shu acupoints and the acupoints of the triple energizer meridian and pericardium meridian such as Xinshu (BL 15), Jueyinshu (BL 14), Shenshu (BL 23), Neiguan (PC 6) and Tongli (HT 5). In the case of lumbar soreness, add Mingmen (GV 4); in the case of aversion to cold and cold limbs, add Guanyuan (CV 4). It is advisable to use the reinforcing method and reducing method simultaneously. Besides, add moxibustion. In the case of deficiency of qi and yin, select Back-Shu acupoints and the acupoints of the heart meridian and spleen meridian like Xinshu (BL 15), Pishu (BL 20), Geshu (BL 17), Shenmen (HT 7) and Sanyinjiao (SP 6). In the case of short breath, add Qihai (CV 6). After acupuncture, add moxibustion. In the case of concurrent phlegm obstruction or qi stagnation, add Fenglong (ST 40) or Ganshu (BL 18).

Ear acupuncture: As for the ear acupuncture therapy, mainly select Xin, Xiaochang (MA-SC 2), Jiaogan (MA-AH 7) and Pizhixia (MA-AT 1), with the auxiliary selection of Naodian, Gan (MA-SC 5), Fei (MA-IC 1), Xiong (MA-AH 11), Jiangyagou, Xingfendian and Zhen. Select three to five acupoints each time and retain the needle for an hour once every other day. Two weeks constitute one course of treatment.

Massage: In the case of yin deficiency intermingled with blood stasis, it is advisable to select Shenshu (BL 23), Ganshu (BL 18), Xinshu (BL 18), Sanyinjiao (SP 6) and Taixi (KI 3) and needle them with the pushing, kneading and pressing manipulations; in the case of yang deficiency intermingled with blood stasis, select Mingmen (GV 4), Pishu (BL 20), Xinshu (BL 18), and Neiguan (PC 6) and needle them with the pressing-kneading manipulation and the additional scrubbing method on Shenshu (BL 23), Dachangshu (BL 25) and Mingmen (GV 4); in the case of deficiency of qi and yin, add Zusanli (ST 36) and Qihai (CV 6) on the basis of the acupoints in case of yin deficiency intermingled with blood stasis. As for the patients who lie in bed for a long time, massage the whole body properly to dredge the general blood vessels, prevent venous thrombosis and bed sore.

8.2.4.2.5 Dietary therapy

In the case of yin deficiency intermingled with blood stasis, select the combined use of Yuzhu Gruel (Gruel of *Rhizoma Polygonati Odorati*) with Shanzha Gruel (Gruel of *Fructus Grataegi*); in the case of yang deficiency intermingled with blood stasis, select the combined use of Xiebai Gruel (Gruel of *Bulbus Allii Macrostemi*) with Taoren Gruel (Gruel of *Semen Persicae*); in the case of deficiency of qi and yin, select the combined use of Renshen Gruel (Gruel of *Radix Ginseng*) with Baihe Gruel (Gruel of *Bulbus Lilii*).

8.2.4.2.6 External therapy

Make the small plaster weighing 1.5 g each with Jianghuang (*Rhizoma Curcumae Longae*), Wutou (*Radix Aconiti*), Xuejie (*Resina Draconis*), Hujiao (*Fructus Piperis Nigri seu Albi*), Sanqi (*Radix Notoginseng*), Guizhi (*Ramulus Cinnamomi*), Shexiang (*Moschus*), Chuanxiong (*Rhizoma Ligustic Chuanxiong*) and Xiebai (*Bulbus Allii Macro*) respectively according to the ratios of 10∶5∶5∶1∶3∶5∶0.1∶5∶10. Apply the plaster on Xinshu (BL 15) and Danzhong (CV 17) once every other day. Fifteen times constitute one course

俞、心俞、心包俞、内关等穴，用按揉手法，并在肾俞、大肠俞、命门穴加用擦法。气阴不足证，则可在阴虚挟瘀证的取穴基础上，加用足三里、气海等穴。对较长时间卧床的患者，可适当按摩全身，以疏通全身血脉，预防静脉血栓和褥疮的形成。

5. 食疗

阴虚挟瘀证，可选用玉竹粥合山楂粥。阳虚挟瘀证，可选薤白粥合桃仁粥。气阴不足证，可选用人参粥合百合粥。

6. 外治

按姜黄 10、乌头 5、血竭 5、胡椒 1、三七 3、桂枝 5、麝香 0.1、川芎 5、薤白 10 的比例，制成每张重 1.5 g 的小膏药，敷贴心俞和膻中穴。隔日 1 次，15 次为 1 个疗程。亦可选用通心膏敷贴。

of treatment. It is also advisable to apply the Tongxin plaster.

8.2.4.2.7 Nursing in daily life

The patients should prevent cold and keep the body warm at usual times. They should be more careful when getting up in the morning or going to WC at night in the very cold winter. Do not hold breathing or strain too much during defecation. In the case of constipation, it is advisable to take proper cathartics.

8.2.5 Chronic obstructive pulmonary disease

"Chronic obstructive pulmonary disease" refers to the disturbances of cardiopulmonary functions and the limitation of physical activities caused by long-term chronic bronchitis, bronchial asthma and pulmonary emphysema with the repeated onset. The following section discusses the rehabilitation measures of the disease at the remission stage.

8.2.5.1 Syndrome differentiation and treatment

8.2.5.1.1 Asthenia of the lung

It manifests spontaneous sweating, aversion to wind, susceptibility to common cold, short breath, low voice, or mild cough with dyspnea, white, clear and thin sputum, thin fur, thready and weak or feeble and large pulse. In the case of concurrent yin deficiency, the commonly-seen manifestations include cough with chocking, scanty and sticky sputum, dry throat and mouth and red tongue. It is advisable to tonify the lung and consolidate defensive qi. The prescription used is the modified Yupingfeng Powder (Jade-Screen Powder). In the case of concurrent yin deficiency, this prescription is used in combination with Shengmai Powder (Pulsation-Promoting Powder) with modification.

7. 起居护理

平素要防寒保暖,特别是严冬季节,清晨起床或夜间用厕时更须多加小心。大便时不可屏气或过分用力,若有便秘者可适当服用通便药物。

五、慢性阻塞性肺病

长期慢性支气管炎、支气管哮喘及肺气肿所导致的心肺功能障碍和体力活动限制,且反复发作,称为"慢性阻塞性肺病"。以下论述其缓解期的康复措施。

【辨证施治】

1. 肺虚

自汗怕风,常易感冒,气短声低,或有轻度咳喘,痰白清稀,苔薄,脉细弱或虚大。若兼阴虚,则见咳呛,痰少质黏,咽干口燥,舌质红。宜补肺固卫。玉屏风散加减,兼阴虚者则当合生脉散加减。

8.2.5.1.2 Asthenia of the spleen

It manifests poor appetite, epigastric fullness, loose stool, or susceptibility to diarrhea due to ingestion of greasy food, short breath with dyspnea, thin and greasy or white and slippery fur, pale tongue, thready and soft pulse. In the case of concurrent yang deficiency, the manifestations include cold body and limbs, cold sensation in the middle abdomen and regurgitation of clear water. It is advisable to strengthen the spleen and resolve phlegm. The prescription used is the modified Liujunzi Decoction (Decoction of Six Ingredients). In the case of concurrent yang deficiency, add Guizhi (*Ramulus Cinnamomi*) and Ganjiang (*Rhizoma Zingiberis*).

8.2.5.1.3 Asthenia of the kidney

It manifests short breath with dyspnea at ordinary times aggravated by activities, unsmooth respiration, palpitation, dizziness, tinnitus, lumbar soreness and flaccidity of knees which easily occur after physical overstrain. In the case of marked yang deficiency, the manifestations include aversion to cold, cold limbs, spontaneous sweating, pale complexion, whitish fur, tender and enlarged tongue, deep and thready pulse; in the case of yin deficiency, the manifestations include flushing of zygomatic region, dysphoria with smothery sensation, sticky sweat, red tongue with a little fur, thready and rapid pulse. It is advisable to strengthen the kidney and regulate inspiration. In the case of marked yang deficiency, use the modified Jinkui Shenqi Bolus; in the case of marked yin deficiency, use the modified Liuwei Dihuang Bolus (Bolus of Six Drugs Including Rehmannia) and Qiwei Duqi Bolus.

8.2.5.2 Rehabilitation methods

8.2.5.2.1 Regulating emotions and recreation therapy

Please refer to the relevant part in the section of

2. 脾虚

食少脘痞,大便不实,或食油腻易于腹泻,倦怠,气短不足以息,苔薄腻或白滑,质淡,脉细软。若伴阳虚,则有形寒肢冷,中脘觉冷,泛吐清水。宜健脾化痰。六君子汤加减,兼阳虚者则可加桂枝、干姜。

3. 肾虚

平素短气息促,动则为甚,吸气不利,心慌,脑转耳鸣,腰酸膝软,劳累后易发作。偏阳虚者,有畏寒、肢冷,自汗,面色㿠白,舌苔淡白,质胖嫩,脉沉细;偏阴虚者,见颧红,烦热,汗出粘手,舌质红少苔,脉细数。宜补肾摄纳。偏阳虚者用金匮肾气丸加减;偏阴虚者用六味地黄丸、七味都气丸加减。

【康复方法】

1. 调节情志和娱乐疗法

参照"冠心病",在其基础

"Coronary heart disease". On this basis, select the singing therapy additionally, or practice singing coordinatively with abdominal breathing.

8.2.5.2.2 Physical training

Select walking and setting-up jogging. At the beginning, it is advisable to walk and jog alternately. Then, extend the time for jogging and shorten the time for walking gradually. Finally, realize the transition from walking to the whole distance jogging completely. Keep the training until mild short breath occurs every time.

Persist in practicing abdominal breathing at usual times. The method is as follows. Relax the shoulder and back, and concentrate the mind. Then, exhale and inhale air in the proper order. Inspire until the cheeks bulge and expire until the cheeks restore the normal state. Next, adopt the flute-playing method of exhaling air. Namely, contract the lips to form the flute-playing posture. At this time, exhale air slowly via the narrowed degree of lip-rounding. Meanwhile, contract the abdominal muscle and push the diaphragm upwards. Keep self training with this method until a perfect command is achieved.

8.2.5.2.3 Bathing

Seawater bath The seawater pressure, seawater lash and swimming movement can deepen breathing to enhance the respiratory function. If the seasonal condition permits, take seawater bath once a day or once every other day. The duration is not advisable to exceed 30 minutes.

Cave bath The air in the cave is fresh and contains a large number of negative oxygenic ions. This can keep the nasopharyngeal mucosa moist, relax the bronchus, improve the pulmonary ventilation function and increase blood oxygen. Accordingly, the method is applicable to the patients with this disease.

上可再选用歌咏疗法,或配合腹式呼吸进行练习。

2. 体育疗法

选择步行和健身跑,开始时可走、跑间歇交替,再逐步延长慢跑时间,缩短步行时间,最终过渡到全程慢跑。每次锻炼以出现轻微气短、气急为度。

平时坚持练习腹式呼吸,方法:放松肩背,思想集中,先呼后吸,吸鼓呼瘪。再用"吹笛样"呼气法,即将嘴唇缩成吹笛状,使气体通过缩窄的口形徐徐呼出,并收缩腹肌,推动膈肌上抬。该法坚持自我训练,直至运用自如。

3. 沐浴疗法

海水浴 海水压力、海水冲击及游泳动作可使呼吸加深,从而提高呼吸功能。条件许可的季节,每日1次或隔日1次。每次以不超过30分钟为宜。

洞穴浴 洞穴内空气清新,含有大量的负氧离子,可使鼻咽部黏膜保持湿润,支气管得到松弛,改善肺的换气功能,提高血氧含量,故适用于本病患者。

Sunbath Adopt the general sunbath, but long duration is not advisable. Besides, it is suitable to apply ultraviolet radiation, first on the whole body, then on the acupoints. As for the latter, apply ultraviolet radiation on the chest [Tiantu (CV 22) and Danzhong (CV 17)], back [Dazhui (GV 20), Feishu (BL 13), Gaohuang (BL 43) and Geshu (BL 17)] and waist [Shenshu (BL 23) and Mingmen (GV 4)] alternately. In the case of profuse sputum, add Zusanli (ST 36) and Fenglong (ST 40); in the case of susceptibility to common cold, add Hegu (LI 4) and Yongquan (KI 1).

8.2.5.2.4 Acumox and massage

Acupuncture: As for acumox, select Feishu (BL 13), Pishu (BL 20), Shenshu (BL 23), Gaohuang (BL 43), Qihai (CV 6), Zusanli (ST 36), Taiyuan (LU 9), Taixi (KI 3) and Mingmen (GV 4). Each time, select three to five acupoints from the above ones, once every other day. Use the reinforcing manipulation. Or select one pair of Jiaji acupoints from the first to sixth thoracic Jiaji acupoints and inject 0.5 to 1 ml of placental injection in each acupoint. Exchange the acupoints from the upper ones to the lower ones.

As for the ear acupuncture therapy, select Fei (MA-IC 1), Pi, Shen, Xin, Qiguan (MA-IC 2), Yanhou (MA-T 3), Ershenmen (MA-TF 1), Sanjiao (MA-IC 4) and Neifenmi (MA-IC 3). Apply the therapy once a week and use the needle-embedding method on three to five acupoints.

Moxibustion: Select Dazhui (GV 14), Fengmen (BL 12), Feishu (BL 13), Danzhong (CV 17), Shenshu (BL 23) and Qihai (CV 6). Apply the moxibustion with the wheat-grain-sized moxa cone in dog days. Use three to five moxa cones for each acupoint. Apply moxibustion once every ten days. Three times make up one course of

日光浴 采用全身日光浴,时间不宜长。亦可用紫外线照射,先全身照射,然后分部穴位照射,即胸部(天突、膻中)、背部(大椎、肺俞、膏肓、膈俞)和腰部(肾俞、命门)轮流照射。痰多则加足三里、丰隆,易感冒则加合谷、涌泉。

4. 针灸、推拿疗法

针灸 取肺俞、脾俞、肾俞、膏肓、气海、足三里、太渊、太溪、命门等穴。每次3~5穴,针用补法,隔日1次。或取胸1~6夹脊穴,每次选穴一对,每穴注射胎盘注射液0.5~1 ml,由上而下,逐日更换。

耳针 取肺、脾、肾、心、气管、咽喉、神门、三焦、内分泌等穴,每星期1次,每次埋针3~5穴。

灸法 取大椎、风门、肺俞、膻中、肾俞、气海等,用麦粒灸,于盛夏三伏天施灸。每穴每次灸3~5壮,10日灸1次,3次为一疗程。

treatment.

Massage: It is advisable to grasp and lift the back and spine, tighten the chest, rub and press the subhypochondriac region, knead Fengchi (GB 20) and Mingmen (GV 4), pinch Hegu (LI 4) and knead Xuehai (SP 10).

Self-massage

Wiping the chest　Wipe the region from one lateral shoulder to the subhypochondriac corner of the other side from the upper part to the lower part in an oblique line with the hands alternately for ten times respectively.

Patting the upper back　Pat the region from the bilateral pulmonary apexes along the thorax from the upper part to the lower part for ten times with the hands alternately and respectively (one time refers to one pat from the upper part to lower part).

Pounding the back　Form empty fists with the hands and then pound the back. When exhaling air, pound the back from the interior part to the exterior part with the empty fists. Simultaneously, bend the back slightly forwards. When inhaling air, pound the back from the exterior part to the interior part. Meanwhile, throw out the chest. This is a cycle. Repeat the cycle for ten times.

Massaging Danzhong (CV 17)　Massage Danzhong (CV 17) clockwise and anticlockwise respectively for 36 times with the palm. Then, massage the relevant acupoints according to the specific concurrent symptoms. In the case of cough and difficult expectoration, knead and press Tiantu (CV 22) [The thumb should knead and press the internal surface of the manubrium of sternum from Tiantu (CV 22) until soreness and distension appear]; in the case of short breath, tap Dingchuan (EX－B 1); in the case of profuse sputum, clench the fist and pound Fenglong (ST 40) with the dorsal parts of the interphalangeal joints

推拿　可用背脊拿提、束胸、摩按季肋下、揉风池、揉命门、捏合谷、揉血海等法。

自我按摩

抹胸　两手交替由一侧肩部由上至下呈斜线抹至另侧肋下角部,各重复10次。

拍肺　两手自两侧肺尖部开始沿胸廓自上而下拍打各 10 次(自上至下拍打算1次)。

捶背　两手握空拳置后背部,呼气时由里向外捶打,同时背稍前屈,吸气时由外向里捶打,同时挺胸,重复10次。

摩膻中穴　用手掌按于膻中穴,作顺、逆时针方向按摩各 36 次。然后,根据具体兼症按摩有关穴位,若咳嗽或喉中痰堵不易咳出,可揉按天突穴(注意拇指要从天突穴向胸骨柄内面揉压,以有酸胀感为宜)。若气急息促,可用指尖扣打定喘穴。若痰多,可用手握成拳状,以指间关节背侧捶打丰隆穴。

of hands.

8.2.5.2.5 Dietary therapy

In the case of pulmonary asthenia, select Huangqi Paste (Paste of *Radix Astragali seu Hedysari*); in the case of splenic asthenia, select Renshen Lianrou Gruel (Gruel of *Radix Ginseng* and *Semen Nelumbinis*); in the case of renal asthenia, select Wuweizi Paste (Paste of *Fructus Schisandrae*) and Thick Soup of Baiyangshen (Thick Soup of *Ren Caprae seu Ovis*) respectively. The prescriptions of the dietary therapy are:

Siren Jizi Gruel (Four-Kernel Gruel with Egg) One share of Baiguoren (*Semen Ginkgo*) and Tianxingren (*Semen Armeniacae*) respectively, two shares of Hutaoren (*Semen Juglandis*) and shelled peanut respectively. Grind the ingredients into powder and mix the powder evenly. Cook a bowl of gruel with 20 g of the powder, one egg and a proper amount of round-grained nonglutinous rice. Drink the gruel in every early morning. The ingestion of this gruel lasts for half a year.

Eggs Soaked in Wuweizi (*Fructus Schisandrae*) Decoction Decoct 250 g of Wuweizi (*Fructus Schisandrae*) in 3 kg of water for 30 minutes. When the decoction becomes cool, soak 20 eggs in it. The eggs will turn soft in six days. Eat one egg respectively in the morning and the evening after soaking the egg in hot water for five minutes to remove the shell.

Stew 50 g of pork with 30 g of Luxiancao (*Herba Pyrolae*) to be eaten at a draught.

8.2.5.2.6 External application of drugs on acupoints

Grind 20 g of Baijiezi (*Semen Sinapis Albae*) and Yanhusuo (*Rhizoma Corydalis*) respectively, 10 g of Gansui (*Radix Euphorbiae Kansui*) and Xixin (*Herba Asari*) respectively into powder. Then, add 0.6 g of

5. 食疗

肺虚证,可选用黄芪膏。脾虚证,用人参莲肉粥。肾虚证,可分别用五味子膏和白羊肾羹。食疗方剂有:

四仁鸡子粥 白果仁、甜杏仁各1份、胡桃仁、花生仁各2份,共研末和匀,每日清晨取20 g,鸡蛋1只,粳米适量,煮一碗服下,连用半年。

五味子蛋 五味子250 g,水3 kg,煮30分钟,待凉时用新鲜鸡蛋20只浸入汤内。6天后待蛋壳变软,即可取服。早晚各一只,热水中浸5分钟后去壳服下。

鹿衔草30 g,猪肉50 g,炖服。

6. 药物穴位敷贴

白芥子、延胡索各20 g,甘遂、细辛各10 g,共为末,加麝香0.6 g,和匀,在夏季三伏分三次用姜汁调敷肺俞、膏

Shexiang (*Moschus*) to the powder and mix them evenly. Mix the drug with fresh ginger juice in three different times of the three ten-dog-day periods respectively and apply the mixed drug on Feishu (BL13), Gaohuang (BL43) and Bailao (EX). Keep the drug on the acupoints for one to two hours, once in every ten days.

8.2.6 Diabetes

Diabetes corresponds to "xiao ke" in TCM. Pathologically, yin deficiency is the primary cause, and dryness and heat are the secondary ones. If the disease involves five zang organs, various complications may occur such as cataract, night blindness, deafness, boil, hypertension and myocardiac infarction.

8.2.6.1 Syndrome differentiation and treatment

8.2.6.1.1 Dryness and heat due to yin deficiency

It manifests dry mouth or thirst with inclination to drink, polyphagia, bulimia, cloudy and sweet urine, soreness and flaccidity of the waist and knees, dizziness, tinnitus, dry skin, red tongue with a little fur, thready and rapid pulse. It is advisable to nourish yin and tonify blood, clear away heat and moisten dryness. The prescription used is the modified Dihuang Decoction (Rehmannia Decoction) in combination with Liuwei Dihuang Bolus (Bolus of Six Drugs Including Rehmannia).

8.2.6.1.2 Deficiency of both yin and yang

It manifests frequent urination, very turbid urine, even urination immediately after drinking in severe cases, feverish palms and soles, dry throat and tongue, wan and sallow complexion, or blackish complexion, soreness and flaccidity of the waist and knees, cold limbs, aversion to cold, even impotency in severe cases, pale tongue with

肓、百劳等穴，约 1~2 小时，每 10 日敷 1 次。

六、糖尿病

糖尿病相当于中医的"消渴"证。病理上以阴虚为本，燥热为标，若损及五脏，则发生多种并发症，如白内障、雀盲、耳聋、痈疽、高血压、心肌梗死等。

【辨证施治】

1. 阴虚燥热

口干或口渴引饮，能食善饥，尿混浊或尿甜，腰膝酸软，头昏耳鸣，皮肤干燥，舌红少苔，脉细数。宜滋补阴血，清热润燥。地黄饮子合六味地黄丸加减。

2. 阴阳两亏

小便频数，混浊如膏，甚则饮一溲一，手足心热，咽干舌燥，面容憔悴，面色黧黑，腰膝酸软，四肢欠温，畏寒，甚则阳痿，舌淡苔白，脉沉细无力。宜温阳滋阴补肾。金匮肾气

whitish fur, deep and thready pulse without force. It is advisable to warm yang, nourish yin and tonify the kidney. The prescription used is the modified Jinkui Shenqi Pill.

8.2.6.1.3 Deficiency of splenogastric qi

It manifests thirst with the inclination to drink, coexistence of polyphagia and loose stool, or reduced appetite, listlessness, lassitude of limbs, pale tongue with whitish fur, thready and weak pulse without force. It is suitable to strengthen the spleen, supplement qi, promote the production of body fluids to quench thirst. The prescription used is the modified Qiwei Baizhu Powder (Seven-Ingredient Powder with Rhizoma Atractylodis Macrocephalae).

If the above syndromes have the complications of cataract, night blindness and deafness, it is suitable to nourish and tonify the liver and kidney, strengthen essence and nourish blood. The selected prescriptions include Mingmu Dihuang Bolus (Sight-Improving Bolus with *Radix Rehmanniae*), Shihu Yeguang Pill (Nyctalopia-Curing Pill with Herba Dendrobii), and Qiju Dihuang Bolus (Bolus of Six Drugs, *Rehmannia* with *Wolfberry* and *Chrysanthemum*), etc. In the case of the complication of boil, it is advisable to clear away heat and remove toxic substances. The prescription used is the modified Wuwei Xiaodu Decoction (Antiphlogistic Decoction of Five Drugs).

8.2.6.2 Rehabilitation Methods

The basic rehabilitation principle of the disease mainly lies in supplementing qi, nourishing yin, clearing away heat and promoting body fluids production. In the case of complications, the treatment should be based on the syndromes accordingly.

丸加减。

3. 脾胃气虚

口渴引饮,能食与便溏并见,或饮食减少,精神不振,四肢乏力,舌淡苔白,脉细弱无力。宜健脾益气,生津止渴。七味白术散加减。

上述各证型若并发白内障、雀盲、耳聋者,宜滋补肝肾,益精养血,方选明目地黄丸、石斛夜光丸及杞菊地黄丸等。并发痈疽者,宜清热解毒,方选五味消毒饮加减。

【康复方法】

本病康复当以益气养阴,清热生津为基本大法。若有并发症,则应随症施治。

8.2.6.2.1 Regulating emotions and recreation therapy

Please refer to the relevant part of the section of "Coronary heart disease".

8.2.6.2.2 Physical training

Physical training can improve the regulatory function of central nervous system, enhance the metabolic function of body, reduce the factors which easily cause diabetes (such as obesity, hyperlipemia and arteriosclerosis), consequently reducing blood-sugar. The patients may select events like walking, jogging, swimming, boating, cycling, Taijiquan and eight-section brocade, of which walking is the most common method. Take a walk once or twice a day, with a daily amount of exercise less than 5 km.

The patients with the administration of insulin should avoid excessive training during the maximal action period. Otherwise, the training may aggravate the hypoglycemic reaction. When having physical training at ordinary times, the patients should take some sweet with them for later use so as to prevent hypoglycemic reaction.

8.2.6.2.3 Acumox and massage

Acumox: In the case of dryness and heat due to yin deficiency, select Shuigou (GV 26), Chengjiang (CV 24), Jinjin (EX－HN 12), Yuye (EX－HN 13), Lianquan (CV 23), Quchi (LI 11), Laogong (PC 8), Taichong (LR 3), Xingjian (LR 2), Shangqiu (KI 7), Rangu (KI 2), Yinbai (SP 1), Sanyinjiao (SP 6), Shenshu (BL 23), Sanjiaoshu (BL 22), etc. Select three to five acupoints each time and adopt the reinforcing method and reducing method simultaneously. In the case of deficiency of both yin and yang, select Mingmen (GV 4) and Guanyuan (CV 4) in addition; in the case of splenogastric qi deficiency, select Pishu (BL 20), Weishu (BL 21), Qihai (CV 6) and Zusanli

1. 调节情志与娱乐疗法

参照"冠心病"。

2. 体育疗法

可改善中枢神经系统的调节功能,加强机体内新陈代谢功能,减少引起糖尿病的易患因素(如肥胖、高血脂和动脉硬化等),从而降低血糖水平。可选择步行、慢跑、游泳、划船、骑自行车、太极拳、八段锦等项目,其中步行是最常用的方法,每日1～2次,一日的总运动量不超过5 km。

使用胰岛素的患者,应避免在胰岛素的最大作用时间内过多运动,否则会使低血糖反应加重。锻炼时应随身带些糖果,以备发生低血糖反应时服用。

3. 针灸、推拿疗法

针灸 阴虚燥热证,取水沟、承浆、金津、玉液、廉泉、曲池、劳宫、太冲、行间、商丘、然谷、隐白、三阴交、肾俞、三焦俞等穴,每次选3～5穴,补泻兼施。若阴阳两亏证,可再配用命门、关元等穴。若脾胃气虚证,配用脾俞、胃俞、气海、足三里等穴。

(ST 36).

In the case of concurrent night blindness, select Chengqi (ST 1), Sibai (ST 2), Juliao (ST 3), Sanyinjiao (SP 6), Zusanli (ST 36) and Neiting (ST 44). Retain the needle for ten minutes. Apply the method once every other day. In the case of concurrent boil, select Quchi (LI 11), Chize (LU 5), Sanyinjiao (SP 6) and Zusanli (ST 36). Retain the needle for 15 minutes or so. Apply the method once every other day.

Ear acupuncture: Select the main acupoints of Yi (MA - SC 6) and Neifenmi (MA - IC 3) and the adjuvant acupoints of Shen, Sanjiao (MA - IC 4), Ermigen, Ershenmen (MA - TF 1), Xin and Gan (MA - SC 5). Apply the therapy with the filiform needle once every other day, or adopt the pill-pressing method. The return visit should be followed once every three to seven days. Select three or four acupoints each time.

In the case of concurrent cataract, select Yanqu and retain the needle for fifteen to thirty minutes. Apply the therapy once every other day. Twenty times make up one course of treatment. Or select the sensitive spots from Yan (MA - SC 5), Gan (MA - SC 6), Shen, Shenshangxian, Xin and Jiaogan (MA - AH 7). Then, apply Wangbuliuxingzi (Semen Vaccariae) on the spots. Select two or three such spots each time. Replace these spots with new ones once every three to five days. Apply the method on the two ears alternately.

Massage: Push the two sides of the spine, rub and scrub the back from the upper part to the lower part, knead the acupoint of the back, pinch and twirl the toes. In the case of concurrent ocular diseases, press, push and rub Shangdantian, digitally press the inner canthi and gently knead the upper and lower eyelids.

Self massage   Ask the patients to massage

Chengjiang (CV 24), Zhongwan (CV 12), Guanyuan (CV4), Qimen (LR 14) and Shenshu (BL 23) regularly. Massage each acupoint for eighteen to thirty-six times with the coordination of abdominal breathing.

8.2.6.2.4 Dietary therapy

Control the intake of sugar. Suddenly or gradually limit the intake of sugar in the staple food. At the beginning of the control over the diet, the patients may feel hungry. Then, they may eat some proper vegetables (except the melons with a high content of carbohydrate). If the conditions permit, it is advisable to eat for more times with less amount of food at a time. This can lessen the burden of islet cells. If the control over the diet alone fails to check the development of the state of illness, adopt other therapeutic methods. The patient should not depend on merely reducing food intake unlimitedly. Otherwise, it may give rise to ketoacidosis.

Eat more coix seeds, bran, pumpkins, red beans, celery, cabbage, chives, packchoi, spinach, wax gourds, tomatoes, soybeans, eggs, lean meat, etc. Onions, ricefield eels, soft-shelled turtles, etc. can help the organism make better use of glucose and have the action of reducing blood sugar. Therefore, eat them regularly.

The prescriptions of the dietary therapy include Thick Soup of Zhuji (*Medulla Suis*), Seamed Crucian Carp with Tea, etc. In the case of marked dryness and heat, select Five-Juice Drink; in the case of concurrent gastric qi deficiency, select Soup of Zhuyi (Pancreas Suis); in the case of concurrent boil and excessive heat, drink Green Gram Gruel regularly; in the case of ulcerated carbuncle with pus, Yiyiren Gruel (Gruel of *Semen Coicis*) is added.

8.2.6.2.5 Empirical recipes

Cut seven pigs' pancreas into pieces and cook the meat well. Then, add 500 g of honey to it to make paste. Take 15 g of the paste each time.

Remove the skin of one live Shuishe (*Creas Enhydris*) and mince the meat. Then, soak 50 snails in water to get rid of the saliva. Make the above two ingredients, together with a small amount of Tianhuafen (*Radix Trichosanthis*) and Shexiang (*Moschus*) respectively into pills. Take the pill with ginger soup.

Steam 30 g of Shanzhuyu (*Fructus Corni*), 20 g of Wuweizi (*Fructus Schisandrae*), 20 g of Wumei (*Fructus Mume*) and 20 g of Cangzhu (*Rhizoma Atractylodis*) in 2,000 ml of water until there is 1,000 ml of water left. Take the warm decoction three times in the morning, at noon and in the evening respectively. It is particularly applicable to deficiency of both yin and yang as well as non-insulin dependent diabetes.

Decoct three to five grams of Xingandujuan (*Cuculus Poliocephalus Xingan*), 3 g of Dingxiang (*Flos Caryophylli*), 12 g of Wuweizi (*Fructus Schisandrae*) and 1.5 g of Ganjiang (*Rhizoma Zingiberis*) in water for oral administration. Or make the above ingredients into granula or tablets. One course of treatment lasts for one month. It is particularly applicable to non-insulin dependent diabetes.

External application of drugs　Grind 5 g of Shigao (*Gypsum Fibrosum*), 2 g of Zhimu (*Rhizoma Anemarrhenae*), 0.6 g of Shengdihuang (*Radix Rehmanniae*), 0.6 g of Dangshen (*Radix Codonopsis Pilosulae*), 1 g of Zhigancao (prepared *Radix Glycyrrhizae*), 1 g of Xuanshen (*Radix Scrophulariae*), 0.2 g of Tianhuafen (*Radix Trichosanthis*), 0.3 g of Huanglian (*Rhizoma Coptidis*) and a bit of Jingmi (*Semen Oryzae*

5. 单方验方

猪胰七具，切碎煮熟，加蜂蜜500 g熬成膏，每次服15 g。

活水蛇一条去皮为末，天花粉末、麝香少许，蜗牛50个水浸去涎，做成丸服，姜汤下。

山茱萸30 g，五味子20 g，乌梅20 g，苍术20 g，加水2 000 ml，蒸至1 000 ml，分早、中、晚3次饭后温服，尤适用于阴阳两虚证。尤适用于非胰岛素依赖型糖尿病。

兴安杜鹃3～5 g，丁香3 g，五味子12 g，干姜1.5 g，水煎服，或制成冲剂、片剂，1个月为一疗程。尤适用于非胰岛素依赖型糖尿病。

药物敷脐　取石膏5 g，知母2 g，生地黄0.6 g，党参0.6 g，炙甘草1 g，玄参1 g，天花粉0.2 g，黄连0.3 g，粳米少许，制成粉剂，放阴处保存备用。每次取粉250 mg，加盐酸二甲双胍40 mg，混合敷脐，上盖以药棉，外用胶布固定。每

Sativae) into powder. Store the powder in the shade for later use. Mix 250 mg of the powder with 40 mg of dimethyldiguanide hydrochloride each time. Then, apply the drug on the navel covered with gauze and fixed with adhesive plaster. Conduct the dressing change once every five to seven days. Six times constitute one course of treatment.

8.2.7 Senile dementia

The main pathological changes of this disease are cerebral atrophia and degeneration mainly manifested by dementia in clinic.

8.2.7.1 Syndrome differentiation and treatment

8.2.7.1.1 Asthenia of the liver and kidney

Apathy, slow reaction, amnesia, insomnia, even asophia, incoherent speech and loss of self viability, red tongue with a little fur and thready pulse. It is advisable to nourish and tonify the liver and kidney, replenish medulla and tonify the brain. The prescription used is the modified Qifu Decoction, or the modified Dabuyin Bolus (Bolus for Replenishing Vital Essence) in combination with Shenrong Dihuang Pill.

8.2.7.1.2 Asthenia of the spleen and kidney

Rigid expression, slow movement, even hypologia and motionlessness, foolish cry and laugh, concurrent palpitation, short breath as well as soreness and cold of the waist and knees, pale tongue with whitish and thin fur, deep and thready pulse. It is advisable to tonify the kidney and strengthen the spleen, promote the production of medulla and tonify the brain. The prescription used is the modified Huanshao Pill (Rejuvenation Pill).

8.2.7.1.3 Obstruction of phlegm intermingled with qi stagnation

Keeping silent all day long, sudden alternate laughing

5～7天换药1次，每6次为一疗程。

七、老年性痴呆

本病以大脑的萎缩和变性为主要病理变化，以痴呆为主要临床表现。

【辨证施治】

1. 肝肾亏虚

神情淡漠，反应迟钝，健忘失眠，甚至发音不清，语无伦次，丧失生活自理能力，舌红少苔，脉细。宜滋补肝肾，填髓健脑。七福饮加减，或大补阴丸合参茸地黄丸加减。

2. 脾肾不足

表情呆板，行动迟缓，甚或终日寡言不动，傻哭傻笑，兼见心悸、气短、腰膝酸冷，舌淡，苔薄白，脉沉细。宜补肾益脾，生髓充脑。还少丹加减。

3. 痰气交阻

终日不言不语，忽笑忽

and anxiety, sudden alternate singing and cry, improper clothing, inability to distinguish good things from bad ones, loss of self viability in critical cases, concurrent chest tightness, heavy sensation of the body, somnolence, whitish and greasy fur, taut and slippery pulse. It is advisable to regulate qi, strengthen the spleen, resolve phlegm and induce resuscitation. The prescription used is the modified Xiaoyao Pill (Ease Pill) in combination with Xixin Decoction.

8.2.7.1.4 Blood stasis due to qi stagnation

Apathy, susceptibility to fright and fear, wild talk, purple tongue or with petechiae and ecchymoses, thready and taut or unsmooth pulse. It is advisable to promote blood circulation and qi flow, induce resuscitation to benefit intelligence. The prescription used is the modified Tongqiao Huoxue Decoction (Resuscitation-Inducing and Blood-Activating Decoction).

8.2.7.2 Rehabilitation methods

8.2.7.2.1 Regulating emotions

Select the method of checking one emotion with another, suggestion therapy or behavior therapy according to the specific conditions of the patients. Encourage and console the patients with depression as well as impetuosity and irascibility respectively and lingually to stabilize their emotions. By means of psychological guidance, encourage the patients to read newspapers, retell the content, tell stories and recite short articles. This can increase their abilities to discern, remember and judge things.

8.2.7.2.2 Recreation therapy

The musical therapy has good therapeutic effects. In the case of depression as the main symptom, select the musical prescriptions of "expressing emotions to remove depression" and the tunes of "inspiring enthusiasm and

愁，忽歌忽哭，衣被不敛，善恶不辨，重症则不能自理生活，伴见胸闷不舒，身重喜睡，苔白腻，脉弦滑。宜理气健脾，化痰宣窍。逍遥丸合洗心汤加减。

4．气滞血瘀

表情淡漠，善惊善恐，妄言离奇，舌质紫暗或有瘀点瘀斑，脉细弦或涩。宜活血行气，宣窍益智。通窍活血汤加减。

【康复方法】

1．调节情志

针对病人不同情况，选择以情制情法、暗示疗法，或行为疗法。对抑郁寡欢和急躁易怒的患者，应分别用语言予以鼓励和安慰，使其保持情绪稳定。可在心理诱导下，鼓励病人读书看报，复述所读内容，以及讲故事，背诵短文，逐步增加其识别、记忆、判断的能力。

2．娱乐疗法

音乐疗法有较好疗效。抑郁为主者，选用"抒情解郁"类、"振奋激昂"类乐曲；急躁易怒者，则选用"宁心安神"

arousing feeling"; in the case of impetuosity and irascibility, select musical prescriptions of "tranquilizing the mind" and tunes of "inhibiting impetuosity and checking anger". But, mainly select the prescriptions and tunes of improving intelligence. It is also advisable to select the songs which the patients were familiar with and liked when they were young. This can help the rehabilitation of the patients with senile dementia. Besides, watch plays, practice calligraphy and painting, play a musical instrument and play chess regularly. All these events may delay decline of intelligence, train the fine movements of hands simultaneously and promote the rehabilitation of the disease.

8.2.7.2.3 Physical training

Applying the setting-up ball is a better method. It is advisable to play the ball from simple movements to complicated and difficult ones. Train the left and right hands alternately with the ball and do not ignore the training of the left hand so as to guarantee the balanced development of the functions of the two cerebral hemispheres. In addition, it is suitable to practice the simplified Taijiquan, eight-section brocade, five mimic-animal games, etc.

8.2.7.2.4 Acumox and massage

Acumox The first group of acupoints includes Dazhui (GV 14), Anmian (EX), Shenmen (HT 7) and Zusanli (ST 36); the second group of acupoints include Yamen (GV 15), Baihui (GV 20), Anmian (EX) and Neiguan (PC 6); the ready-for-use acupoints include Shenshu (BL 23), Xinshu (BL 15), Fenglong (ST 40) and Taichong (LR 3). Puncture the two groups of acupoints alternately with strong stimulation, once a day. Ten days constitute one course of treatment. The next course of treatment is assumed in three to four days.

Ear acupuncture: Select Ershenmen (MA-TF 1),

Pizhixia (MA‑AT 1), Shen, Naodian, Zhen and Xin. Apply the method once a day. Select two to three acupoints each time. Twenty times make up one course of treatment. It is also advisable to attach anode and cathode of the electric stimulator to the two Shenmen acupoints of the ears respectely (use DC impulse generator with maximal voltage of 50 V, the frequency of 3 times per second and sine wave). Ask the patients or their relatives to control the current stimulation at ordinary times. Remove the stimulator only when the patients sleep at night. At the beginning, the time of current stimulation lasts for ten minutes each time in the daytime with an interval of ten minutes. After a week, electrify the ear acupoints four times a day. Each time lasts for thirty minutes.

Massage: Mainly apply self massage. It is advisable to use the methods of wiping the forehead, pressing the nape, beating the Tiangu (ear drum), rubbing the hands against each other to bathe the face, kneading Neiguan (PC6) and patting the vertex.

8.2.7.2.5 Dietary therapy

In the case of hepatorenal asthenia, select the combined use of Tianmendong Paste (Paste of *Radix Asparagi*) Stewed with Pork Liver and Xuanshen (*Radix Scrophulariae*); in the case of splenorenal asthenia, select Thick Soup of Baiyangshen (*Ren Caprae seu Ovis*); in the case of phlegm stagnation intermingled with qi stagnation, select Meihua Gruel (Gruel of *Flos Mume*); in the case of blood stasis due to qi stagnation, select Shanzha Gruel (Gruel of *Fructus Grataegi*) and Taoren Gruel (Gruel of *Semen Persicae*).

8.2.8 Senile pruritus

Senile pruritus mainly manifests skin irritation without primary skin rash. Its pathogenesis lies in generation

8 Rehabilitation Examples of Commonly Seen Diseases

of wind due to blood deficiency or stagnation of six exogenous factors in skin. General pruritus and localized itching are both common.

8.2.8.1 Syndrome differentiation and treatment

8.2.8.1.1 External attack by wind and cold

It manifests general pruritus without definite site and dry skin covered with squamae which mostly occur in winter or after attack by wind and cold, and of which pruritus is relieved by warmth, or concurrent aversion to cold and wind, whitish and thin fur, floating and tense or floating and slow pulse. It is advisable to eliminate wind, dispel cold and check itching. The prescription used is the modified Wind-Dispelling Powder. In the case of wet scratch and oozing of water due to scratching, add Cangzhu (*Rhizoma Atractylodis*), Zexie (*Rhizoma Alismatis*) and Baixianpi (*Cortex Dictamni Radicis*); in the case of spontaneous sweating due to exterior syndrome of deficiency, add Huangqi (*Radix Astragali seu Hedysari*) and Baizhu (*Rhizoma Atractylodis Macrocephalae*).

8.2.8.1.2 Excessive wind due to blood heat

It manifests itching, red skin with calor aggravated by warmth, drinking and eating pungent food, relieved by cold, or concurrent fever and aversion to wind, vexation, dry mouth, yellowish and thin fur, red tongue, floating and slippery or taut and rapid pulse. It is advisable to eliminate wind, clear away heat, cool blood and check itching. The prescription used is the modified Pruritus-Checking and Wind-Dispelling Decoction which is composed of Shengdihuang (*Radix Rehmanniae*), Danggui (*Radix Angelicae Sinensis*), Mudanpi (*Cortex Moutan Radicis*), Huangqin (*Radix Scutellariae*), Lianqiao (*Fructus Forsythiae*), Baijili (*Fructus Tribuli*), Jingjie (*Herba Schizonepetae*), Fangfeng (*Radix Ledebouriellae*), Bo-

病机为血虚生风,或六淫郁遏肌肤。全身性瘙痒、局限性瘙痒均可见到。

【辨证施治】

1. 风寒外袭

周身瘙痒无定处,皮肤干燥,上覆鳞屑,多发于冬季或受风寒后,温暖时瘙痒减轻;或伴畏寒恶风。舌苔薄白,脉浮紧或浮缓。宜祛风散寒止痒。消风散加减。搔抓引起湿烂、渗水,加苍术、泽泻、白鲜皮;表虚自汗者,加黄芪、白术。

2. 血热风盛

瘙痒,皮肤色红,扪之灼热,遇热或饮酒食辣后加重,遇冷减轻。或兼发热、恶风,心烦口干。舌苔薄黄,舌质红,脉浮滑或弦数。宜祛风清热,凉血止痒。止痒熄风汤(生地黄、当归、牡丹皮、黄芩、连翘、白蒺藜、荆芥、防风、薄荷、龙骨、甘草)加减。热甚,加紫草、栀子;便秘,加大黄、芒硝。

he (*Herba Menthae*), Longgu (*Os Draconis*) and Gancao (*Radix Glycyrrhizae*). In the case of severe heat, add Zicao (*Radix Arnebiae seu Lithospermi*) and Shanzhi (*Radix Pittospori*); in the case of constipation, add Dahuang (*Radix et Rhizoma Rhei*) and Mangxiao (*Natrii Sulfas*).

8.2.8.1.3 Dyness of blood due to yin deficiency

It manifests susceptibility to onset in autumn and winter, dry skin covered with squamae, wide-spread scratches, severe nocturnal itching, thickened skin in the scratched area, or concurrent palpitation, insomnia, red or reddish tongue, taut and thready pulse. It is advisable to nourish yin and blood, moisten dryness and check itching. The prescription used is the modified Yangxue Runfu Decoction (Blood-Nourishing and Skin-Moistening Decoction). In the case of purple skin scratches and deep purple tongue, add Sumu (*Lignum Sappan*), Taoren (*Semen Persicae*) and Zaojiaoci (*Spina Gleditsiae*); in the case of itching worsened by emotional changes, add Tianma (*Rhizoma Gastrodiae*), Gouteng (*Ramulus Uncariae cum Uncis*), Longgu (*Os Draconis*) and Muli (*Choncha Ostreae*).

8.2.8.1.4 Downward flow of dampness and heat

It manifests pruritus mostly occurring around the anus and pudenda suddenly, secondary skin rash, pustulae, oozing of water and pain after scratching, concurrent foul leukorrhea with yellowish colour, red tongue with yellowish and greasy fur, taut, slippery and rapid pulse. It is advisable to clear away heat, promote diuresis, expel wind and check itching. The prescription used is Longdan Xiegan Decoction (Decoction of Gentiana for Purging the Liver Fire) with additional Muli (*Concha Ostreae*),

3. 阴虚血燥

多发于秋冬，皮肤干燥，上覆鳞屑，遍布抓痕，夜间痒甚，搔抓处皮肤增厚。或兼心慌失眠。舌红或淡红，脉弦细。宜滋阴养血，润燥止痒。养血润肤饮加减。如皮肤抓痕色紫，舌紫黯者，加苏木、桃仁、皂角刺；瘙痒遇情绪波动而加重者，加天麻、钩藤、龙骨、牡蛎。

4. 湿热下注

瘙痒多发于肛门、阴部，常突然发作，搔抓后继发丘疹、脓疱、渗水、疼痛，妇女伴带下腥臭色黄。舌质红，苔黄腻，脉弦滑数。宜清热利湿，祛风止痒。龙胆泻肝汤加牡蛎、黄柏、白蒺藜、白鲜皮。女阴瘙痒，带下腥臭者，加土茯苓、蛇床子；肛门瘙痒者，加苦

Huangbai (*Cortex Phellodendri*), Baijili (*Fructus Tribuli*) and Baixianpi (*Cortex Dictamni Radicis*). In the case of pruritus vulvae and fishy leukorrhea, add Tufuling (*Rhizoma Smilacis Glabrae*) and Shechuangzi (*Fructus Cnidii*); in the case of anal pruritus, add Kushen (*Radix Sophorae Flavescentis*) and Difuzi (*Fructus Kochiae*); in the case of scrotal pruritus, add Chantui (*Periostracum Cicadae*).

8.2.8.2 Rehabilitation Methods

8.2.8.2.1 Regulating emotions

The disease is closely related to emotional factors. Therefore, the patients should remain a cheerful frame of mind and avoid being in an anxious state of mind.

8.2.8.2.2 Recreation therapy

Please refer to the relevant part of the section of "Coronary heart disease".

8.2.8.2.3 Acumox

Acupuncture Select Quchi (LI 11), Hegu (LI 4), Xuehai (SP 10), Zusanli (ST 36), Fengchi (GB 20), Sanyinjiao (SP 6), Yinlingquan (SP 9) and Fengfu (GV 16). Puncture two to four acupoints each time. In the case of sthenia syndrome, use the reducing manipulation; in the case of asthenia syndrome, use the reinforcing manipulation. Retain the needle for ten to twenty minutes. Puncture the acupoints once a day. Ten times constitute one course of treatment.

Ear acupuncture: Select Ershenmen (MA-TF 1), Jiaogan (MA-AH 7), Shenshangxiang, Neifenmi (MA-IC3), Feiqu and Yangdian. Each time, select two to three acupoints with the method of embedding the needle on one ear. Change the ears alternately in one week.

8.2.8.2.4 Dietary therapy

In the case of downward flow of dampness and heat, select Yiyiren Gruel (*Gruel of Semen Coicis*); in the

参、地肤子；阴囊瘙痒者，加蝉蜕。

【康复方法】

1. 调节情志

本病与精神因素较为密切，应保持精神愉快，防止情绪波动。

2. 娱乐疗法

参见"冠心病"。

3. 针灸疗法

针灸　取曲池、合谷、血海、足三里、风池、三阴交、阴陵泉、风府，每次2～4穴，实证用泻法，虚证用补法，留针10～20分钟，每日1次，10次为1疗程。

耳针　取神门、交感、肾上腺、内分泌、肺区、痒点，每次选2～3穴，单耳埋针，两侧交替，1星期后轮换。

4. 食疗

湿热下注者，选薏苡仁粥；血热风盛者，用米醋、红糖

case of excessive wind due to blood heat, decoct 30 g of rice vinegar and brown sugar respectively and take the decoction in two different times; in the case of dryness of blood due to yin deficiency, select Thick Soup of Wushe (*Zao-cys*) or Chanchu Shuishe Gruel (Gruel of *Bufo* and *Creas Enhydris*); in the case of external attack by wind and cold, pound 500 g of fresh chives to juice and take 100 ml of the juice orally while applying the rest on the itching part.

At ordinary times, abstain from pungent food, smoking and drinking as well as seafood and fishy foods such as hot pepper, Chinese prickly ash, Chinese green onion, garlic, fish, shrimp, soft-shelled turtle, milk, mushroom, red bayberry, pot herb mustard, rape, three-colored amaranth, coriander, meat of pork head and cock. Besides, pay attention to the pathogenic foods and avoid eating them.

8.2.8.2.5 Empirical recipes

Decoct 30 g of Fuping (*Herba Spirodelae*) and Difuzi (*Fructus Kochiae*) in water for oral administration; or decoct 30 g of Shengdihuang (*Radix Rehmanniae*), 10 g of Danggui (*Radix Angelicae Sinensis*), 15 g of Baijili (*Fructus Tribuli*), Kushen (*Radix Sophorae Flavescentis*), Baixianpi (*Cortex Dictamni Radicis*) and Bohe (*Herba Menthae*) respectively in water. Use the decoction to fumigate and wash the affected part.

8.3 Rehabilitation for malignant tumor

The rehabilitation of the patients with malignant tumor is mainly to lessen the injury, toxic and side effects in the patients due to the antitumor treatment like operation, chemotherapy and radiotherapy, increase the immunity of the body, control the metastasis and recurrence, promote the restoration of the health. The rehabilitation may prolong the life and relieve pain of the patients in the middle and late stages.

8.3.1 Cancer of digestive tract

Cancer of digestive tract includes the malignant tumor such as esophageal cancer, gastric cancer, carcinoma of colon and rectal cancer, the clinical symptoms of which are related to the position of the tumor. The tumor is removed or controlled by means of the antitumor treatment. However, the healthy qi of the human body is often impaired to various degrees because of the operation, chemotherapy and radiotherapy. As a result, the healthy qi is consumed and becomes deficient. In addition, the operational complications or the reactions of chemotherapy and radiotherapy are again related to qi stagnation, blood stasis and the unsmooth circulation of qi and blood. These form the pathogenesis of asthenia in origin and sthenia in superficiality.

8.3.1.1 Syndrome differentiation and treatment

8.3.1.1.1 Blood stasis due to qi stagnation

It manifests stabbing pain with distenison of esophageal, epigastric and abdominal regions, of which the painful sites mostly correspond to the pathological sites, thoracic and abdominal hardness or hard massees, or occasional eructation, blackish stool, deep red tongue or with ecchymoses, thready and unsmooth pulse. It is advisable to promote blood circulation to remove blood stasis. The prescription used is the modified Xuefu Zhuyu Decoction (Decoction for Removing Blood Stasis in the Chest) or Gexia Zhuyu Decoction (Decoction for Dissipating Blood

Stasis under Diaphram). In the case of severe qi stagnation, add Yujin (*Radix Curcumae*), Quangualou (*Fructus Trichosanthis*), Muxiang (*Radix Aucklandiae*) and Sharenke (*Pericarpium Amomi*); in the case of severe blood stasis, add Zhechong (*Eupolyhage seu Steleophaga*), Qianglangchong (*Catharsius*), Jixingzi (*Semen Impatientis*), Zicao (*Radix Arnebiae seu Lithospermi*) and Danshen (*Radix Salviae Miltiorrhizae*).

8.3.1.1.2 Internal accumulation of dampness and heat

It manifests thoracic and epigastric calor and discomfort worsened by ingestion, concurrent pain, thirst, red tongue, yellowish and greasy fur, taut and rapid or taut and slippery pulse, congestion of fistulous mouth with pain or oozing of liquid when it is pressed after fistulation due to carcinoma of colon. It is advisable to clear away heat and dry dampness. The prescription used is the modified Huanglian Jiedu Decoction (Antidotal Decoction of Coptis). In the case of consumption of yin and body fluids due to dampness and heat, add Shengdihuang (*Radix Rehmanniae*), Xuanshen (*Radix Scrophulariae*), Maimendong (*Radix Ophiopogonis*) and Tianhuafen (*Radix Trichosanthis*); in the case of concurrent qi stagnation, add Qingpi (*Pericarpium Citri Reticulatae Viride*), Chenpi (*Pericarpium Citri Reticulatae*), Chaihu (*Radix Bupleuri*), Zhike (*Fructus Aurantii*) and Baishaoyao (*Radix Paeoniae Alba*); in the case of excessive heat, add Baihuasheshecao (*Herba Hedyotis Diffusae*), Longkui (*Herba Solani Nigri*), Banzhilian (*Herba Scutellariae Barbatae*) and Shemei (*Herba Duchesneae Indicae*); in the case of profuse fluid oozing from the fistulous mouth of carcinoma of colon, add Ermiao Powder (Two Wonderful Drugs Powder).

2. 湿热内蕴

胸脘灼热不适,进食时尤为明显,并可伴有疼痛,口渴,舌红,苔黄腻,脉弦数或弦滑。若结肠癌造瘘手术后,可见瘘口红肿,触之疼痛,或有液体渗出。当清热燥湿。黄连解毒汤加减。若阴液为湿热所伤,可加用生地黄、玄参、麦门冬、天花粉等;如伴有气机郁滞者,可加用青皮、陈皮、柴胡、枳壳、白芍药等;如热毒较盛者,可加用白花蛇舌草、龙葵、半枝莲、蛇莓等。结肠、直肠癌瘘口渗液较多,可加用二妙散。

8.3.1.1.3 Incoordination between the liver and stomach

It manifests dysphagia, epigastric tightness and fullness, frequent vomiting and regurgitation or eructation, occasional inclination to sigh, distending pain of hypochondriac regions, vexation, irascibility, thin fur and taut pulse. It is advisable to disperse the liver and regulate the stomach. The prescription used is the modified Chaihu Shugan Decoction (Bupleurum Decoction for Dispersing the Liver). In the case of severe adversely rising gastric qi and lingering vomiting and nausea, add Xuanfuhua (*Flos Inulae*), Daizheshi (*Haematitum*), Zhuru (*Caulis Bambusae in Taeniam*), Huanglian (*Rhizoma Coptidis*), Wuzhuyu (*Fructus Euodiae*) and Jiangbanxia (prepared *Rhizoma Pinelliae*).

8.3.1.1.4 Obstruction of phlegm stagnation intermingled with blood stasis

It manifests hardness and pain of thoracic, epigastric and abdominal tumorous regions, pain with definite site or lumps, thoracic and diaphragmatic distension and tightness, vomiting of sputum and saliva, or blackish stool, dyschezia or stool with pus and blood as well as foul odor, dark red tongue with purple spots or ecchymoses, thready and unsmooth, or thready, slippery and rapid pulse. It is advisable to resolve phlegm and remove blood stasis. In the case of esophageal carcinoma, use the modified Qige Powder in combination with Taohong Decoction; in the case of gastric carcinoma, use the modified Haizao Yuhu Decoction; in the case of colonic carcinoma and rectal carcinoma, use the modified Yiyi Fuzi Baijiang Powder (Powder of *Semen Coicis*, *Radix Aconiti Praeparata* and *Herba Patriniae*) in combination with Rhubark Powder. In the case of severe vomiting of sputum and saliva, add Quanguanlou (*Fructus Trichosanthis*), Fabanxia

3. 肝胃不和

吞咽不利,胃脘闷满,时时呕逆或嗳气,时欲叹息,两胁胀痛,心烦易怒,苔薄,脉弦。宜疏肝和胃。柴胡疏肝汤加减。如胃气上逆,呕恶不止,可加用旋覆花、代赭石、竹茹、黄连、吴茱萸、姜半夏等。

4. 痰瘀交阻

胸、脘、腹肿瘤部位痞硬疼痛,痛有定处,或有肿块,胸膈胀闷,泛吐痰涎,或有黑便,大便细而艰难,或便脓血,有恶臭气味,舌质暗红有紫气或瘀斑,脉细涩,或脉细滑而数。宜化痰散瘀。食道癌用启膈散合桃红饮加减,胃癌用海藻玉壶汤加减,结肠、直肠癌用薏苡附子败酱散合大黄汤加减。如泛吐痰涎较甚,可加用全瓜蒌、法半夏、白芥子、代赭石等。若呕如赤豆汁或黑便,可加用仙鹤草、白及、参三七等。若患处扪及肿块,或痰核累累,可加用龙葵、肿节风、铁树叶、菝葜等。

(*Rhizoma Pinellinae Praeparata*), Baijiezi (*Semen Sinapis Albae*) and Daizheshi (*Ochra Haematitum*); in the case of vomiting like red bean juice or in the case of blackish stool, add Xianhecao (*Herba Agrimoniae*), Baiji (*Rhizoma Bletillae*) and Shensanqi (*Radix Notoginseng*); in the case of lump in the affected part or subcutaneous phlegm nodules, add Longkui (*Herba Solani Nigri*), Zhongjiefeng (*Folium et Ramulus Sarcandrae*), Tieshuye (*Folium Cycadis Revolutae*) and Baqia (*Rhizoma Smilacls Chinensis*).

8.3.1.1.5 Yin consumption of the lung and stomach

It manifests emaciation, dry mouth and throat, thirst with inclination to drink, or foul breath, dysphoria with feverish sensation of the chest, palms and soles, thoracic, dorsal and epigastric burning pain, constipation, uncoated and smooth tongue, thready and rapid pulse. It is advisable to nourish yin and fluid of the lung and stomach. In the case of esophageal carcinoma, use the modified Shashen Maidong Decoction (Decoction of *Glehnia* and *Ophiopogon*); in the case of gastric carcinoma, use the modified Zhuye Shigao Decoction (Lophatherum and Gypsum Decoction). In the case of yin consumption and severe heat, add Shandougen (*Radix Sophoare Subprostratae*), Pugongying (*Herba Taraxaci*), Jinyinhua (*Flos Lonicerae*), Baihuasheshecao (*Herba Hedyotis Diffusae*) and Banzhilian (*Herba Scutellariae Barbatae*). In the case of consumption involving hepatorenal yin, use the modified Yiguan Decoction (An Ever Effective Decoction for Nourishing the Liver and Kidney) or Pulsation-Promoting Decoction.

8.3.1.1.6 Deficiency of both qi and blood

It manifests emaciation, lustreless complexion, lassitude, hypodynamia, short breath, palpitation, dull pain of

5. 肺胃阴伤

形体消瘦，口干咽燥，渴欲饮水，或口中有臭秽之气，五心烦热，胸背、胃脘灼痛，大便干结，舌红苔光剥，脉细数。宜滋养肺胃阴液。食道癌用沙参麦冬汤加减，胃癌用竹叶石膏汤加减。若阴伤而热毒尤甚，可加用山豆根、蒲公英、金银花、白花蛇舌草、半枝莲等。如已耗竭肝肾真阴，则可用一贯煎或加减复脉汤加减。

6. 气血两亏

形体消瘦，面色无华，倦息乏力，气短心悸，肿瘤患处

neoplastic part, pale tongue, thready and weak pulse. It is advisable to supplement qi and tonify blood. The prescription used is the modified Bazhen Decoction (Eight Precious Ingredients Decoction). In the case of concurrent deficiency of yang qi, add Shufuzi (*Radix Aconiti Praeparata*) and Danganjiang (*Rhizoma Zingiberis*).

8.3.1.1.7 Digestive cancer after radiotherapy and chemotherapy

In the case of arrest of bone marrow, marked leukopenia and thrombocytopenia after the treatment of carcinoma of digestive tract with radiotherapy and chemotherapy, decoct Dangshen (*Radix Codonopsis Pilosulae*), Danggui (*Radix Angelicae Sinensis*), Huangqi (*Radix Astragali seu Hedysari*), Gouqizi (*Fructus Lycii*), Gusuibu (*Rhizoma Drynariae*), Cebaiye (*Cacumen Biotae*), Tianmendong (*Radix Asparagi*), Dongguazi (*Semen Benincasae*), Heidou (*Semen Sojae Nigrum*) and Huzhang (*Rhizoma Polygoni Cuspidati*).

8.3.1.2 Rehabilitation methods

8.3.1.2.1 Regulating emotions

Teach the patients how to control their emotions by themselves and cultivate the mind. In the case of anxiety, restlessness, pessimism and depression, guide them to relax themselves mentally by means of conversation, reading books and newspapers, recreation, etc.

8.3.1.2.2 Recreation therapy

Guide the patients to participate in recreational activities with joyous atmosphere according to the patients' abilities and specific conditions of anticancer therapies. If the patients are in a depressed state, let them listen to more lively, beautiful and elegant music, arrange them to receive convalescence in the beautiful wooded mountains and seasides.

隐痛,舌淡,脉细弱。宜补益气血。八珍汤加减。若兼有阳气虚衰者,可加用熟附子、淡干姜等。

7. 消化道癌症放疗、化疗

有骨髓抑制,白细胞、血小板等显著减少者,可用党参、当归、黄芪、枸杞子、骨碎补、侧柏叶、天门冬、冬瓜子、黑豆、虎杖等制方煎服。

【康复方法】

1. 调节情志

教会病人自我控制情绪,涵养精神。如出现焦躁、悲观、抑郁情绪,要指导其通过交谈、阅读书报、娱乐等方法来松弛精神。

2. 娱乐疗法

根据病人的能力和接受抗癌疗法的具体情况,指导其参加具有喜悦气氛的娱乐活动,如病人心情抑郁,可以多听一些旋律欢快、优美、悠扬的音乐,安排到风景优美的山林、海边疗养等。

8.3.1.2.3 Acumox and massage
(1) Esophageal carcinoma

Acumox: In the case of anastomotic inflammation, edema and stenosis after the operation, select Zusanli (ST 36), Xiajuxu (ST 39), Danzhong (CV 17), Zhongting (CV 16), Yutang (CV 18) and Neiguan (PC 6) and needle them with the reducing manipulation; in the case of the patients with weak constitution, apply the reinforcing method and reducing method simultaneously and retain the needles for twenty minutes, once a day; in the case of severe reactions of digestive tract after the chemotherapy or radiotherapy, select Neiguan (PC 6), Zusanli (ST 36), Neiting (ST 44) and Zhongwan (CV 12) with concurrent use of the reinforcing and reducing methods and retain the needles for fifteen minutes once a day; in the case of failure to receive a radical cure in the patients with late cancer, select Tiantu (CV 22), Danzhong (CV 17), Zusanli (ST 36), Shenzhu (GV 12), Lingtai (GV 10), Zhiyang (GV 9), Geshu (BL 17), Pishu (BL 20), Weishu (BL 21) and Huatuojiaji (EX) with the concurrent use of the reinforcing and reducing methods and retain the needles for twenty to thirty minutes once a day; in the case of deficiency of yang qi, apply moxibustion on Qihai (CV 6) in addition.

Ear acupuncture: Apply the therapy mainly on Shidao (MA - IC 6), Wei, Jiaogan (MA - AH 7) and Xiong (MA - AH 11). Select two or three acupoints each time and retain the needles for an hour. Apply the method once every other day. Or adopt the needle-embedding with the intradermal needles. Embed the needle in each acupoint for five days.

Gastric carcinoma

Acumox: In the case of the patients with the manifestations of dumping syndrome, select Zusanli (ST 36), Zhongwan (CV 12), Xiawan (CV 10), Liangmen (ST 21)

3. 针灸、推拿疗法
食管癌

针灸 手术后吻合口炎症、水肿、狭窄者，取足三里、下巨虚、膻中、中庭、玉堂、内关等穴，可用泻法，如患者体质较差，用补泻兼施法，留针20分钟，每日1次。如化疗或放疗后消化道反应严重，取内关、足三里、内庭、中脘等穴，多用补泻兼施法，留针15分钟，每日1次。对于未能作根治治疗的晚期患者，取天突、膻中、足三里、身柱、灵台、至阳、膈俞、脾俞、胃俞以及华佗夹脊穴等，手法宜补泻兼施，留针20~30分钟，每日1次。如阳气衰微者，可加灸气海穴。

耳针 以食道、胃、交感、胸为主，每次取2~3穴，留针1小时，隔日1次，或用皮内针埋针，每穴埋五天。

胃癌
针灸 表现为倾倒综合征者，取足三里、中脘、下脘、梁门、内庭等穴，用补泻兼施

and Neiting (ST 44) with the simultaneous use of reinforcing and reducing methods. Besides, additional moxibustion is applicable to Zusanli (ST 36), Weishu (BL 21) and Qihai (CV 6). In the case of severe reaction of digestive tract after the chemotherapy, select Zusanli (ST 36), Neiguan (PC 6), Waiguan (TE 5) and Neiting (ST 44). Adopt the reducing method and retain the needles for fifteen to twenty minutes. The therapy is pre-ferred two to four hours before the chemotherapy. In the case of severe gastralgia in the patients with late gastric cancer, select Zusanli (ST 36) and Zhongwan (CV 12) with concurrent use of reinforcing and reducing methods. Besides, the reducing method or the cupping therapy is applicable to Gongsun (SP 4). These methods have better analgesic effect. In the case of splenogastric asthenic cold and vomiting, select Qihai (CV 6), Guanyuan (CV 4), Zusanli (ST 36) and Geshu (BL 17). Moxibustion is applicable to all the above acupoints additionally.

Ear acupuncture: As for the ear acupuncture therapy, mainly select Fei (MA-IC 1), Pi, Jiaogan (MA-AH 7) and Gan (MA-SC 5). Select two or three acupoints each time and retain the needles for an hour. Apply the therapy once every other day. Or adopt the needle-embedding method with the intradermal needles. Embed each acupoint for five days.

(2) Colonic cancer and rectal cancer

Acumox: Select Zusanli (ST 36), Dachangshu (BL 25), Guanyuan (CV 4), Tianshu (ST 25), Shangjuxu (ST 37), Xiajuxu (ST 39) and Changqiang (GV 1) with the simultaneous application of the reinforcing and reducing methods. Retain the needles for twenty minutes once a day. In the case of severe nausea and vomiting, add Neiguan (PC 6) and needle it with the reducing method; in the case of severe abdominalgia, Gongsun (SP 4) with the reducing method; in the case of general weakness and hypodynamia, apply moxibustion on Qihai (CV 6) and Guanyuan (CV 4) additionally.

Ear acupuncture: As for the ear acupuncture therapy, mainly select Dachang, Xiaochang, Fu, Jiaogan and Pixia. Select two or three acupoints each time and retain the needles for an hour. Or adopt the needle-embedding therapy with the intradermal needles, or apply Wangbuliuxingzi (Semen Vaccariae) on the acupoint and press it.

Massage: Mainly press the acupoints of stomach meridian of foot-yangming, spleen meridian of foot-taiyin, large intestine meridian of hand-yangming and conception vessel. Besides, it is advisable to adopt the manipulations of horizontally rubbing the upper abdomen, obliquely rubbing the abdomen and rubbing the periumbilical region. For the patients failing to receive a radical cure, massage is not advisable on the local part of tumor. But it is advisable to digitally press, scrub and knead the relevant acupoints on the abdomen, back and limbs such as Zusanli (ST 36), Weishu (BL 21), Pishu (BL 20), Qihai (CV 6), Neiguan (PC 6), Waiguan (TE 5), Danzhong (CV 17) and Tiantu (CV 22). The patients may select Zusanli (ST 36), Shangwan (CV 13), Zhongwan (CV 12) and Xia-wan (CV 10) to apply self massage. Rub the acupoints with the palm for fifteen minutes one hour after the meals every day.

8.3.1.2.4 Dietary therapy

In the case of postoperational anastomotic inflammation and edema, select Shanyao Lianyi Gruel (Gruel of *Rhizoma Discoreae*, *Semen Nelumbinis* and *Semen Coicis*) and Lizhi Biandou Decoction (Decoction of Lychee and Hyacinth Bean); in the case of yin consumption of the lung and stomach or yin deficiency occurring in other syndromes, select Five-Juice Drink and Mulberry Paste; in the case of the patients with late cancer failing to receive

耳针 以大肠、小肠、腹、交感、皮质下为主。每次取2～3穴，留针1小时。或用皮内针埋针，或用王不留行子穴位贴压。

推拿 重点按足阳明、足太阴、手阳明、任脉等经脉穴位经穴，并可选用上腹横摩法、腹部斜摩法、脐周围摩法等。未作根治术的患者，在肿瘤局部不宜进行推拿，但可在腹部、背部、四肢有关穴位上进行点按擦揉，如足三里、胃俞、脾俞、气海、内关、外关、膻中、天突等。病人也可进行自我按摩法，取足三里及上、中、下脘穴，每日饭后1小时用掌心按摩15分钟。

4. 食疗

手术后吻合口有炎症、水肿者，可选用怀山药莲薏粥、荔枝扁豆汤。对于肺胃阴伤证或其他证型中出现阴虚者，可选用五汁饮、桑椹子膏。对于未获根治的晚期病人，可选用菱角薏苡仁粥、鲜鱼冻。

a radical cure, select Lingjiao Yiyiren Gruel (Gruel of *Fructus Trapae Bispinosae* and *Semen Coicis*) and fresh fish jelly.

The patients with esophageal cancer and gastric cancer may select Dysphagia Paste or drink goose's blood (draw five to ten ml of blood from the vessel under the wing of the goose and drink it while it is warm with rice wine). In the case of dysphagia, swallow fresh chives juice (or add milk to it) slowly, 200 to 300 ml each day. Besides, it is advisable to eat Egg Stewed with Hetaozhi (Ramulus Juglandis). In the case of gastric cancer due to asthenic cold, cook one Zhudu (*Ventriculus Suis*), 30 g of Hujiao (*Fructus Piperis Nigri seu Albi*) and a proper amount of condiment until the meat is thoroughly cooked. Eat the meat. In the case of gastric heat consuming yin, use 50 g of fresh lotus root, 200 ml of fresh milk, 50 g of shelled peanuts and 30 ml of honey. First, pound the shelled peanut and fresh lotus root to paste. Then, add milk and honey to the paste. Finally, decoct all the ingredients together. Take 30 to 50 ml every evening. In the case of colonic cancer and rectal cancer complicated by stool with pus and blood, cut 200 g of Machixian (*Herba Portulacae*) into pieces and pound the pieces to paste to extract the juice. Then, add a proper amount of brown sugar to the juice. Finally, stew the juice in a pot for 20 minutes for oral administration.

In the case of carcinoma of digestive tract with severe qi stagnation, decoct 10 g of Xuanfuhua (*Flos Inulae*), Laifuzi (*Semen Raphani*) and Shashen (*Radix Adenophorae*) respectively. Then, keep the decoction and remove the dregs. Next, add 30 g of Yiyiren (*Semen Coicis*) to the decoction to cook gruel for ingestion. One dose is for a day and 15 to 20 days constitute one course of treatment. In the case of severe blood stasis, fry Yubiao

食道癌、胃癌可选用噎膈膏或饮用鹅血（用针管抽取鹅翅下血管血液5～10 ml，趁热用米酒冲饮）。吞咽困难者，可用鲜韭菜汁或加牛奶缓缓咽下，每日200～300 ml。也可服用核桃枝鸡蛋。胃癌属虚寒者，可用猪肚1个，胡椒30 g，适当加入调料煮烂服用。如表现为胃热阴伤者，可用鲜藕50 g、鲜牛奶200 ml、花生仁50 g、蜂蜜30 ml，将花生仁、鲜藕捣烂，加牛奶、蜂蜜共煮，每晚服30～50 ml。结肠、直肠癌大便带脓血者，可用鲜马齿苋200 g切碎捣烂挤汁，加适量红糖上锅内炖20分钟，取服。

消化道癌症患者如气滞较甚者，可用旋覆花、莱菔子、沙参各10 g，煎取汤，去渣，加入薏苡仁30 g煮粥服，每日1剂，15～20日为1疗程。如瘀血较甚者，可用黄花鱼鳔以香油炸脆，研末，每次5 g，加参三七末3 g，用黄酒冲服，每日

(*Pneumatophorus Pseudosciaenae*) of the yellow croaker with sesame oil until it is crisp. Then, grind it into powder. Each time, use 5 g of the powder and additional 3 g of the powder of Sanqi (*Radix Notoginseng*) to be mixed with millet wine for oral administration, one dose a day and 15 to 20 days make up one course of treatment. In the case of severe deficiency of qi and blood, wash one live crucian carp clean. Then, cut one garlic into thin slices. Next, place the slices inside the abdomen of the crucian carp. At this time, wrap the crucian carp in a piece of paper and cover the whole crucian carp with mud. Afterwards, roast it till the mud is dry. Take out the crucian carp and ground it into fine powder. Take 3 g of the powder each time by mixing it in the decoction of ten jujubes, 12 g of Dangshen (*Radix Codonopsis Pilosulae*) and 6 g of Chenpi (*Pericarpium Citri Reticulatae*), one dose a day. In the case of severe nausea due to yin deficiency, it is advisable to drink goat's milk; in the case of constipation and abdominal distension, eat 250 g of spinach and 6 garlics, or drink Laifuzi Gruel (Gruel of *Semen Raphani*); in the case of hematochezia, use Huaihua Decoction (Decoction of *Flos Sophorae*); or Wumei Gruel (Gruel of *Fructus Mume*) and Stewed Egg with Lotus Juice and Sanqi (*Radix Notoginseng*); in the case of the patients with late cancer, weak constitution and poor appetite, it is advisable to select Stewed Rabbit's Meat with Jujubes, Jujube Nutrition Gruel, Sweet Thick Soup of Yin'er (*Tremella*) and Stewed Egg with Hetaozhi (*Ramulus Juglandis*).

Regulating the diet is of vital importance for nursing the patients with carcinoma of digestive tract. After the operation, the patients should mainly ingest the liquid and semiliquid diet, and decrease the amount of each intake and increase the times of intakes. The food should be

1剂，15～20日为1疗程。如气血虚甚者，可用活鲫鱼一尾洗净，加大蒜一头去皮切细填入鱼腹，纸包泥封煨干取出，研细，每次3g，另用大枣10枚、党参12g、陈皮6g煎汤冲服，每日1剂。如阴虚泛吐较甚者，可用羊乳饮。如便秘腹胀者，可每天食用菠菜250g，大蒜头6个，或用莱菔子粥。如便血者可用槐花饮，或用乌梅粥、藕汁三七蛋。对于晚期患者体质虚弱，进食较少者，可选用红枣炖兔肉、大枣营养粥、银耳甜羹、核桃枝鸡蛋等。

消化道癌症的饮食护理至关重要。施行根治手术后，应以流质、半流质为主，并做到少食多餐。食物要清淡易消化，且有较丰富的营养。多

bland, light and nutritious. Eat more melons, fruits, vegetables, coix seed, edible fungus, mushrooms, lily, water chestnut, Chinese yam, squid, Cishen (*Radix Morinae Delavayi*), carrot, etc. These things can not only strengthen the spleen, supplement qi, nourish yin and body fluids, but also have anticancer action to a certain degree. Meanwhile, avoid eating strongly irritative food, eat less pungent, sour, rotten, dry- and hot-natured, hard and heavy foods. It is not advisable to eat more chocolate and condensed milk products like extract of malt. This can avoid giving rise to discomfort in the patients due to the production of acid from these foods after fermentation. In addition, the patients should abstain from meat of pig's head, goose, cock, strong spirit and smoking.

8.3.1.2.5 External treatment with drugs

Dust the Cancer-Eliminating and Pain-Relieving Plaster with the powder of 1 g of Shexiang (*Moschus*) and 1 g of Xuejie (*Restina Draconis*). Then, apply the plaster on Danzhong (CV17) in the case of carcinoma of esophageal tract and the affected part in epigastric region in the case of gastric tumor. Conduct the dressing change once every three days.

In the case of colonic cancer and rectal cancer with prolonged puric, bloody and mucous stool, as well as down-bearing anal pain, the patients may take the hip bath in the decoction of Kushen (*Radix Sophorae Flavescentis*) twice a day; in the case of accumulation of dampness, heat and toxic substance with profuse oozing of fluid from the fistulous mouth, wash the body locally and externally with the decoction of Jinyinhua (*Flos Lonicerae*) and Gancao (*Radix Glycyrrhizae*) or the decoction of Huangbai (*Cortex Phellodendri*). Then, apply Huashifen (Powder of *Talcum*) on the part washed.

8.3.2 Pulmonary carcinoma

Pulmonary carcinoma is also called "primary bronchial cancer". The location of the disease lies in the lung. But it is closely related to the spleen, stomach, kidney, etc. The operative treatment may cause the decline of pulmonary function and serious deficiency of qi and yin. The chemotherapy or radiotherapy may give rise to local stimulation, pain, swelling and necrosis, consequently impairing the healthy qi of the human body.

8.3.2.1 Syndrome differentiation and treatment

8.3.2.1.1 Deficiency of both qi and yin

It manifests lassitude, hypodynamia, short breath, chest tight-ness, dry cough with scanty sputum, dry mouth and tongue, thin and small tongue with little fur, thready and rapid pulse. It is advisable to supplement qi and nourish yin. The prescription used is the modified integration of Baihe Gujin Decoction (Lily Decoction for Strengthening the Lung) with Pulsation-Promoting Powder. In the case of severe pulmonary yin deficiency, add Yuzhu (*Rhizoma Polygonati Odorati*) and Beishashen (*Radix Glehniae*); in the case of severe pulmonary qi deficiency, add Huaishanyao (*Rhizoma Dioscoreae*) and Fuling (*Poria*).

8.3.2.1.2 Qi deficiency of the lung and spleen

It manifests lassitude, hypodynamia, lustreless complexion, short breath, disinclination to speak, cough with low voice, clear and thin sputum, anorexia, or nausea and vomiting, pale tongue with white fur or with marginal dental marks, thready and weak pulse. It is advisable to supplement qi of the lung and spleen. The prescription used is the modified Sijunzi Decoction (Decoction of Four Noble Drugs). In the case of severe nausea and vomiting,

二、肺癌

肺癌又称"原发性支气管癌",病位在肺,但与脾胃、肾等脏腑有较密切的联系。手术治疗造成肺的正常功能减退,气阴不足之虚象较重。化疗或放疗,引起局部刺激,造成疼痛、肿胀、坏死,损伤人体正气。

【辨证施治】

1. 气阴两虚

倦怠乏力,气短胸闷,干咳痰少,口干舌燥,舌体瘦小,苔少,脉细数。宜益气养阴。百合固金汤合生脉散加减。若肺阴虚甚,可加玉竹、北沙参,若肺气虚甚,可加怀山药、茯苓。

2. 肺脾气虚

倦怠乏力,面色无华,气短懒言,咳声无力,吐痰清稀,不思饮食,或有恶心呕吐,舌淡苔白,或边有齿痕,脉细弱。宜补益肺脾之气。四君子汤加味。若恶心呕吐较甚,可加用姜半夏、川黄连、吴茱萸。

add Jiangbanxia (prepared *Rhizoma Pinelliae*), Chuanhuanglian (*Rhizoma Polyonati*) and Wuzhuyu (*Fructus Euodiae*).

8.3.2.1.3 Qi deficiency of the lung and kidney

It manifests chest tightness, occasional cough, short breath, even asthma on exertion, deep and thready pulse. It is advisable to strengthen the lung and kidney. The prescription used is the modified combination of Liuwei Dihuang Bolus (Bolus of Six Drugs Including Rehmannia) with Sijunzi Decoction (Decoction of Four Noble Drugs). In the case of profuse sweat, it is advisable to add Huangqi (*Radix Astragali seu Hedysari*), Wuweizi (*Fructus Schisandrae*), Muli (*Concha Ostreae*) and Dongchongxiacao (*Cordyceps*).

8.3.2.1.4 Yin impairment of the lung and stomach

It manifests dry cough, scanty sputum with difficult expectoration, hectic fever, night sweat, dry mouth and throat, hoarse voice, scanty urine, dry stool, red tongue with scanty body fluid, a little fur, thready and rapid pulse. It is advisable to nourish the lung and stomach. The prescription used is the modified Shashen Maidong Decoction (Decoction of Glehnia and Ophiopogon). In the case of yin impairment of the lung and kidney, the prescription is used in combination with the modified Baihe Gujin Decoction (Lily Decoction for Strengthening the Lung).

8.3.2.1.5 Dryness and heat scorching the lung

It manifests dry cough with paroxysmal onset, scanty sputum or bloody sputum, thoracic pain, short breath, or fever, dry mouth and tongue, red tongue, thready and rapid pulse. It is advisable to clear away heat and moisten the lung. The prescription used is the modified Qingzao Jiufei Decoction (Decoction for Relieving Dryness of the

3. 肺肾气虚

胸闷,时有咳嗽,气急,动则喘促,脉沉细。宜补肺益肾。六味地黄丸合四君子汤加减。若汗出淋漓,可加黄芪、五味子、牡蛎、冬虫夏草。

4. 肺胃阴伤

干咳痰少难咯,潮热,盗汗,口干咽燥,发音嘶哑,尿少便干,舌红少津,苔少,脉细数。宜滋养肺胃。沙参麦冬汤加减。如属肺肾阴伤证,可合百合固金汤加减。

5. 燥热灼肺

干咳阵作,痰少或痰中带血,胸痛,气急,或有发热,口舌干燥,舌红,脉细数。宜清热润肺。清燥救肺汤加减。若大便干结,可加用生地黄、玄参。

Lung). In the case of constipation, it is advisable to add Shengdihuang (*Radix Rehmanniae*) and Xuanshen (*Radix Scrophulariae*).

8.3.2.1.6 Internal stagnation of phlegm and heat

It manifests cough with forceful voice, short breath, yellowish, thick and sticky sputum, thoracic pain and tightness, or fever, dry mouth, red tongue with yellowish and greasy fur, slippery and rapid pulse. It is advisable to clear away heat and resolve phlegm. The prescription used is the modified Qingqi Huatan Bolus (Bolus for Clearing away Heat and Resolving Phlegm). In the case of thoracic tightness and pain and expectoration, it is advisable to add Quangualou (*Fructus Trichosanthis*), Baihuasheshecao (*Herba Hedyotis Diffusae*), Banzhilian (*Herba Scutellariae Barbatae*) and Shengnanxing (unprepared *Rhizoma Arisaematis*).

8.3.2.1.7 Internal accumulation of blood stasis and heat

It manifests cough, chest tightness, expectoration of yellowish sputum, or bloody sputum with deep red colour, thoracic stabbing pain, dry mouth without inclination to drink, deep purple tongue or with ecchymoses, thready and unsmooth pulse. It is advisable to remove blood stasis and clear away heat. The prescription used is Taohong Siwu Decoction in combination with Yuxingcao (*Herba Houttuyniae*), Baihuasheshecao (*Herba Hedyotis Diffusae*), Baijiangcao (*Herba Patriniae*), etc.

8.3.2.2 Rehabilitation methods

8.3.2.2.1 Regulating emotions and recreation therapy

Please refer to the relevant part in the section of "Carcinoma of digestive tract".

6. 痰热内郁

咳嗽声重,气急,痰黄稠胶粘,胸痛作闷,或有发热,口干,舌质红,苔黄腻,脉滑数。宜清化痰热。清气化痰丸加减。若胸闷痛咯痰,可加用全瓜蒌、白花蛇舌草、半枝莲、生南星。

7. 瘀热内蕴

咳嗽胸闷,吐黄痰,或痰中带血,色暗红,胸痛如刺,口干不欲饮,舌质紫暗或有瘀斑,脉细涩。宜化瘀清热。桃红四物汤合鱼腥草、白花蛇舌草、败酱草等。

【康复方法】

1. 调节情志和娱乐疗法

参见"消化道癌症"。

8.3.2.2.2 Acumox and massage

Acumox: In the case of cough, short breath and expectoration as the main manifestations, select Feishu (BL 13), Xinshu (BL 15), Kongzui (LU 6), Taiyuan (LU 9) and Lieque (LU 7); in the case of profuse sputum, add Fenglong (ST 40); in the case of concurrent failure to inspire due to renal asthenia, add Guanyuan (CV 4), Qihai (CV 6) and Shenshu (BL 23); in the case of concurrent yin consumption, add Zusanli (ST 36), Taixi (KI 3) and Sanyinjiao (SP 6). In the case of poor appetite, vomiting and nausea as the main manifestations, select Zusanli (ST 36), Neiting (ST 44) and Zhongwan (CV 12). In the case of severe expectoration, add Neiguan (PC 6). In the case of the patients with late cancer, select Feishu (BL 13), Gaohuang (BL 43), Chize (LU 5), Pishu (BL 20), Bailao (EX) and Taiyuan (LU 9). In the case of short breath, add Qihai (CV 6), Guanyuan (CV 4) and apply moxibustion after acupuncture; in the case of yellowish and thick sputum or concurrent fever, add Quchi (LI 11) and Hegu (LI 4).

Ear acupuncture: In the case of marked cough and thoracic pain, select Fei (MA - IC 1), Jiaogan (MA - AH 7) and Xiong (MA -AH 11) as the main acupoints; in the case of severe short breath, select Fei (MA - IC 1), Pingchuan and Migen as the major acupoints.

Massage: In the case of cough, short breath and thoracic pain as the main manifestations, select Feishu (BL 13), Shenzhu (BL 23), Zhongfu (LU 1) and Quchi (LI 11) as the main acupoints. The manipulations may include the manipulations of relieving chest oppression, relaxing the shoulder, tightening the chest, kneading Feishu (BL 13) and Gaohuang (BL 43), parting-pushing the back, pushing the scapular area with the palm, digitally pressing the back and spine, kneading Chize (LU 5) and pushing Yuji (LU 10).

8.3.2.2.3 Dietary therapy

In the case of deficiency of qi and yin, use Stewed Pork Lung with Chuanbeimu (*Bulbus Fritillariae Cirrhosae*) and snow Pear; in the case of pulmonary and splenic qi deficiency, use Renshen Dazao Gruel (Gruel of *Radix Ginseng* and *Fructus Ziziphi Jujubae*); in the case of pulmonary and renal qi deficiency, steam or stew ten to fifteen grams of Dongchongxiacao (*Cordyceps*), a proper amount of duck meat and lean pork respectively. Eat the meat and drink the soup. Besides, it is advisable to use Piba Hetao Paste (Paste of *Folium Eriobotryae* and *Semen Juglandis*). In the case of pulmonary and gastric yin consumption, use Five-Juice Drink; in the case of pulmonary and renal yin consumption, use Xingou Baili Drink, or Stewed Edible Bird's Nest with Baiji (*Rhizoma Bletillae*) that is particularly applicable to hemoptysis.

Daily diet In the case of deficiency of qi and yin, it is advisable to eat the foods for moistening the lung and supplementing qi such as water chestnut, apricot seed, pear, lily, Chinese yam, wolfberry and jellyfish; in the case of pulmonary and splenic qi deficiency, it is advisable to eat the foods for strengthening the lung and spleen such as sweet apricot seed, Chinese cabbage, lotus seed and Chinese yam; in the case of pulmonary and gastric yin consumption, it is advisable to eat foods for nurishing yin and promoting body fluid production like spinach, water chestnut, edible bird's nest, snow pear, loquat root, white edible fungus and sugarcane juice; in the case of pulmonary and renal yin deficiency, it is advisable to eat the foods for nourishing the lung and kidney such as turtle meat, mussel and jellyfish.

It is not advisable to eat fried, extremely salty and

按背脊法、揉尺泽法、推鱼际法。

3. 食疗

气阴两虚证可用川贝雪梨炖猪肺。肺脾气虚证可用人参大枣粥。肺肾气虚证可取冬虫夏草10~15 g,鸭和瘦猪肉适量,蒸或炖烂,食肉和汤;也可用枇杷核桃膏。肺胃阴伤证可用五汁饮。肺肾阴伤可用杏藕白梨饮,或用白及炖燕窝,对咳血者尤为适用。

日常饮食 气阴两虚者,宜食荸荠、杏仁、白梨、百合、怀山药、枸杞子、海蜇等润肺益气的食物。肺脾气虚者,宜食白萝卜、百合、甜杏仁、白菜、莲子、怀山药等补益肺脾的食物。肺胃阴伤者,宜食菠菜、荸荠、燕窝、白梨、枇杷、白木耳、蔗汁等养阴生津的食物。肺肾阴伤者,宜食鳖肉、淡菜、海参等滋养肺肾的食物。

不宜食用油煎炙煿、过咸

greasy foods, or pungent and hot-natured, pungent and irritative foods like uncooked green onion and hot pepper. This can prevent dampness from generating phlegm. The patients with this disease should abstain from drinking and smoking.

8.3.2.2.4 External therapy with drugs

It is advisable to apply Ruyi Jinhuang Powder externally in the case of local pain, swelling and hardness and necrosis due to intravenous injection; it is suitable to apply Tumor-Eliminating and Pain-Relieving Plaster on the painful part once every three days.

8.3.3 Cerebroma

Cerebroma is also called "intracranial tumor" (including two types of benign one and malignant one). The patients have healthy qi deficiency after the operative, chemical and radiation therapies, mostly manifested as asthenia of the liver and kidney and deficiency of qi and blood. Asthenia in origin and sthenia in superficiality exists in the patients with cerebral tumor at the stage of recovery.

8.3.3.1 Syndrome differentiation and treatment

8.3.3.1.1 Yin deficiency of the liver and kidney

It manifests continuous headache, frequent vertigo, tinnitus, vexation, feverish palms and soles, dry mouth and eyes, red tongue with scanty body fluid, thready and rapid pulse. It is advisable to tonify the liver and kidney. The prescription used is the modified Qiju Dihuang Bolus (Bolus of Six Drugs, Rehmannia with Wolfberry and Chrysanthemum). In the case of asthenic wind disturbing the upper orifices, and subsequent severe headache and dizziness, add Gouteng (*Ramulus Uncariae cum*

Uncis), Shijueming (*Concha Haliotidis*), Mingtianma (*Rhizoma Gastrodiae*), Biejia (*Carapax Trionycis*), Muli (*Concha Ostreae*) and Guiban (*Plastrum Testudinis*); in the case of incoordination between the kidney and heart, restless sleep, add Yejiaoteng (*Caulis Polygoni Multiflori*), Suanzaoren (*Se men Ziziphi Spinosae*), Baiziren (*Semen Biotae*), Hehuanpi (*Cortex Albiziae*) and Lianxin (*Plumula Nelumbinis*); in the case of night sweat due to asthenic heat forcing body fluid to come out of the body, add Wumei (*Fructus Mume*), Bietaogan, Fuxiaomai (*Fructus Tritici Levis*) and Wubeizi (*Galla Chinensis*).

合欢皮、莲子；若虚热迫津外泄而盗汗，可加用乌梅、瘪桃干、浮小麦、五倍子。

8.3.3.1.2 Deficiency of qi and blood

It manifests lassitude, hypodynamia, lustreless complexion, palpitation, short breath, poor appetite, insomnia, amnesia, pale tongue with whitish fur, thready and weak pulse. It is advisable to supplement qi and tonify blood. The prescription used is the modified Bazhen Decoction (Eight Precious Ingredients Decoction). In the case of splenogastric asthenia and anorexia, add Baibiandou (*Semen Dolichoris Album*), Chaoguya (parched *Fructus Oryzae*), Chaogumaiya (*Fructus Hordei*) and Chenpi (*Pericarpium Citri Reticulatae*); in the case of nausea and vomiting due to adversely rising gastric qi, add Jiangbanxia (prepared *Rhizoma Pinelliae*), Chaozhuru (parched *Caulis Bambusae in Taeniam*), Suye (*Folium Perillae*) and Huanglian (*Rhizoma Coptidis*); in the case of palpitation and insomnia, add Suanzaoren (*Semen Ziziphi Spinosae*), Longchi (*Dens Draconis*), Hehuanpi (*Cortex Albiziae*) and Zhufushen (*Poria cum Ligno Hospite*).

2. 气血不足

倦怠乏力，面色无华，心悸气短，食欲不振，失眠健忘，舌质淡苔白，脉细弱。宜补益气血。八珍汤加减。若脾胃虚弱，不思饮食，可加白扁豆、炒谷麦芽、陈皮；胃气上逆而恶心呕吐，可加姜半夏、炒竹茹、苏叶、黄连等；心悸失眠，可加用酸枣仁、龙齿、合欢皮、朱茯神。

8.3.3.1.3 Internal obstruction of turbid phlegm

It manifests severe headache, vertigo, nausea, vom-

3. 痰浊内阻

头痛如裹，眩晕，恶心呕

iting, thoracic and epigastric stuffiness and tightness, greasy fur, taut and slippery pulse. It is advisable to eliminate phlegm and dredge collaterals. The prescription used is the modified Huatan Qingnao Decoction (Phlegm-Resolving and Brain-Refreshing Decoction). In the case of severe dizziness, distension and pain of the head, add Chuanbeimu (*Bulbus Fritillariae Cirrhosae*), Huoxiang (*Herba Agastachis*), Jianbanxia (prepared *Rhizoma Pinelliae*) and Dilong (*Lumbricus*); in the case of thoracic stuffiness and nausea, add Zhuru (*Caulis Bambusae in Taeniam*), Huashi (*Talcum*), Chenpi (*Pericarpium Citri Reticulatae*), Zhike (*Fructus Aurantii*) and Foshoupian (*Fructus Citri Sarcodatylis*).

8.3.3.1.4 Blood stasis due to qi stagnation

It manifests stabbing pain of the head with definite site worsened at night, dry mouth with disinclination to swallow water, occasional vomiting and nausea, deep red tongue or with ecchymoses and petechiae, deep and unsmooth pulse. It is advisable to regulate qi, activate blood circulation and dredge collaterals. The prescription used is the modified Tongqiao Huoxue Decoction (Decoction for Activating Blood Circulation). In the case of severe headache, add Tufuling (*Rhizoma Smilacis Glabrae*), Quanxie (*Scorpio*), Wugong (*Scolopendra*) and Dilong (*Lumbricus*).

8.3.3.1.5 Accumulation of toxic heat

It manifests severe distending pain of the head, flushed complexion, dysphoria with feverish chest, palms and soles, thirst with inclination to cool drink, constipation, yellowish urine, slippery and rapid pulse. It is advisable to clear away heat, cool blood and dredge collaterals. The prescription used is the modified Xijiao Dihuang Decoction (Decoction of *Cornu Rhinoceri Asiatici* and *Radix Rehmanniae*). In the case of dysphoria with smoth-

吐,胸脘痞闷,苔腻,脉弦滑。宜祛痰通络。化痰清脑汤加减。若头昏闷胀痛甚,可加用川贝母、藿香、姜半夏、地龙;胸痞呕恶,可加用竹茹、滑石、陈皮、枳壳、佛手片。

4. 气滞血瘀

头痛如刺,固定不移,夜间为甚,口干饮水不欲咽,时作呕恶,舌质暗红,或有瘀斑瘀点,脉沉涩。宜理气活血通络。通窍活血汤加减。若头痛较甚,可加用土茯苓、全蝎、蜈蚣、地龙。

5. 热毒蕴结

头胀痛如劈,面目红赤,五心烦热,口渴欲凉饮,便秘尿黄,脉滑数。宜清热凉血通络。犀角地黄汤加减。若烦热口渴,可加用生石膏、知母、栀子、天花粉、玄参。

ery sensation and thirst, add Shengshigao (*Gypsum Fibrosum*), Zhimu (*Rhizoma Anemarrhenae*), Zhizi (*Fructus Gardeniae*), Tianhuafen (*Radix Trichosanthis*) and Xuanshen (*Radix Scrophulariae*).

8.3.3.1.6 Endogenous liver wind

It manifests dizziness, headache, restlessness, irascibility, numbness of limbs, repeated and sudden onset of clonic convulsion and tremor followed by paralysis, bitter taste, red tongue, yellowish and thin fur, taut and rapid pulse. It is advisable to calm the liver to stop wind. The prescription used is the modified Lingjiao Gouteng Decoction (Decoction of Antelope's Horn and Uncaria Stem). In the case of numbness of limbs, tremor and clonic convulsion, add Tufuling (*Rhizoma Smilacis Glabrae*), Shijueming (*Concha Haliotidis*), Quanxie (*Scorpio*), Wugong (*Scolopendra*), Cishi (*Magnetitum*) and Daizheshi (*Ochra Haematitum*); in the case of blurred vision, distending pain of the head, add Daizheshi (*Ochra Haematitum*), Chuanbeimu (*Bulbus Fritillariae Cirrhosae*), Chongweizi (*Fructus Leonuri*) and Cheqianzi (*Semen Plantaginis*).

8.3.3.2 Rehabilitation methods

8.3.3.2.1 Regulating emotions and recreation therapy

Please refer to the relevant part of the section of "Carcinoma of digestive tract".

8.3.3.2.2 Physical training

Select Taijiquan, five mimic-animal games, eight-section brocade, etc. according the specific conditions of the patients' physical strength. For instance, certain disturbances in the movement or feeling of limbs may exist in the patients with cerebroma who have not received a radical cure. At this time, their physical training should be moderate and their movements should not be necessarily

6. 肝风内动

头晕痛,烦躁易怒,肢体麻木,反复突然发作抽搐震颤,发后可伴有肢体瘫痪,口苦,舌红,苔薄黄,脉弦数。宜平肝熄风。羚角钩藤汤加减。若肢体麻木,震颤抽搐,可加用土茯苓、石决明、全蝎、蜈蚣、磁石、代赭石;视物昏花,头胀痛,可加用代赭石、川贝母、茺蔚子、车前子。

【康复方法】

1. 调节情志和娱乐疗法

参见"消化道癌症"。

2. 体育疗法

根据体力状况选练太极拳、五禽戏、八段锦等。如脑肿瘤未根治者,在肢体运动或感觉上可能有一定的障碍,此时应注意适可而止,动作不必强求符合标准。恶性脑肿瘤病人在采用传统体育康复法

standardized. The patients with malignant cerebroma should avoid extremely strenuous movements and overfatigue.

8.3.3.2.3 Acumox and massage

(1) **Acumox** In the case of headache and dizziness, select Baihui (GV 20), Taiyang (EX - HN 5), Fengchi (GB 20), Yintang (EX - HN 3), Xiaguan (ST 7), Yanglingquan (GB 34), Neiting (ST 44), Waiguan (TE 5) and Lieque (LU 7) with the simultaneous use of the reinforcing and reducing manipulations in acupuncture; in the case of numbness of limbs and tremor, select the acupoints mostly related to limbs such as Jianyu (LI 15), Jianliao (TE 14), Quchi (LI 11), Shousanli (LI 10), Waiguan (TE 5) and Hegu (LI 4) for the treatment of upper limbs; Huantiao (GB 30), Yinmen (BL 37), Weizhong (BL 40), Yanglingquan (GB 34), Chengshan (BL 57), Taixi (KI 3) and Kunlun (BL 60) for the treatment of lower limbs; in the case of vomiting and nausea, select Zhongwan (CV 12), Zusanli (ST 36), Neiting (ST 44) and Neiguan (PC 6).

(2) **Massage** In the case of hepatorenal yin deficiency, deficient qi and blood, select Touwei (ST 8), Shenmen (HT 7), Ganshu (BL 18), Shenshu (BL 23) and Yongquan (KI 1); in the case of phlegm stagnation obstructing collaterals, Danzhong (CV 17), Zhongwan (CV 12), Fenglong (ST 40), Sanyinjiao (SP 6), Yintang (EX - HN 3) and Taiyang (EX - HN 5), with the pushing, grasping and rubbing methods as the main manipulations and pressing and wiping methods as accessary manipulations in massage. In the case of numbness and tremor of limbs, select the acupoints for simultaneous acupuncture and moxibustion. Meanwhile, use kneading, pressing and pushing manipulations as the main methods and grasping, twirling and foulage manipulations as the accessory

时,应注意避免过分激烈的动作和过度疲劳。

3. 针灸、推拿疗法

针灸 头痛、头晕者,取百会、太阳、风池、印堂、下关、阳陵泉、内庭、外关、列缺等穴。针法宜补泻兼施。肢体麻木、震颤者,多取有关肢体的穴位,如上肢取肩髃、肩髎、曲池、手三里、外关、合谷等;下肢取环跳、殷门、委中、阳陵泉、承山、太溪、昆仑等。呕吐、恶心者,取中脘、足三里、内庭、内关等穴。

推拿 肝肾阴亏、气血不足证,取头维、神门、肝俞、肾俞、涌泉等穴。痰瘀阻络证,取膻中、中脘、丰隆、三阴交、印堂、太阳等穴,以推、拿、摩为主,按、抹等为辅。肢体麻木震颤者,取穴同针灸,推拿手法以揉、按、推为主,拿、捻、搓为辅。对于晚期卧床不起的病人,则可适当按摩全身,以疏通血脉,预防褥疮。

methods. As for the patients with paralysis at the late stage of the disease, massage the whole body properly to dredge blood vessels and prevent bed sore.

8.3.3.2.4 Dietary therapy

In the case of hepatorenal yin deficiency, select Steamed Yangnao (*Cerebrum seu Ovis*) with Gouqizi (*Fructus Lycii*); in the case of deficient qi and blood, select Longyanrou Gruel (Gruel of *Arillus Longan*) or Stewed Chicken with Danggui (*Radix Angelicae Sinensis*) and Renshen (*Radix Ginseng*); in the case of amnesia and slow reaction after the operation, select Heizhima Sangshen Paste (Paste of *Semen Sesami Nigrum* and *Fructus Mori*); in the case of splenogastric asthenia after the operation or chemotherapy and radiotherapy, select Yiyiren Gruel (Gruel of *Semen Coicis*) and Huaishanyao Gruel (Gruel of *Rhizoma Dioscoreae*).

Abstain from smoking, drinking, the pungent and irriative foods like uncooked green onion, hot pepper and mustard as well as the meat of pig's head. Eat more Chinese yam, lotus root, wax gourd, tremella, Xianggu mushroom, wild rice stem, celery, beef, fishes and turtle.

8.3.4 Mammary cancer

Mammary cancer is one of the most commonly-seen malignant tumor in women. Asthenia in origin and sthenia in superficiality coexist after radical operative cure or chemotherapy and radiotherapy. At the late stage, visceral functions decline increasingly and a series of symptoms of healthy qi deficiency may occur such as deficiency of the spleen yang, deficiency of qi and blood, and yin deficiency of the liver and kidney.

4. 食疗

肝肾阴虚证,可选用枸杞子蒸羊脑。气血不足证,可选用龙眼肉粥,或用归参炖母鸡。术后健忘、反应迟钝,可选用黑芝麻桑椹子糊。术后或化疗、放疗后,脾胃虚弱,可食用薏苡仁粥、怀山药粥等。

忌烟酒、生葱、辣椒、芥末之类辛辣走窜的食品,忌猪头肉。应多食怀山药、藕、冬瓜、银耳、香菇、茭白、芹菜、牛肉、鱼类、鳖等食物。

四、乳腺癌

乳腺癌女性最常见的恶性肿瘤之一。手术根治或放疗、化疗后,本虚与标实并存。至晚期,脏腑功能日渐减退,可出现脾阳虚衰、气血两亏、肝肾阴虚等一系列正虚证候。

8.3.4.1 Syndrome differentiation and treatment

8.3.4.1.1 Blood and water obstructing collaterals

It manifests swelling and distension of unilateral upper limb as well as certain degree of disturbance in movement after the operative treatment of mammary cancer, deep red tongue, thready and unsmooth pulse. It is advisable to promote blood circulation and promote diuresis. The prescription used is Huoluo Xiaoling Pill (Effective Collateral-Activating Pill) with additional Fuling (*Poria*), Jianghuang (*Rhizoma Curcumae Longae*), Guizhi (*Ramulus Cinnamomi*), Sangzhi (*Ramulus Mori*), Chishaoyao (*Radix Paeoniae Rubra*) and Chuanxiong (*Rhizoma Ligustici Chuanxing*).

8.3.4.1.2 Qi stagnation and phlegm stasis

It manifests hard swelling lump of breast with normal color, thoracic stuffiness, inclination to sigh, deep red tongue with thin fur, thready and taut or thready and unsmooth pulse. It is advisable to regulate qi, resolve phlegm and dispel stasis. The prescription used is the modified Chaihu Shugan Decoction (Bupleurum Decoction for Relieving the Liver Qi). In the case of severe mammary distending pain, add Chuanshanjia (*Squama Manitis*), Wangbuliuxingzi (*Semen Vaccariae*), Gualou (*Fructus Trichosanthis*) and Danshen (*Radix Salviae Miltiorrhizae*); in the case of hard lump with gradual enlargement, add Tubeimu (*Rhizoma Bolbostemmatis*), Shancigu (*Rhizoma Pleionis*), Kunbu (*Thallus Laminariae seu Eckloniae*) and Haizao (*Sargassum*).

8.3.4.1.3 Accumulation of toxic heat

It manifests gradual enlargement of mammary lump with congestion and pain, even severe ulceration, filthy water with foul odor, vexation, dry mouth, constipation,

【辨证施治】

1. 血水阻络

乳腺癌术后,患侧上肢肿胀,活动有一定障碍,舌质暗红,脉细涩。宜活血利水。活络效灵丹加茯苓、姜黄、桂枝、桑枝、赤芍药、川芎等。

2. 气滞痰瘀

乳房肿块,质硬,皮色正常,胸闷欲叹息,舌质暗红苔薄,脉细弦或细涩。宜理气化痰逐瘀。柴胡疏肝汤加减。乳房胀痛较甚,加穿山甲、王不留行子、瓜蒌、丹参;肿块发硬而渐增大,加土贝母、山慈姑、昆布、海藻。

3. 热毒蕴结

乳房肿块日渐增大,红肿疼痛甚则破溃翻花,污水恶臭,心烦口干,便秘尿黄,舌质

yellowish urine, deep red tongue with yellowish greasy fur, taut and rapid pulse. It is advisable to clear away heat, remove toxic substance and dispel accumulation. The prescription used is the modified Lianqiao Jinbei Decoction with additional ingredients. In the case of diabrotic lump with flowing blood and fluid, it is advisable to add Shenghuangqi (unprepared *Radix Astragali seu Hedysari*), Bailian (*Radix Ampelopsis*), Pugongying (*Herba Taraxaci*) and Lianqiao (*Fructus Forsythiae*).

8.3.4.1.4 Adverse qi flow due to qi deficiency of the middle energizer

It manifests anorexia after the radiotherapy and chemotherapy, nausea, vomiting, abdominalgia, reddish tongue or with dental marks, thready and taut pulse. It is advisable to supplement qi and lower the adversely rising qi. The prescription used is the modified Xiangsha Liujunzi Decoction (Decoction of Cyperus and Amomum with Six Noble Ingredients). In the case of severe vomiting, it is advisable to use the modified Xuanfu Daizhu Decoction (Decoction of Inula and Hematitum), or add Jiangbanxia (prepared *Rhizoma Pinelliae*), Zisuye (*Folium Perillae*) and Huanglian (*Rhizoma Coptidis*).

8.3.4.1.5 Obstruction of dampness due to asthenia of the spleen

It manifests general tiredness with heavy sensation, thoracic and epigastric mass, anorexia, edema of the face or lower limbs, tender and enlarged tongue, white, thick and greasy or white and slippery fur, thready and slippery pulse. It is advisable to warm the spleen and promote diuresis. The prescription used is the modified Shiwei Liuqi Decoction.

8.3.4.1.6 Deficiency of both qi and blood

It manifests lustreless complexion, lassitude, hypodynamia, spontaneous sweating, palpitation, short

暗红，苔黄腻，脉弦数。宜清热解毒散结。加味连翘金贝煎加减。肿块破溃流血水，可加用生黄芪、白蔹、蒲公英、连翘等。

4. 中虚气逆

放疗、化疗后不思饮食，恶心呕吐，腹痛，舌质淡红，或有齿痕，脉细弦。宜补气降逆。香砂六君子汤加减。呕吐较甚，可用旋覆代赭汤加减，或加姜半夏、紫苏叶、黄连。

5. 脾虚湿阻

全身困重，胸脘痞满，纳食不香，面目或下肢浮肿，舌胖嫩，苔白厚腻或白滑，脉细滑。宜温脾利湿。十味流气饮加减。

6. 气血两亏

面色无华，倦怠无力，自汗，心悸气短，或手术后创面

breath, or prolonged healing of wound after the operation, pale tongue, thready and weak pulse. It is advisable to supplement qi and tonify blood. The prescription used is the modified Shiquan Dabu Decoction (Decoction of Ten Powerful Tonics). In the case of prolonged healing of wound due to deficiency of qi and blood, add Danshen (*Radix Salviae Miltiorrhizae*), Xueyutan (*Crinis Carbonisatus*) and Ercha (*Catechu*).

8.3.4.1.7 Asthenia of the liver and kidney

It manifests grey complexion, soreness and flaccidity of the waist and knees or pain of the waist and limbs, dizziness, tinnitus, dysphoria with feverish chest, palms and soles, dry and deep red or flaccid tongue, thready and rapid pulse. It is advisable to nourish the liver and kidney. The prescription used is the modified Yiguan Decoction (An Ever Effective Decoction for Nourishing the Liver and Kidney).

The oral administration of Xihuang Pill (Pill of Rhinoceros Horn and Rehmannia) can be coordinatively used in all the above syndromes.

8.3.4.2 Rehabilitation methods

8.3.4.2.1 Regulating emotions and recreation therapy

Please refer to the relevant part of the section of "Carcinoma of digestive tract".

8.3.4.2.2 Physical training

Start exercising the limb of the affected side three to five days after the operation. At first, exercise the elbow. Then, train the movements of shoulder after a week and increase the amount of exercise gradually. Guide the patients to train the wall-climbing movement with the fingers and comb the hair with the affected limb. The movements of upper limbs in Taijiquan have better effects on limbering up thoracic muscles and joints and eliminating

久不愈合,舌淡,脉细弱。宜补益气血。十全大补汤加减。若气血不足而术后创口久不愈合者,加丹参、血余炭、儿茶。

7. 肝肾亏虚

面色灰暗,腰膝酸软或腰肢疼痛,头晕耳鸣,五心烦热,舌干暗红或萎软,脉细数。宜滋补肝肾。一贯煎加减。

上述各证均可配合犀黄丸内服。

【康复方法】

1. 调节情志和娱乐疗法

参见"消化道癌症"。

2. 体育疗法

手术后3~5日即可锻炼患侧肢体,先从肘部开始,1星期后可练习肩部活动,并逐步加大活动量。指导患者作手指爬墙活动,用患肢梳理头发等。太极拳中的上肢动作,对于舒展胸部筋骨,消除上肢肿胀有较好的效果,可以反复练

swelling of upper limbs. Therefore, it is advisable to practice the movement repeatedly. Besides, other events like eight-section brocade and five mimic-animal games can be accordingly selected.

8.3.4.2.3 Acumox and massage

Acumox: In the case of swelling of upper limbs of the affected side and disturbance of activity, select Jianyu (LI 15), Binao (LI 14), Quchi (LI 11), Waiguan (TE 5), Hegu (LI 4), etc. of the same side. Adopt the simultaneous use of the reinforcing and reducing manipulations, and retain the needles for fifteen to twenty minutes, once a day or once every other day; in the case of deficient qi and blood or prolonged healing of wound, select Guanyuan (CV 4), Qihai (CV 6) and Zusanli (ST 36), mainly use moxibustion for ten to twenty minutes each time, once a day or once every other day; in the case of adverse qi flow due to qi deficiency of the middle energizer, select Zhongwan (CV 12), Pishu (BL 20), Weishu (BL 21), Zusanli (ST 36) and Neiguan (PC 6). Adopt the reinforcing manipulation and reducing one simultaneously on Neiguan (PC 6). But use the reinforcing manipulation on all the other acupoints.

Massage: In the case of non-operative treatment, all the manipulations are contraindicated on the local part of the mammary lump; in the case of disturbance of activity of the upper limbs of the affected side after the operation, adopt some manipulations to massage the periscapular part such as rubbing and pressing the periscapular part, pressing Jianyu (LI 15), pinching the upper limbs, shaking the shoulder, pushing the three yang meridians of upper limbs and pushing the three yin meridians of forearms; in the case of the patients with late mammary cancer, it is advisable to digitally press Geshu (BL 17), Zhiyang (GV 9) and Zusanli (ST 36), press and knead

习。其他如八段锦、五禽戏等都可以酌情选用。

3. 针灸、推拿疗法

针灸 手术后患侧上肢肿胀，活动障碍者，可取同侧肩髃、臂臑、曲池、外关、合谷等穴，行补泻兼施法，留针15～20分钟，每日或隔日1次。术后气血不足，或创面久不愈合者，取关元、气海、足三里等，以灸为主，每次灸10～20分钟，每日或隔日1次。中虚气逆证，可取中脘、脾俞、胃俞、足三里、内关等，针法除内关穴补泻兼施外，均行补法。

推拿 如未经手术者，乳房肿块局部忌用推拿诸法。术后患侧上肢活动功能障碍者，可采用肩周围的一些推拿手法，如摩按肩周法、按肩髃法、捏上臂法、摇肩法、推上臂三阳法、推前臂三阴法等。晚期病人，可点按膈俞、至阳、足三里，按揉膻中、期门、三阴交等穴。

Danzhong (CV 17), Qimen (LR 14) and Sanyinjiao (SP 6).

8.3.4.2.4 Dietary therapy

In the case of postoperative deficiency of qi and blood, drink wolfberry tea regularly and ingest Rice of Shenzao (*Radix Ginseng* and *Fructus Ziziphi Jujubae*), Gruel of Renshen (*Radix Ginseng*) and Gruel of Huangqi (*Radix Astragali seu Hedysari*); in the case of adversely rising qi of the stomach, heat and toxic pathogens consuming yin during the radiotherapy, it is advisable to take Tree-Juice Drink (pear juice, apple juice and a small amount of fresh ginger juice); in the case of severe reaction of digestive tract during the chemotherapy, eat Gruel of Yiyiren (*Semen Coicis*) and Gruel of Huaishanyao (*Rhizoma Dioscoreae*); in the case of the patients with late mammary cancer, it is advisable for them to eat Jujube Steamed with Langdu (*Radix Euphorbiae Ebracteolatae*) [Decoct 250 g of Langdu (*Radix Stellerae seu Euphorbiae*) in a pot with water and place a food steamer in the pot. Then, put 500 g of jujubes on the food steamer. Steam the jujubes until they are thoroughly cooked. Eat seven jujubes each time, twice or three times a day].

In daily life, eat more fresh vegetables and fruits like carrots, water chest nuts, tomatoes, lotus roots, towel gourds, lemons, oranges and tangerines, haws and pears.

8.3.4.2.5 External treatment with drugs

In the case of postoperative disunion of wound surface or ulceration of mammary cancer, it is advisable to apply Shengji Yuhong Plaster on the affected part; in the case of skin swelling or blister and erosion, use the decoction of Huajiao (*Pericarpium Zathoxyli*) and Kufan (*Alumen Exsiccatum*) to wash the affected part externally, and then apply Ruyi Jinhuang Powder on the part; in the case of erosion, dust the affected part with Jiuyi Pill externally.

4. 食疗

术后气血不足者,可常服枸杞茶,并可食用参枣米饭、人参粥、黄芪粥等。放疗期间若有胃气上逆、热毒伤阴表现,可服三汁饮(白梨汁、苹果汁、少量鲜姜汁)。化疗时消化道反应较重,可服薏苡仁粥、怀山药粥等。晚期患者可试服狼毒蒸枣(狼毒250 g,放入锅内加水煮,上放蒸笼,蒸笼上置大枣500 g,蒸熟为度。取枣服,每次7枚,每日2～3次)。

日常多食新鲜蔬菜和水果,如胡萝卜、荸荠、番茄、藕、丝瓜、柠檬、柑橘、山楂、梨等。

5. 局部外治

术后创口不愈合或乳腺癌已破溃者,可外用生肌玉红膏。在放疗后皮肤红肿或有水泡、糜烂者,可用花椒、枯矾煎水清洗,外敷如意金黄散;已有糜烂者,外撒九一丹。

8.4 Rehabilitation for commonly-seen internal diseases

8.4.1 Chronic nephritis

Chronic nephritis mostly results from acute nephritis that is lingering without cure. The disease may have latent onset as well. It can develop into chronic renal failure eventually. Therefore, people should attach great importance to the rehabilitation at remission stage.

8.4.1.1 Syndrome differentiation and treatment

8.4.1.1.1 Excessive dampness due to splenic asthenia

It manifests mild edema worsened after physical overstrain, mental fatigue, hypodynamia, anorexia, facial edema with yellowish complexion, reddish tongue with white and thin fur, deep and slow pulse. It is advisable to strengthen the spleen to promote diuresis. The prescription used is the modified Shenling Baizhu Powder (Power of *Ginseng*, *Poria* and *Bighead Atractylodes*). In the case of urinary protein, use more Huangqi (*Radix Astragali seu Hedysari*) and add Chixiaodou (*Semen Phaseoli*) and Chantui (*Periostracum Cicadae*).

8.4.1.1.2 Asthenia of both the spleen and kidney

It manifests pale complexion, listlessness, lassitude, hypodynamia, aching pain of the waist, edema of lower limbs which does not restore to the original state when pressed, white and thin fur and thready pulse. It is advisable to strengthen the spleen and kidney. The prescription used is the modified Bupi Yishen Decoction (Spleen-Strengthening and Kidney-Benefiting Decoction).

第四节 常见内科病症的康复

一、慢性肾炎

慢性肾炎多由急性肾炎迁延不愈而致,也可隐匿起病,最终发展为慢性肾功能衰竭,故应重视缓解期的康复治疗。

【辨证施治】

1. 脾虚湿重

轻度浮肿,劳累后加重,神疲乏力,纳差,面色浮黄,舌淡红,苔薄白,脉沉缓。宜健脾利湿。参苓白术散加减。有尿蛋白者重用黄芪,加赤小豆、蝉蜕。

2. 脾肾两虚

面色㿠白,精神不振,倦怠无力,腰部酸痛,下肢浮肿,按之凹陷不易恢复,苔薄白,脉细。宜培补脾肾。补脾益肾汤加减。

8.4.1.1.3 Yin deficiency of the spleen and kidney

It manifests dizziness, headache, dry eyes blurred vision, tinnitus, hyposomnia, red complexion dry throat and mouth, red tongue with a little fur and taut pulse. It is advisable to nourish the liver and kidney. The prescription used is the modified Qiju Dihuang Bolus (Bolus of Six Drugs, Rehmannia with Wolfberry and Chrysanthemum). In the case of hypertension, add Zhenzhumu (*Concha Margaritifera Usta*), Xixiancao (*Herba Siegsbeckiae*) and Juemingzi (*Semen Cassiae*); in the case of purple tongue, add Taoren (*Semen Persicae*), Honghua (*Flos Carthami*) and Danggui (*Radix Angelicae Sinensis*).

8.4.1.1.4 Internal accumulation of dampness and heat

It manifests sticky mouth with bitter taste, vexation, or sore throat, epigastric oppression, anorexia, dry mouth with scanty water intake, yellowish and scanty or yellowish urine, red tongue with yellowish and greasy fur, slippery and rapid pulse. It is advisable to clear away heat and promote diuresis. The prescription used is the modified Ganlu Xiaodu Pill(Sweet Dew Detoxication Pill). In the case of scanty urine, add Zexie (*Rhizoma Alismatis*), Fuling (*Poria*) and Zhuling (*Polyporus Umbellatus*); in the case of sore throat, add Tuniuxi (*Radix et Rhizoma Achyranthis*), Xuanshen (*Radix Scrophulariae*) and Mabo (*Lasiosphaera seu Calvatia*).

8.4.1.2 Rehabilitation methods
8.4.1.2.1 Recreation therapy

It is advisable to appreciate music, calligraphy and painting, grow flowers, raise birds, go fishing and outing. As for the musical therapy, in the case of low spirits, select the musical prescriptions of "inspiring the enthusiasm and arousing the feeling"; in the case of dysphoria,

3. 肝肾阴虚

头晕头痛,目涩视糊,耳鸣少寐,面易升火,咽干口燥,苔少舌红,脉弦。宜滋养肝肾。杞菊地黄丸加减。血压高加珍珠母、豨莶草、决明子;舌质紫加桃仁、红花、当归。

4. 湿热内蕴

口黏口苦,心烦,或有咽痛,脘闷纳差,口干而饮水不多,尿少色黄或黄赤,舌质红,苔黄腻,脉滑数。宜清热利湿。甘露消毒丹加减。尿少加泽泻、茯苓、猪苓;咽喉肿痛加土牛膝、玄参、马勃。

【康复方法】
1. 娱乐疗法

欣赏音乐,观赏书画,种花养鸟,钓鱼郊游等均宜。如音乐疗法,情绪低落时,可选"振奋激昂"类;情绪烦躁时,可选"宁心安神"类;有水肿

select the prescriptions of "tranquilizing the mind"; in the case of edema, appreciate the natural sounds like flowing water and peaceful and happy music.

8.4.1.2.2 Physical training

It is suitable to take a walk on the flat ground for fifteen to twenty minutes in the morning or at dusk. In addition, it is advisable to select Taijiquan, five mimic-animal games and eight-section brocade.

8.4.1.2.3 Acumox and massage

Acumox: Select Shenshu (BL 23), Pishu (BL 20) and Sanjiaoshu (BL 22). In the case of splenic asthenia, add Shuifen (CV 9), Qihai (CV 6), Zusanli (ST 36) and Sanyinjiao (SP 6); in the case of renal asthenia, add Mingmen (GV 4), Pangguangshu (BL 28), Guanyuan (CV 4) and Yingu (KI 10). Apply acupuncture once every other day. After acupuncture, apply moxibustion, or moxibustion with the warming needle.

Acupoint injection: Inject 2 ml of Bannangen (*Radix Isatidis*) injection and 2 ml Yuxingcao (*Herba Houttuyniae*) injection into Shenshu (BL 23) (*bilateral*) and Zusanli (ST 36) (*bilateral*) alternately once a day and 20 times constitute one course of treatment. Or inject 0.5 ml of 5% Danggui (*Radix Angelicae Sinensis*) injection into one to two acupoints of Jingmen (GB 25), Pangguangshu (BL 28), Shuidao (ST 28), Zusanli (ST 36) and Fuliu (KI 7) once a day and seven to ten times make up one course of treatment.

As for the ear acupuncture, select Shenqu and Pangguang (MA-SL 8), with the puncturing method, or the needle-embedding method of thumb-tack needle. It is also advisable to apply Wangbuliuxingzi (*Semen Vaccariae*) on acupoints externally.

Massage: Select the acupoints in the light of acupoint selection and adopt the pushing, kneading, pressing and scrubbing manipulations to massage the acupoints several times a day. It is also advisable to rub the costal regions, Shenshu (BL 23), sulcus auriculae posterior and Yongquan (KI 1) respectively for one hundred times or so with the palm in the morning and evening. In the case of hypertension, scrub and knead Yongquan (KI 1) or Taixi (KI 3) respectively for one hundred times in the morning and evening every day; in the case of nausea and vomiting, press and knead Zusanli (ST 36) and Neiguan (PC 6); in the case of scanty urine or anuria, press and knead Guanyuan (CV 4) and Sanyinjiao (SP 6) to dredge the water passage.

8.4.1.2.4 Dietary therapy

In the case of excessive dampness due to splenic asthenia, select Spleen-Benefiting Cake, Gruel of Baibiandou (*Semen Dolichoris Album*), Eight-Treasure Gruel and Gruel of Huaishanyao (*Rhizoma Dioscoreae*); in the case of splenorenal asthenia, select Gruel of Lizi (*Semen Castaneae*), Soup of Dongchongxiacao (*Cordyceps*) and Gruel of Powder of Qianshi (*Semen Euryales*); in the case of hepatorenal yin deficiency, select Gruel of Shengdihuang (*Radix Rehmanniae*) and Paste of Tianmendong (*Radix Asparagi*); in the case of internal accumulation of dampness and heat, select Gruel of Huoxiang (*Herba Agastachis*), Gruel of Yiyiren (*Semen Coicis*) and Gruel of Pibaye (*Folium Eriobotryae*). Besides, it is advisable to select Gruel of Mahetao (*Rhizoma Gastrodiae* and *Semen Juglandis*) and Steamed Crucian Carp with Tea.

Drinking fresh goat's milk on an empty stomach every early morning is extremely beneficial to the treatment of the disease. Each time, cook 250 to 1,500 ml of goat's milk until it boils and take it in two different times by adding a bit of white sugar or honey. Abstain from salt during the milk-drinking period. Drink the milk continu-

次。亦可用掌心早晚摩两胁、肾俞、耳根、涌泉各100次左右。血压偏高时,每日早晚擦揉涌泉穴或太溪穴各100次。恶心呕吐时,可按揉足三里和内关。尿少或无尿时,可按揉丹田和三阴交,以疏通水道。

4. 食疗

脾虚湿重证,可选用益脾饼、白扁豆粥、八宝粥、怀山药粥等。脾肾两虚证,可选用栗子粥、冬虫夏草汤、芡实粉粥等。肝肾阴虚证,可选用生地黄粥、天门冬膏等。湿热内蕴证,可选用藿香粥、薏苡仁粥、枇杷叶粥等。此外,麻核桃粥、清蒸茶鲫鱼均可选用。

每天早晨空腹服鲜羊奶对本病极有好处,每次250～1 500 ml,煮沸后分次服用,可加入少量白糖或蜂蜜,服羊乳期间忌盐,连服1个月。日常饮食应补充优质蛋白质,如鸡

ously for one month. Supplement high-quality protein in the daily diet such as egg, fresh fish, duck meat, lean pork. As for fats, it is suitable to eat vegetable oil. Eat green grams, red beans, wax gourds, watermelons, carrots, rapes and kelps at ordinary times. Abstain from seafoods, allergenic products, pungent, fat and greasy foods like beef, mutton, dog meat, chicken meat, fresh jellyfish and shrimp. Control salt intake and abstain from salt in the case of edema. Do not overeat sugar so as to prevent renal diabetes. If the disease develops into renal insufficiency, it is advisable to select the diet with the low phosphorus and low protein.

8.4.1.2.5 Nursing in daily life

Prevent common cold or other infectious diseases of respiratory tract strictly. Keep the oral cavity and skin clean at ordinary times. Moderate sexual life so as to prevent impairment of renal qi.

Be sure to use drugs with caution to prevent renal injury due to drug toxicity. Drugs that harm the kidney should be absolutely contraindicated such as kanamycin, gentamycin and some antipyretic and analgesic tablets.

8.4.2 Chronic hepatitis and cirrhosis

After the development of acute hepatitis into chronic hepatitis, the prolonged hepatic failure to regulate qi and blood may give rise to blood stasis due to qi stagnation. If blood stasis lasts long, it will accumulate in the subhypochondriac region, developing into cirrhosis in the case of prolonged state. The pathogenesis of the diseases mainly lies in asthenia of the liver and kidney, dampness obstruction due to asthenia of the spleen and blood stasis due to qi stagnation.

蛋、鲜鱼、鸭肉、瘦猪肉等。脂肪类以植物油为宜,可常食绿豆、赤小豆及冬瓜、西瓜、胡萝卜、油菜、海带等食品。忌食牛肉、羊肉、公鸡肉、新鲜海蟹、虾等海腥发物以及辛辣肥腻之品。控制盐的摄入量,如有水肿则需忌盐,勿过食糖类,以防肾性糖尿病。若发展到肾功能不全阶段,则宜选用低磷低蛋白饮食。

5. 起居护理

严防感冒或其他上呼吸道感染,要经常保持口腔清洁和皮肤清洁。注意节制房事,以防伤败肾气。

用药务必谨慎,以防药物毒性损伤肾脏。卡那霉素、庆大霉素、某些退热止痛片等对肾脏有损害的药物绝对禁用。

二、慢性肝炎和肝纤维化

急性肝炎转入慢性期后,肝失疏泄日久,可由气郁而成血瘀,血瘀留着日久不去,结于胁下,日久则渐成肝纤维化。其病机以肝肾不足,脾虚湿阻,气滞血瘀为主。

8.4.2.1 Syndrome differentiation and treatment

8.4.2.1.1 Residual dampness and heat

It manifests heavy sensation of the body, insufficient food intake, anorexia, thoracic and hypochondriac distension, nausea, aversion to oil, dry mouth and bitter taste, vexation, dark and scanty urine, dry or loose stool, red lingual margin, yellowish and greasy or white and greasy fur, slippery and rapid, soft and rapid or taut and slippery pulse. It is advisable to clear away heat and remove dampness. The prescription used is the modified Three-Kernel Decoction. In the case of relatively excessive heat, add Daqingye (*Folium Isatidis*) and Pugongying (*Herba Taraxaci*).

8.4.2.1.2 Stagnation of the liver and asthenia of the spleen

It manifests thoracic tightness and discomfort, restlessness or depression, mental fatigue, distending or wandering pain of right hypochondrium with the right back or chest and breast or underbelly involved occasionally, bitter taste, eructation, anorexia, loose stool, pale or reddish tongue with white and thin or white and greasy fur, taut or taut and slippery pulse. It is advisable to soothe the liver and strengthen the spleen. The prescription used is the modified Xiaoyao Powder (Ease Powder). In the case of marked hypochondriac pain, add Chuanlianzi (*Fructus Meliae Toosendan*) and Yanhusuo (*Rhizoma Corydalis*).

8.4.2.1.3 Hepatorenal yin deficiency

It manifests tiredness, hypodynamia, light-headedness, insomnia, dream-disturbed sleep, soreness of the waist and flaccidity of legs, feverish palms and soles, vexation, dull hypochondriac pain, dry mouth, anorexia, seminal emission, irregular menstruation, red tongue or red

【辨证施治】

1. 湿热未尽

身重体倦,食少,纳呆,胸胁胀满,恶心厌油,口干口苦,心烦,尿短赤,大便或结或溏,舌边红,苔黄腻或白腻,脉滑数、濡数或弦滑。宜清热祛湿。三仁汤加减。若热邪偏盛,加大青叶、蒲公英。

2. 肝郁脾虚

胸闷不舒,烦躁或抑郁,精神疲倦,右胁胀痛或窜痛,有时痛连右背或胸乳,或痛引少腹,口苦,嗳气,纳呆,便溏,舌质淡或淡红,苔薄白或白腻,脉弦或弦滑。宜舒肝健脾。逍遥散加减。胁痛明显者,加川楝子、延胡索。

3. 肝肾阴虚

疲倦乏力,头晕目眩,失眠多梦,腰酸腿软,手足心热,心烦,胁部隐痛,口干,纳呆,男子遗精,女子月经失调,舌或舌尖红,苔薄或无苔,脉弦

tongue tip with thin fur or without fur, taut, thready and rapid or taut and thready pulse, weak pulse in the two chi regions. It is advisable to nourish the liver and kidney. The prescription used is the modified Yiguan Decoction (An Ever Effective Decoction for Nourishing the Liver and Kidney).

8.4.2.1.4 Blood stasis due to qi stagnation

It manifests dim or blackish complexion, distending pain or stabbing pain of the hypochondriac region which has the wandering or definite site, anorexia, epigastric and abdominal distending pain, difficult defecation, enlargement of the liver and spleen, dull-colored tongue or with ecchymoses, thin fur, taut and unsmooth pulse. It is advisable to regulate qi and remove blood stasis. The prescription used is the modified Xuanfuhua Decoction (Decoction of *Flos Inulae*). Replace Xinjiang in the prescription with Qiancao (*Radix Rubiae*) and add Danggui (*Radix Angelicae Sinensis*), Danshen (*Radix Salviae Miltiorrhizae*), Taoren (*Semen Persicae*) and Jixueteng (*Caulis Spatholobi*) accordingly. In the case of subhypochondriac mass, add Renshen (*Radix Ginseng*), Honghua (*Flos Carthami*) and Chuanshanjia (*Squama Manitis*).

8.4.2.2 Rehabilitation methods

8.4.2.2.1 Regulating emotions

The patients with hepatic disease are liable to get excited. Accordingly, it is particularly important to regulate their emotions and check their anger. The doctors may adopt the methods of straightening out the patients psychologically, checking one emotion with another, suggestion and diverting emotions in combination with the color therapy and flower therapy to help the regulation of emotions of the patients.

细数或弦细，两尺脉多无力。宜滋补肝肾。一贯煎加减。

4. 气滞血瘀

肝病日久，面色晦暗或黧黑，胁肋胀痛或刺痛，窜走或固定不移，食欲不振，脘腹胀痛，大便难，肝脾肿大，舌质暗淡或有瘀斑，苔薄，脉弦涩。宜理气化瘀。旋覆花汤加味。方中新绛改用茜草，酌加当归、丹参、桃仁、鸡血藤。若肋胁下有痞块，加人参、红花、穿山甲等。

【康复方法】

1. 调节情志

肝病患者情绪易于激动，达理怡情和忍耐制怒尤为重要。医者应针对患者的各种不良情绪，采用谈心说理开导、情志相胜、暗示移情等方法，结合色彩疗法、香花疗法，帮助患者调节情志。

8.4.2.2.2 Recreation therapy

Take part in the activities of appreciating music, practicing calligraphy and painting, playing a musical instrument, dancing, flying a kite, fishing and outing accordingly. In the case of depression, select classical music; in the case of hypochondriac pain, select the music from the musical prescriptions of "inhibiting restlessness and checking anger" of the musical therapy.

8.4.2.2.3 Physical training

Select several independent movements from Taijiquan accordingly. Then, increase the amount of exercise and the content of movements gradually. It is also advisable to select the corresponding postures from eight-section brocade. In the case of thoracic tightness and discomfort, restlessness and irascibility, select "stretching both hands upwards to regulate the triple energizer, bending a bow with alternate hands to shoot a vulture."; in the case of anorexia and abdominal distension, it is advisable to practice "stretching one hand upwards to regulate the spleen and stomach". Besides, five mimic-animal games and Yijinjing may be selected in combination with the above techniques.

8.4.2.2.4 Acumox and massage

Acumox: The acupoints are divided into two groups. The first group includes Zhiyang (GV 9) and Zusanli (ST 36) and the second group Danshu (BL 19) and Taichong (LR 3). Use the two groups alternately once a day with the moderate stimulation. In the case of hepatalgia, add Qimen (LR 14), Yanglingquan (GB 34) and Qiuxu (GB 40); in the case of increased transaminase, add Dazhui (GV 14), Ganshu (BL 18), Yanglingquan (GB 34), Taichong (LR 3) and Zhongfeng (LR 4); in the case of various hepatic functional changes, add Ganyan (two cun above the tip of the medial ankle) and Taichong (LR 3);

2. 娱乐疗法

音乐、书画、琴棋、舞蹈、风筝、钓鱼、郊游等，均可酌情参加。如心情忧郁者，可选听古典音乐；胁痛时，可选音乐疗法中的"抑躁制怒"类。

3. 体育疗法

酌情先从太极拳中选择几个单独动作，再逐步加大运动量和动作内容。亦可选择八段锦相应术式，如胸闷不舒，急躁易怒，选"二手托天理三焦，左右开弓似射雕"；纳呆腹胀，宜练"调理脾胃须单举"。此外，五禽戏、易筋经亦可配合选练。

4. 针灸、推拿疗法

针灸 取穴分2组。第1组为至阳、足三里；第2组为胆俞、太冲。两组交替选用，每日1次，中度刺激。肝区疼痛加期门、阳陵泉、丘墟；转氨酶高加大椎、肝俞、阳陵泉、太冲、中封。各项肝功能均有异常的加肝炎穴（内踝尖上2寸）、太冲。肝脾肿大加痞根（第1腰椎棘突下旁开3.5寸，肝脏肿大针右侧，脾脏肿大针

in the case of hepatosplenic enlargement, add Pigen (3.5 cun lateral to the spinous process of the first lumbar vertebra, puncture the right side in the case of hepatic enlargement and the left side in the case of splenic enlargement), Pishu (BL 20) and Ganshu (BL 18).

Acupoint injection: Select Ganshu (BL 18), Zhongdu (LR 6), Riyue (GB 24) and Qimen (LR 14). Inject vitamin B_1 or Bannangen (*Radix Isatidis*) into the above acupoints, 1 ml each acupoint, once a day. Ten to fifteen times constitute one course of treatment.

Ear acupuncture: As for the ear acupuncture, select Ganyandian (between Weixue and Ganzhongda), Gan (MA-SC 5), Sanjiao (MA-JC 4), Jiaogan (MA-AH 7), Ganyang, Dan (MA-SC 6), Pi and Ershenmen (MA-TF 1).

Massage: Rubbing the abdomen: Go to number one first. Then, assume the supine position and flex the knees. If the patient is weak, put a pillow under the popliteal fossa to relax the abdominal muscle. Massage the abdomen with one hand or both. At first, use the pressing and stroking manipulations to massage the abdomen from the right upper side of the abdomen to the centre of the abdomen. Afterwards, adopt the kneading-pinching and vibrating methods. In addition, it is advisable to use the kneading-pinching method with the palm or rubbing-scrubbing method with the palm. The patients may practice self massage as well. First, scrub-rub the periumbilical region with the right hand in an increasingly large circle for 20 times. Then, use the left hand to massage in the same way for 20 times. Rubbing the back: Place the left hand on the back and rub the back gently upwards and downwards for 20 times. Then, use the right hand to massage the back in the same way for 20 times. Meanwhile, digitally press Ganshu (GB 18), Danshu (BL 19) and Weishu (BL 21).

左侧)、脾俞、肝俞。

穴位注射 选穴肝俞、中都、日月、期门,用维生素 B_1 或板蓝根注射液,每穴 1 ml,每日 1 次,10~15 次为 1 疗程。

耳针 选穴肝炎点(胃穴与右肝肿大区之间)、肝、三焦、交感、肝阳、胆、脾、神门。

推拿 摩腹部:先解小便,仰卧,两膝屈曲。若患者体弱,须用枕头垫在腘部,使腹部肌肉放松,用单手或双手进行操作。先行按抚法,自右上腹侧面起向腹中部推进,继而用揉捏法、颤动法。还可用掌揉捏法或掌摩擦法。亦可自我按摩,先用右手围绕肚脐周围轻轻逐渐扩大回旋擦摩 20 次,再换用左手围绕肚脐周围轻轻回旋擦摩 20 次。摩后背:可先将左手伸于后背上下轻摩 20 次,再换右手轻摩 20 次。注意点按肝俞穴、胆俞穴、胃俞穴。

8.4.2.2.5 Dietary therapy

In the case of residual dampness and heat, select Celery Gruel, Gruel of Yiyiren (*Semen Coicis*) and Gruel of Heye (*Folium Nelumbinis*); in the case of hepatic stagnation and splenic asthenia, select Gruel of Meihua (*Flos Mume*), Gruel of Meigui (*Flos Rosae*) and Yiyiren and Chinese dates Gruel (Gruel of *Semen Coicis* and *Fructus Ziziphi Jujubae*); in the case of hepatorenal yin deficiency, select Stewed Pork Liver with Xuanshen (*Radix Scrophulariae*), Paste of Wuweizi (*Fructus Schisandrae*) and Thick Soup of Yiner (*Tremella*); in the case of blood stasis due to qi stagnation, select Gruel of Taoren (*Semen Persicae*) and Gruel of Shanzha (*Fructus Crataegi*).

The prescriptions of dietary therapy Raise 2,000 g of live loaches in clear water for a day so that they can discharge all the intraintestinal waste. On the next day, put the loaches into an oven (100℃ is advisable) to make them dry. Then, grind them into powder and store the powder in a bottle. Take the powder with warm boiled water three times a day, ten grams each time. Fifteen days make up one course of treatment while the longest duration does not exceed four courses.

In the case of hepatic stagnation and splenic asthenia, it is advisable to eat the foods for strengthening the spleen and nourishing the liver such as Huaishanyao (*Rhizoma Dioscoreae*) and Dazao (*Fructus Ziziphi Jujubae*), and abstain from uncooked, cold-and cool-natured foods; in the case of residual dampness and heat, accumulation of residual pathogenic factors in the liver and gallbladder, eat foods for clearing away heat and removing dampness like water melon, wax gourd, shepherd's purse, and abstain from pungent and hot-natured foods, smoking and drinking.

5. 食疗

湿热未尽证,可选用芹菜粥、薏苡仁粥、荷叶粥等。肝郁脾虚证,可选用梅花粥、玫瑰粥、薏苡仁红枣粥等。肝肾阴虚证,可选用玄参炖猪肝、五味子膏、银耳羹等。气滞血瘀证,可选用桃仁粥、山楂粥等。

食疗方 活泥鳅2 000 g,放清水中养24小时,排尽肠内废物,次日放干燥箱内(100℃为宜)烘干,研末装瓶,每日3次,每次10 g,温开水送服。15日为1个疗程,最多不超过4个疗程。

如属肝郁脾虚,宜食健脾养肝类食物,如怀山药、大枣等,禁忌生冷凉性食物;如属湿热未清,余邪蕴积肝胆,宜食清热利湿类食物,如西瓜、冬瓜、荠菜等,忌食辛辣热性食物。力戒烟酒。

8.4.2.2.6 External treatment with drugs

Crush a proper amount of Kuxingren (*Semen Armeniacae Amarum*), Shengtaoren (unprepared *Semen Persicae*), Shengzhizi (unprepared *Fructus Gardeniae*) and Sangshenzi (*Fructus Mori*) respectively to paste. Then, mix the paste with glutinous millet and vinegar evenly. Finally, apply the prepared drug on the navel. One dose can be applied for three times. Replace the used drug with the new one once every other day.

8.4.2.2.7 Nursing in daily life

Abstain from sexual life in the case of chronic hepatitis at the active stage and marked injury of hepatic functions; moderate sexual life at the stationary phase as well. Married women should take care not to become pregnant.

8.4.3 Gastroptosis

Gastroptosis results from the weak lifting and holding power of the middle energizer qi due to the unhealthy spleen and stomach. The pathogenesis at the stage of recovery mainly lies in qi deficiency of the middle energizer and concurrent stagnation and blood stasis.

8.4.3.1 Syndrome differentiation and treatment

8.4.3.1.1 Sunken qi of the middle energizer

It manifests declining appetite, anorexia, even unconsciousness of starvation, concurrent postcibal epigastric and abdominal oppression and distension, inclination to vomiting in the case of excessive or insufficient food intake, short breath, disinclination to speak, lassitude, hypodynamia, pale tongue with white and thin fur, slow and weak pulse. It is advisable to strengthen the middle energizer and supplement qi. The prescription used is the modified Buzhong Yiqi Decoction (Decoction for Strengthening the Middle Energizer and Supplementing Qi).

8.4.3.1.2 Qi stagnation due to asthenia of the middle energizer

It manifests epigastric mass and abdominal distension which are relieved in the case of an empty stomach, defecation, wind from bowels or eructation and aggravated after the meals, thin fur and taut pulse. It is advisable to strengthen the middle energizer and regulate qi. The prescription used is the modified combination of Buzhong Yiqi Decoction (Decoction for Strengthening the Middle Energizer and Supplementing Qi) with Zhizhu Decoction (Decoction of Immature Bitter Orange and Bighead Atractylodes).

8.4.3.1.3 Blood stasis due to asthenia of the middle energizer

It manifests anorexia, short breath, disinclination to speak, lassitude of limbs, epigastric and abdominal distending pain with definite site, purple tongue in most cases, thready and unsmooth pulse. It is advisable to strengthen the middle energizer and remove blood stasis. The prescription used is Buzhong Yiqi Decoction (Decoction for Strengthening the Middle Energizer and Supplementing Qi) with additional Taoren (*Semen Persicae*), Honghua (*Flos Carthami*), Danggui (*Radix Angelicae Sinensis*) and Chuanxiong (*Rhizoma Ligustici Chuanxiong*).

In addition, grind 30 g of Renshen (*Radix Ginseng*) and 60 g of Cangzhu (*Rhizoma Atractylodis*) into fine powder. Put the powder into capsules. Take 1 g each time, three times a day. This administration and dosage are applicable to all the above syndromes.

8.4.3.2 Rehabilitation methods

8.4.3.2.1 Regulating emotions and recreation therapy

Adopt the method of checking one emotion with another to keep free from worries and use the method of

2. 中虚气滞

脘痞腹胀,空腹痞胀轻,食后痞胀重,得大便、矢气或嗳气则为快,舌苔薄,脉弦。宜补中理气。补中益气汤合枳术汤加减。

3. 中虚血瘀

饮食无味,少气懒言,四肢乏力,脘腹胀痛,痛位固定,舌质多有紫气,脉细涩。宜补中化瘀。补中益气汤加桃仁、红花、当归、川芎。

各证型均可选用人参30 g,苍术60 g,共研细末,装入胶囊,每次1 g,日服3次。

【康复方法】

1. 调节情志与娱乐疗法

用情志相胜法以舒畅情志,用说理开导以安神逸志,

straightening out the patients to tranquilize the mind in combination with the color therapy and flower therapy. As for the musical therapy, select the music for strengthening the spleen and stomach. In the case of constipation due to qi deficiency, it is advisable to select the beautiful, gentle and sweet tunes of classical music.

8.4.3.2.2 Physical training

Practice two or three postures or a dozen of postures of Taijiquan in the light of the state of illness and physical conditions of the patient. It is also advisable to practice the section of "Stretching One Hand Upward to Regulate the Functions of the Stomach and Spleen".

8.4.3.2.3 Acumox and massage

Acumox: Select Qihai (CV 6), Zusanli (ST 36), Guanyuan (CV 4), Zhongwan (CV 12), Weishang (bilaterally, two cun above the navel and four cun lateral to the anterior midline), Neiguan (PC 6), Zhangmen (LR 13), Liangmen (ST 21), Gongsun (SP 4) and Jianli (CV 11). Puncture two to four acupoints each time with the twirling manipulation once a day. Retain the needles for fifteen to twenty minutes.

Penetration needling: Penetrate more acupoints on the upper abdomen along the skin with a longer thick filiform needle. Twirl the needle to one direction mostly so that the muscle fibre twines around the body of the needle. Then, adopt the lifting-pulling manipulation to produce the full, convulsive and tight sensation in the stomach.

Acupoint injection: Mix 100 mg of vitamin B_1 injection with 0.1 mg of vitamin B_{12} injection. Inject the mixed injection into the two groups of the bilateral Zhangmen (LR 13) acupoints and Zusanli (ST 36) acupoints as well as the bilateral Pishu (BL 20) acupoints and Weishu (BL 21) acupoints alternately once a day, 0.5 ml each acupoint.

并可配合色彩疗法、香花疗法。音乐疗法可选健脾强胃的乐曲。若有气虚便秘，则宜选古典音乐中优美动听、节拍柔和悦耳的曲目。

2. 体育疗法

可根据病情和身体条件，有针对性地练习太极拳中的两三式或十几式。亦可选练八段锦中"调理脾胃须单举"等。

3. 针灸、推拿疗法

针灸　选气海、足三里、关元、中脘、胃上穴（双侧，脐上2寸，旁开4寸）、内关、章门、梁门、公孙、建里，每次选2～4穴，每日1次，每次捻转留针15～20分钟。

长针透刺　用较长的粗毫针，多选用上腹部俞穴沿皮透刺，并常采用向一个方向搓针，使肌纤维缠绕于针身上，然后再采用提拉针的手法，使胃部产生饱满、抽紧感。

穴位注射　以维生素B_1注射剂100 mg与维生素B_{12}注射剂0.1 mg混合，分双侧章门、足三里及双侧脾俞、胃俞2组穴位，交替注射，每日1次，每次每穴注射0.5 ml。

Ear acupuncture: Select Wei, Jiaogan (MA-AH 7), Pizhixia (MA-AT 1) and Gan (MA-SC 5).

Massage: Massage Zhongwan (CV 12), Xiawan (CV 10), Shimen (CV 5), Tianshu (ST 25), Qihai (CV 6), Guanyuan (CV 4), Pishu (BL 20), Weishu (BL 21), Weicang (BL 45), Zusanli (ST 36) and Fenglong (ST 40) with the digital pressing, pressing, kneading and vibrating manipulations and with moderate strength once every other day. Ten times make up one course of treatment.

8.4.3.2.4 Dietary therapy

In the case of sunken middle energizer qi due to asthenia, select Gruel of Renshen (*Radix Genseng*), Gruel of Huangqi (*Radix Astragali seu Hedysari*) and Asthenia-Curing and Qi-Strengthening Gruel; in the case of qi stagnation due to asthenia of the middle energizer, select Renshen Lianrou Soup (Decoction of *Radix Ginseng* and *Semen Nelumbinis*), Jubing Soup (Orange Cake Soup) and Damai Soup (Soup of *Fructus Hordei*); in the case of blood stasis due to asthenia of the middle energizer, select Gruel of Renshen (*Radix Ginseng*), Gruel of Huangqi (*Radix Astragali seu Hedysari*), Gruel of Shanzha (*Fructus Crataegi*) and Gruel of Taoren (*Semen Persicae*).

In addition, wrap 30 g of Huangqi (*Radix Astragali seu Hedysari*) and 15 to 20 g of Zhike (*Fructus Aurantii*) in a piece of gauze. Then, place it into a clean-washed Zhudu (*Ventriculus Suis*). Next, stew the meat and drugs with slow fire until the meat is done. At this time, remove the dregs of drugs to eat the meat and drink the soup. Finish the administration of one dose within two to three days, three times a day. Take two doses a week. Altogether, take ten doses continuously in the same way.

8.4.3.2.5 External treatment with drugs

Make medicinal cakes with 98% Bimaziren (*Semen*

耳针 胃、交感、皮质下、肝。

推拿 以中等强度的点、按、揉及震颤等法,按摩中脘、下脘、石门、天枢、气海、关元、脾俞、胃俞、胃仓、足三里、丰隆。隔日1次,10次为1疗程。

4. 食疗

中虚下陷证,可选用人参粥、黄芪粥、补虚正气粥等。中虚气滞证,可选用人参莲肉汤、橘饼汤、大麦汤等。中虚血瘀证,可选用人参粥、黄芪粥、山楂粥、桃仁粥等。

此外,可取猪肚1个(洗净),黄芪30 g,枳壳15~20 g。将两药用纱布包扎好,置于猪肚内,温火炖熟,去药渣,吃肚喝汤,2天或3天服完,每天3次,服时可加少量盐作调味剂。每周服两剂,如法连服10剂。

5. 药物外治

用蓖麻子仁98%、五倍子

Ricini) and 2% Wubeizi (*Galla Chinensis*). Then, apply the cake on Baihui (GV20) and iron the cake for ten minutes in the morning and evening every day. It is also advisable to pound two shares of Bimaziren (*Semen Ricini*) and one share of Wubeizi (*Galla Chinensis*) to paste and apply the paste on the navel. Fix the drug externally with several pieces of Analgesic Plaster. Iron the drug once in the morning, at noon and in the evening respectively. Remove the drug on the fourth day in general. The drug is commonly ironed for six times.

8.4.4 Pulmonary tuberculosis

The basic pathogenesis of pulmonary tuberculosis mainly lies in excessive fire due to yin deficiency. In the case of prolonged duration of disease, it may cause deficiency of qi and yin, even deficiency of yin and yang in severe cases. The pathogenesis at the stage of recovery mainly exists in asthenia of the lung and kidney.

8.4.4.1 Syndrome differentiation and treatment

8.4.4.1.1 Pulmonary yin deficiency

It manifests dry cough or expectoration of a bit of white and sticky sputum, short and urgent cough, occasional occur-rence of blood-tinged sputum, feverish palms and soles after noon, dry mouth and throat, or occasional dull pain of the chest, tiredness, hypodynamia, thin fur, red lingual margin and tip, thready and rapid pulse. It is advisable to nourish yin and moisten the lung. The prescription used is the modified Yuehua Pill. In the case of thoracic pain, add Guangyujin (*Radix Curcumae*).

8.4.4.1.2 Deficiency of qi and yin

It manifests cough without force, short breath, low voice, expectoration of white, clear and thin sputum, hectic fever, aversion to cold, spontaneous sweating,

2%制成药饼贴敷百会穴，每日早晚在药饼上热熨约10分钟。亦可用蓖麻子仁2份，五倍子1份共捣烂制成药团敷脐部，外以关节镇痛膏数张固定之，每日早、中、晚各热熨1次，一般于第4天末取掉，通常敷6次。

四、肺结核

肺结核基本病理以阴虚火旺为主，病程日久，可导致气阴两虚，甚则阴阳两虚。康复期病机以肺肾虚亏为主。

【辨证施治】

1. 肺阴不足

干咳，或咯少量粘白痰，咳声短促，痰中偶带血丝，午后手足心热，口燥咽干，或偶有胸部隐痛，疲乏少力，舌苔薄，边尖质红，脉细带数。宜滋阴润肺。月华丸加减。胸痛加广郁金。

2.气阴两虚

咳嗽无力，气短声低，咯痰清稀色白，潮热，畏风，自汗，饮食少进，大便溏薄，神疲

insufficient food intake, loose stool, mental fatigue, hypodynamia, pale complexion, flushing of zygomatic region, dry mouth, smooth and pale tongue without fur and with scanty fluid, or oral erosion, thready and rapid or feeble, large and weak pulse. It is advisable to supplement qi and nourish yin. The prescription used is the modified Baozhen Decoction. In the case of consumptive fever, spontaneous sweating and aversion to wind, add Guizhi (*Ramulus Cinnamomi*), Chinese dates (*Fructus Ziziphi Jujubae*), Bietaogan, Fuxiaomai (*Fructus Tritici Levis*) and Biejia (*Carapax Trionycis*).

8.4.4.1.3 Deficiency of yin and yang

It manifests cough with hoarse voice, consumptive fever, hectic fever due to yin deficiency, spontaneous sweating, night sweat, weak physique, cold body, aversion to cold, cold limbs, asthma, short breath, insufficient food intake, seminal emission, red and smooth tongue with scanty fluid, or pale and enlarged tongue with dental marks, indistinct and thready pulse. It is advisable to strengthen essence and blood, warm and tonify the spleen and kidney. The prescription used is Baozhen Decoction with additional Ziheche (*Placenta Hominis*), Lujiaojiao (*Colla Cornus Cervi*), Dongchongxiacao (*Cordyceps*) and Zishiying (*Fluoritum*).

8.4.4.2 Rehabilitation methods

8.4.4.2.1 Recreation therapy

The musical therapy: In the case of depression and pessimism, select the musical prescriptions of "expressing the emotions and removing depression" and "inspiring the enthusiasm and arousing the feeling"; in the case of impetuosity, select the musical prescriptions of "tranquilizing the mind" and "inhibiting impetuosity and checking anger". The singing therapy: It has good therapeutic effects on grief and melancholy impairing the lung as well

乏力,面色㿠白,颧红、口干,舌质光淡,苔剥少津,或见口糜,脉细数或虚大无力。宜益气养阴。保真汤加减。劳热,自汗,畏风,加桂枝、红枣,瘪桃干、浮小麦、鳖甲。

3. 阴阳两虚

咳嗽声嘶,劳热骨蒸,自汗盗汗,形体羸弱,形寒恶风,肢冷,喘息气短,饮食少进,遗精,舌光质红少津,或舌淡胖有齿痕,脉象微细。宜填补精血,温补脾肾。保真汤加紫河车、龟版胶、鹿角胶、冬虫夏草、紫石英。

【康复方法】

1. 娱乐疗法

音乐疗法:情绪郁闷悲观者,可选"抒情解郁"类、"振奋激昂"类;心情急躁者,可选"宁心安神"类、"抑躁制怒"类。歌咏疗法对悲忧伤肺,气结不散者,有良好效果。

as prolonged qi stagnation.

8.4.4.2.2 Physical training

Select the traditional sports events like Taijiquan, Taiji sword and eight-section brocade at the resolving stage.

8.4.4.2.3 Acumox and massage

Acumox: Select Chize (LU 5), Feishu (BL 13), Gaohuang (BL 38) and Zusanli (ST 36). In the case of anorexia, add Pishu (BL 20) and Zhongwan (CV 12); in the case of hectic fever, add Dazhui (GV 14) and Taixi (KI 3); in the case of night sweat, add Yinxi (HT 6) and Fuliu (KI 7); in the case of hemoptysis, add Yuji (LU 10) and Kongzui (LU 6); in the case of vexation and insomnia, add Shenmen (HT 7); in the case of cough, add Taiyuan (LU 9); in the case of seminal emission, add Zhishi (BL 47), Guanyuan (CU 4) and Sanyinjiao (SP 6); in the case of amenorrhea, add Xuehai (SP 10) and Pishu (BL 20). Apply the therapy once a day and retain the needles for twenty minutes.

Acupoint injection: Select Jiehexie (3.5 cun lateral to Dazhui), Zhongfu (LU 1), Feishu (BL 13), Dazhui (GV 14), Gaohuang (BL 38), Quchi (LI 11) and Zusanli (ST 36). Each time, inject 100 mg of vitamin B_1 into two or three acupoints of the above acupoints once a day. Use all the above acupoints alternately. Ten times constitute one course of treatment.

Ear acupuncture: Select Fei (MA - IC 1), Zhen (MA), Jiaogan (MA - AH 7), Ershenmen (MA - TF 1) and Pingchuan (MA).

Massage: Massage limbs at the stationary phase. It is also advisable to practice self massage on the chest. The method is as follows: Rub the palms against each until they get warm. Then, put the palms on the prothorax and massage it gently for twenty times along the muscles be-

2. 体育疗法

进入好转期时,可选练太极拳、太极剑、八段锦等传统体育项目。

3. 针灸、推拿疗法

针灸 取尺泽、肺俞、膏肓、足三里。若纳呆,加脾俞、中脘;潮热,加大椎、太溪;盗汗,加阴郄、复溜;咯血,加鱼际、孔最;心烦失眠,加神门;咳嗽,加太渊;遗精,加志室、关元、三阴交;经闭,加血海、脾俞。每日1次,留针20分钟。

穴位注射 结核穴(大椎旁开3.5寸)、中府、肺俞、大椎、膏肓、曲池、足三里,用维生素 B_1 注射液 100 mg 穴位注射,每次2~3穴,交替使用。每日1次,10次为1疗程。

耳针 肺、枕、交感、神门、平喘。

推拿 稳定期时,可按摩四肢。亦可自我按摩胸部,方法是先将两手掌搓热,然后贴于前胸,十指顺骨缝轻轻摩20次,重点按摩膻中穴、云门穴。

tween bones with the ten fingers. Mainly massage Danzhong (CV 17) and Yunmen (LU 2).

Besides, it is advisable to press and knead the auricle, digitally press Fei (MA - IC 1), Jiaogan (MA - AH 7), Zhen (MA) and Ershenmen (MA - TF 1), apply Wanbuliuxingzi (*Semen Vaccariae*) on auricular acupoints as well.

8.4.4.2.4 Dietary therapy

In the case of pulmonary yin deficiency, select Gruel of Baihe (*Bulbus Lilii*), Gruel of Yuzhu (*Rhizoma Polygonati Odorati*) and Autumnal Pear Paste; in the case of deficiency of qi and yin, select Soup of Edible Bird's Nest, Thick Soup of Yiner (*Tremella*) and powder of human placenta (3 g each time, three times a day).

Besides, dry an otter's liver over a slow fire and grind it into fine powder. Take 3 g of the powder each time with rice soup, twice a day. Or dry several eels over a slow fire and grind them into fine powder. Take 5 g of the powder each time, twice a day. The course of treatment is not limited.

8.4.4.2.5 External treatment with drugs

Grind 15 g of Wulingzhi (*Faeces Trogopterorum*), 15 g of Baijiezi (*Semen Sinapis Albae*) and 6 g of Gancao (*Radix Glycyrrhizae*) into powder. Then, mix the powder with 15 g of garlic paste and pound the two ingredients evenly. Next, add a bit of vinegar to the above ingredients. At this time, spread the prepared paste on a piece of gauze. Finally, apply the drug with the gauze on the region which is 1.5 cun lateral to the cervical vertebrae and Jiaji of the lumbar vertebrae for about one to two hours. Remove it when burning heat sensation appears on the skin. Apply the drug once every seven days and two months make up one course of treatment.

8.4.5 Posthemorrhagic syndromes

The rehabilitation on the basis of syndrome differentiation is needed due to dysfunctions of viscera and tissues and complicated symptoms after various types of hemorrhage like hemoptysis, haematemesis, hematuria, hematochezia, epistaxis, gingival hemorrhage, hematohidrosis, metrorrhagia and metrostaxis.

8.4.5.1 Syndrome differentiation and treatment

8.4.5.1.1 Deficiency of yin and body fluids

It manifests hectic fever, flushing of zygomatic region, night sweat, dry mouth and throat, dizziness, tinnitus, lumbar soreness, flaccidity of knees, restlessness due to asthenia, inadequat sleep, constipation, dry skin, red tongue with a litte fur, thready and rapid pulse. It is advisable to nourish yin and body fluids. In the case of pulmonary yin deficiency and concurrent dry cough and scanty sputum, use the modified Baihe Gujin Decoction (Lily Decoction for Strengthening the Lung); in the case of thirst with inclination to drink due to pulmonary heat and yin deficiency, use the modified Yunü Decoction (Gypsum Decoction); in the case of soreness and flaccidity of waist and knees due to hepatorenal yin deficiency, use the modified Liuwei Dihuang Bolus (Bolus of Six Drugs Including Rehmannia) in combination with Pulsation-Restoring Decoction.

8.4.5.1.2 Deficiency of qi and blood

It manifests pale or sallow complexion, light-headedness, palpitation, short breath, lassitude, hypodynamia, poor appetite, numbness of hands and feet, pale lips and tongue, thready and weak pulse. It is advisable to supplement qi and nourish blood. In the case of deficiency of qi and blood, use the modified Maidong Yangrong Decoction;

五、失血后诸证

咳血、吐血、尿血、便血、鼻衄、齿衄、肌衄及崩漏等各种出血后,脏腑组织功能失调,证候繁杂,需辨证康复。

【辨证施治】

1. 阴液亏虚

潮热颧红,盗汗,口燥咽干,头晕耳鸣,腰酸膝软,虚烦少寐,大便干结,皮肤干燥,舌红少苔,脉细数。宜滋养阴液。肺阴虚而兼见干咳少痰者,百合固金汤加减;胃阴虚而口渴欲饮者,玉女煎加减;肝肾阴虚而腰膝酸软者,六味地黄丸合加减复脉汤加减。

2. 气血虚弱

面色㿠白或萎黄,头昏目眩,心悸气短,倦怠乏力,食欲不振,手足麻木,唇舌俱淡,脉细弱。宜补气养血。气血虚弱证,麦冬养荣汤加减。心脾两虚者,归脾汤加减;虚劳萎

in the case of cardiosplenic asthenia, use the modified Guipi Decoction (Decoction for Invigorating the Spleen and Nourishing the Heart); in the case of consumptive diseases and sallow complexion, use the modified Guiqi Jianzhong Deoction (Decoction of *Radix Angelicae Sinensis* and *Radix Astragali seu Hedysari* for Strengthening the Middle Energizer).

8.4.5.1.3 Internal retention of blood stasis

It manifests general or local pain, or headache, or thoracic and hypochondriac stabbing pain with definite site, or low fever at dusk, restless nocturnal sleeping, blackish eyelids, cyanotic tongue with ecchymoses, thready and unsmooth pulse. It is advisable to activate blood circulation to remove blood stasis and promote generation of new blood. The prescription used is the modified Xuefu Zhuyu Decoction (Decoction for Removing Blood Stasis in the Chest). It is also advisable to select Resuscitation-Inducing and Blood-Activating Decoction, Decoction for Dissipating Blood Stasis Under Diaphragm, Decoction for Removing Blood Stagnation in the Lower Abdomen and Decoction for Relieving Pantalgia Due to Blood Stagnation according to the different sites of blood stagnation. In the case of concurrent qi deficiency or blood deficiency, use the modified Buyang Huanwu Decoction (Decoction of Invigorating Yang for Recuperation) or Taohong Siwu Decoction respectively.

8.4.5.2 Rehabilitation methods

8.4.5.2.1 Regulating emotions

Guide the patients to learn how to regulate and relax themselves and establish the good psychological state.

8.4.5.2.2 Recreation therapy

As for those who tend to be emotionally stable, guide them to participate in recreational activities such as appre-

黄者,归芪建中汤加减。

3. 瘀血内停

全身或局部疼痛,或头痛,或胸胁痛,或腹痛,痛如针刺而有定处,或入暮低热,夜寐不安,两目黯黑,舌质青紫,兼有瘀斑,脉细涩。宜活血化瘀,祛瘀生新。血府逐瘀汤加减。根据瘀血部位的不同,亦可用通窍活血汤、膈下逐瘀汤、少腹逐瘀汤、身痛逐瘀汤等;若兼气虚或血虚者,则分别选用补阳还五汤或桃红四物汤加减。

【康复方法】

1. 调节情志

指导患者学会自我调节、松弛的方法,建立良好的心理状态。

2. 娱乐疗法

情绪趋向稳定者,指导其参加娱乐活动,如欣赏音乐、

ciating music, calligraphy and painting, practicing calligraphy, reciting and composing poems, growing flowers and raising birds. The musical therapy: for the patients with mental stress and anxiety, select the tunes of tranquilizing the mind; for the patients with mental depression, select the tunes of removing mental depression; for the patients with susceptibility to excitement and anger, select the sorrowful tunes.

8.4.5.2.3 Acumox and massage

Acumox: In the case of deficiency of yin and body fluids, select Ganshu (BL 18), Shenshu (BL 23), Neiguan (PC 6), Taixi (KI 3) and Sanyinjiao (SP 6) and needle them with the reinforcing manipulation. In the case of insomnia, add Shenmen (HT 7); in the case of concurrent residual heat, add Feishu (BL 13), Dazhui (GV 14) and Hegu (LI 4) and needle with them the uniform reinforcing-inducing manipulation; in the case of deficiency of qi and blood, select Zusanli (ST 36), Pishu (BL 20), Guanyuan (CV 4), Qihai (CV 6) and Baihui (GV 20) with the reinforcing manipulation, and moxibustion is applicable additionally; in the case of poor appetite, add Zhongwan (CV 12) and Weishu (BL 21); in the case of internal accumulation of blood stasis, add Qimen (LR 14), Geshu (BL 17), Qihai (CV 6), Xuehai (SP 10) and Taichong (LR 3) with the reducing manipulation, and the mild moxibustion is applicable to the local blood stasis.

Massage: Mainly use the health care massage. In addition to massaging the waist, back and abdomen, digitally press the acupoints in the light of the acupoint selection in acumox, and mainly press and knead the acupoints of the five zang organs as well as Zusanli (ST 36), Sanyinjiao (SP 6) and Xuehai (SP 10). It is advisable to use gentle and slow manipulations. The massage lasts for about thirty minutes. Ten to fifteen times constitute one

观赏书画、练习书法、吟诗作赋、种花养鸟等。音乐疗法：精神紧张焦虑者，可选具有安神作用的乐曲；精神抑郁者，可选具有开郁作用的乐曲；情绪易冲动、愤怒者，可选音调悲哀的乐曲。

3. 针灸、推拿疗法

针灸 阴液亏虚证，取肝俞、肾俞、内关、太溪、三阴交等穴，针刺用补法。失眠者加神门；兼余热者，加肺俞、大椎、合谷，用平补平泻法。气血虚弱证，取足三里、脾俞、关元、气海、百会，针刺用补法，并可加灸。食欲差者加中脘、胃俞。瘀血内停证，取期门、膈俞、气海、血海、太冲，针刺用泻法，并可对局部瘀血施以温灸法。

推拿 以保健按摩法为主。除按摩腰背部及腹部外，并参照针灸取穴点揉穴位，重点按揉五脏之俞穴及足三里、三阴交、血海等穴，手法宜轻柔缓慢。每次约30分钟，一般10～15次为1疗程。

course of treatment in general.

8.4.5.2.4 Dietary therapy

In the case of deficiency of yin and body fluids, select Gruel of Huangjing (*Rhizoma Polygonati*); in the case of pulmonary yin deficiency, select Gruel of Baihe (*Bulbus Lilii*); in the case of gastric yin deficiency, select Gruel of Maimendong (*Radix Ophiopogonis*); in the case of renal yin deficiency, selcect Gruel of Shanyurou (*Fructus Corni*); in the case of deficiency of qi and blood, select Buxu Zhengqi Gruel (Deficiency-Curing and Qi-Strengthening Gruel); in the case of internal accumulation of blood stasis, select Gruel of Yimucaozhi (Juice of *Herba Leonuri*) or Gruel of Taoren (*Semen Persicae*) respectively according to the specific state of disease.

4. 食疗

阴液亏虚证,可选用黄精粥。肺阴虚用百合粥,胃阴虚用麦门冬粥,肝肾阴虚用山萸肉粥。气血虚弱证,可选用补虚正气粥。瘀血内停证,可根据病情的轻重,分别选用益母草汁粥或桃仁粥。

Postscript

The compilation of *A Newly Compiled Practical English-Chinese Library of TCM* was started in 2000 and published in 2002. In order to demonstrate the academic theory and clinical practice of TCM and to meet the requirements of compilation, the compilers and translators have made great efforts to revise and polish the Chinese manuscript and English translation so as to make it systematic, accurate, scientific, standard and easy to understand. Shanghai University of TCM is in charge of the translation. Many scholars and universities have participated in the compilation and translation of the Library, i.e. Professor Shao Xundao from Xi'an Medical University (former Dean of English Department and Training Center of the Health Ministry), Professor Ou Ming from Guangzhou University of TCM (celebrated translator and chief professor), Henan College of TCM, Guangzhou University of TCM, Nanjing University of TCM, Shaanxi College of TCM, Liaoning College of TCM and Shandong University of TCM.

The compilation of this Library is also supported by the State Administrative Bureau and experts from other universities and colleges of TCM. The experts on the Compilation Committee and Approval Committee have directed the compilation and translation. Professor She

Jing, Head of the State Administrative Bureau and Vice-Minister of the Health Ministry, has showed much concern for the Library. Professor Zhu Bangxian, head of the Publishing House of Shanghai University of TCM, Zhou Dunhua, former head of the Publishing House of Shanghai University of TCM, and Pan Zhaoxi, former editor-in-chief of the Publishing House of Shanghai University of TCM, have given full support to the compilation and translation of the Library.

With the coming of the new century, we have presented this Library to the readers all over the world, sincerely hoping to receive suggestions and criticism from the readers so as to make it perfect in the following revision.

Zuo Yanfu
Pingju Village, Nanjing
Spring 2002

专家对编写工作提出了指导性的意见和建议。尤其是卫生部副部长、国家中医药管理局局长佘靖教授对本书的编写给予了极大的关注，多次垂询编撰过程，并及时进行指导。上海中医药大学出版社社长兼总编辑朱邦贤教授，以及原社长周敦华先生、原总编辑潘朝曦先生及全体编辑对本书的编辑出版工作给予了全面的支持，使《文库》得以顺利面世。在此，一并致以诚挚的谢意。

在新世纪之初，我们将这套《文库》奉献给国内外中医界及广大中医爱好者，恳切希望有识之士对《文库》存在的不足之处给予批评、指教，以便在修订时更臻完善。

左言富
于金陵萍聚村
2002年初春

A Newly Compiled Practical English-Chinese Library of Traditional Chinese Medicine

(英汉对照)新编实用中医文库

Basic Theory of Traditional Chinese Medicine	中医基础理论
Diagnostics of Traditional Chinese Medicine	中医诊断学
Science of Chinese Materia Medica	中药学
Science of Prescriptions	方剂学
Internal Medicine of Traditional Chinese Medicine	中医内科学
Surgery of Traditional Chinese Medicine	中医外科学
Gynecology of Traditional Chinese Medicine	中医妇科学
Pediatrics of Traditional Chinese Medicine	中医儿科学
Traumatology and Orthopedics of Traditional Chinese Medicine	中医骨伤科学
Ophthalmology of Traditional Chinese Medicine	中医眼科学
Otorhinolaryngology of Traditional Chinese Medicine	中医耳鼻喉科学
Chinese Acupuncture and Moxibustion	中国针灸
Chinese Tuina (Massage)	中国推拿
Life Cultivation and Rehabilitation of Traditional Chinese Medicine	中医养生康复学

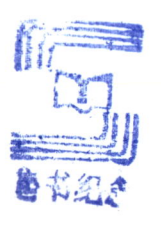